P9-DDW-988

YOU CAN FIGHT
CANCER
AND WIN

Also by Jane E. Brody
SECRETS OF GOOD HEALTH (with Richard Engquist)

YOU CAN FIGHT CANCER AND WIN

Jane E. Brody
The New York Times
with
Arthur I. Holleb, M.D.
The American Cancer Society

Quadrangle/The New York Times Book Co.

Third printing, August 1977.

Copyright © 1977 by Jane E. Brody. All rights reserved, including the right to reproduce this book or portions thereof in any form. For information, address: Quadrangle/The New York Times Book Co., Inc., Three Park Avenue, New York, New York 10016. Manufactured in the United States of America. Published simultaneously in Canada by Optimum Publishing Company Limited, Montreal.

Book design: Beth Tondreau

Library of Congress Cataloging in Publication Data

Brody, Jane E
　　You can fight cancer and win.

　　Includes index.
　　1. Cancer.　 I. Holleb, Arthur I., joint author.
II. Title.　[DNLM:　1. Neoplasms—Popular works.
QZ201　B864y]
RC263.B67　1977　　　616.9′94　　　76-9693
ISBN 0-8129-0659-4

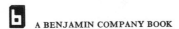 A BENJAMIN COMPANY BOOK

Contents

Acknowledgments

This book is largely the product of the insights, courage, persistence, and painstaking efforts of thousands of physicians and scientists who for decades have been whittling away at the mysteries of cancer, making slow but steady gains toward conquering this killer. While their job is hardly completed, thanks to their progress so far in deciphering the causes of cancer, devising tests to detect hidden cancers, and working out curative therapies, each year countless thousands are spared from dying of this disease.

Progress toward preventing cancer deaths is also the result of the devoted efforts of many thousands of nonprofessionals—the American Cancer Society volunteers—who help to educate the public about cancer and its causes, guide the patient to legitimate sources of care, restore cancer patients to normal lives, and raise money for continuing research. Since 1971, following the passage of the National Cancer Act, the National Cancer Institute (a division of the United States Public Health Service) has bolstered the efforts of the American Cancer Society to educate the public and health professionals, provide direct services to cancer patients, and translate the gains of research into practical, life-saving programs. The successes to date of these efforts, plus the promise of continuing— even accelerating—progress, have made it possible now to write a book about how to fight cancer and win.

I am grateful to my collaborator, Dr. Arthur I. Holleb, senior vice president for medical affairs and research of the American Cancer Society, for his prompt and incisive review of the manuscript throughout its preparation. With his sensitivity and his thorough knowledge of cancer as both a medical and a social problem, he provided invaluable assistance in making this book a useful and accurate guide to the general reader. Thanks, too, to Diane Lynch of the American Cancer Society, whose extraordinary picture files were the source of most of the illustrations in this book, and to the National Cancer Institute's Office of Cancer Communications, which supplied several illustrations and most of the lists in the appendix to help guide cancer patients to the best sources of treatment.

But the biggest "thank you" must go to my husband, Richard Engquist, whose unflagging support, patience, encouragement, and hard work during the last fifteen months made it possible for me to complete this book despite a full-time job at The New York Times. Richard, himself a writer and editor, did far more than put professional touches on the manuscript and type it. He prepared delicious meals every night, cared for our six-year-old sons Lorin and Erik, and attended to our extended family and friends while I devoted the better part of my spare time and attention to researching and writing the book. I could not have done it, Richard, without you.

Jane E. Brody
June 1976

To the Reader

We have tried in this book to compile the most reliable, up-to-date facts about cancer—its causes and management—that were available at the time this manuscript was completed. While no book this size could possibly mention all the important findings in cancer research, we have put together representative results and give you guidance on how to find out more should you want to.

You should not be surprised if progress beyond what this book describes is made by the time you read this, since new facts are accumulating at an ever-increasing rate. It would be disappointing, in fact, if at least some of the information contained within were not extended by new insights in the months it takes to publish a book.

The facts in the book are derived from a wide variety of sources: studies and data that were gathered and analyzed by the National Cancer Institute, which is directing the nation's cancer program; research findings and educational material prepared by the American Cancer Society, the nation's largest voluntary health organization; reports published in the medical and scientific literature and presented at professional meetings; interviews with scores of cancer experts and researchers; interviews with cancer patients and their families; and reports from books, magazines, and newspapers.

Most of the cancer statistics used reflect the latest available national data, or estimates derived from actual data, gathered and analyzed by the National Cancer Institute and the Epidemiology and Statistics Department of the American Cancer Society. Where the statistics represent the results of individual studies, they are so identified. In some cases, improvements in cancer treatment described in the book are so new that there hasn't yet been time for them to be reflected in national statistics. Thus, it can be assumed generally that the results of cancer treatment are better now than when the national statistics were collected.

The anecdotes in the book are based on actual cases, but only when the individual has been publicly identified as a cancer patient is his full, real name used. In all other cases, only a first name is used to protect the individual's privacy.

The information and views expressed in the book are the sole responsibility of the authors. They do not represent official statements of either The New York Times or the American Cancer Society.

Jane E. Brody
Arthur I. Holleb, M.D.

Part I
KNOW THINE ENEMY

1. Why This Book

Cancer has been a big part of my life. When I was 17—four weeks before my graduation from high school and a week before my 13-year-old brother was to assume the responsibilities of manhood as prescribed by Jewish law—cancer claimed the life of our mother. Three years earlier her mother had also died of cancer, but Grandma was 68, had led a full life, and the course of her disease was swift.

Mom, on the other hand, was only 49 and looked and acted ten years younger. She had worked very hard, supporting herself and much of her family from the age of 17. Not two months before her disease was diagnosed, she and my father had taken their first vacation alone together since I was born. It was to be her last.

Her illness, cancer of the ovary, was progressively debilitating, painful, and protracted. It turned a once-stalwart, highly spirited, and jovial person into a shadow of a woman who alternated between empty smiles and tearful despair. When death finally came eleven months later, both she and her family were ready to believe it was a blessing.

Ironically, eleven years later, in 1969, Dr. David Karnofsky, the brilliant, compassionate doctor who had tried so hard to wipe out my mother's disease with the most powerful drugs then known to medicine, and who had devoted his career to humane and modern cancer treatment throughout the world, also died of cancer. He was only 55. At the time of his death, he was chief of medical oncology and director of chemotherapy research at Memorial Sloan-Kettering Cancer Center in New York. It is to his memory—to his achievements, his inspiration, and his intense humanity—that this book is dedicated.

There is hardly a person alive who has not been personally touched by cancer. As the nation's second leading killer, cancer strikes one in four persons, affecting two in three American families. When the victim of cancer is young, a child or young adult, the tragedy of the disease is especially profound. One half of the nation's cancer deaths occurs before the age of 65 and cancer causes more deaths among children between the ages of 1 and 15 than any other disease. When the victim of cancer is old, it is still tragic, for it is hardly a peaceful way to pass out of this life.

But not all cancer need end in tragedy. Through early detection and modern treatment, many patients can be cured. In fact, cancer is far more curable than most people realize. Public attitudes about cancer are a generation or more behind the times; as progress continues to be made in conquering this disease, feelings of hopelessness become less and less justifiable. Through recent advances in therapy, many persons are being cured today of cancers that were considered hopeless just five or ten years ago—including Hodgkin's disease and acute leukemia in children. In part, false expectations of a miracle cancer cure have stood in the way of public realization that genuine, significant progress has already been made in preventing cancer deaths.

The American Cancer Society estimates conservatively that there are at least one and a half million Americans alive today who have been cured of cancer (not counting the millions cured of superficial skin cancers and precancer of the uterine cervix), and each year another 200,000 are saved from the ravages of this dread disease. The Society further estimates that another 100,000 or more persons might be saved each year if their cancers were diagnosed early and promptly and thoroughly treated, using modern therapies. Or, to summarize this progress another way: in 1913 when the American Cancer Society was formed (as the American Society for the Control of Cancer), cancer claimed the lives of more than 90 percent of those it attacked. By the 1930s, mainly through better surgical methods, one in five cancer patients was saved, and in the 1950s, one in four was alive and well five years after a diagnosis of cancer.

Today, through early cancer detection and treatment by surgery, modern radiation therapy, and an ever-expanding array of anticancer drugs (chemotherapy), one in three is cured of cancer, and if all patients got the best available diagnosis and treatment, one in two could be saved. Moreover, many cancers—perhaps one-quarter of the more than 665,000 life-threatening cancers that strike Americans each year—can be prevented entirely by following simple health-saving advice. For example, cigarette smoking is the main cause of nearly a third of the cancer deaths among American men, so the avoidance of just this one habit could theoretically prevent the deaths from cancer of at least 60,000 men and thousands of women each year.

By far the best defense against cancer is an offense. But it is hard to deal effectively with something that is shrouded in secrecy, shame, guilt, and fear. In recent years, more and more public figures—including the wives of the President and Vice President of the United States and a former Vice President himself—have chosen to speak openly and honestly about their bouts with cancer, a sure sign that at last the disease is beginning to come out of the closet. A more straightforward and open approach to cancer can go a long way toward reducing the disease's tragic toll.

My personal experiences with cancer made a tremendous impact on me and how I conduct my life. I might have responded with fear, avoidance, ignorance, and a sense of inevitability. I might have said, "Cancer runs in my family. I'm sure to get it. So why not just accept my fate?" But I realized that fear is cancer's greatest ally. Fear blocks the acquisition of life-saving knowledge. Fear keeps people from adopting sensible living habits, getting periodic checkups, recognizing and acting upon early suspicious symptoms —taking the very steps that can make the difference between winning and losing the battle against cancer.

Instead of retreating in fear and ignorance, I chose the path of information and action, and I do everything within my power to protect myself and my family from an untimely death due to cancer. I am hardly what one would call a health nut or hypochondriac—I lead a very full and pleasure-filled life—but at the same time I am mindful of unnecessary risks and protective health measures. I may or may not be successful, but at least I will know that I tried my best to overcome the threat of cancer.

This book is intended to help you do the same. By understanding what cancer is, its known causes, how it can be detected early enough for cure or prevented entirely, and how even in an advanced stage it can often be treated to optimize the chances for cure or long-term abatement, you too will have the tools to fight cancer and win.

2. Cancer Is Conquerable

Joe is a 55-year-old carpenter who takes great pride in fine workmanship. Ten years ago, as he was making a stereo cabinet that was to be a surprise Christmas present for his wife, Marie, and their three sons, Joe was bothered by a sore on the inside of his lip that just wouldn't heal. He noticed it especially when he was working because he had a habit of pursing his lips when he concentrated and this habit irritated the sore.

A month after he first noticed the irritation, Joe mentioned it to his family doctor, who took one look at it and sent him immediately for a biopsy, a sampling of tissue from the area. The biopsy report took all the joy out of Joe's holiday preparations, for it showed that he had cancer of the mouth. The cancer was removed surgically, and Joe's mouth was reconstructed so that he looked just about as good as new. Fortunately, the surgeon found no sign that the cancer had spread.

Joe spent Christmas day in the hospital and was a little late in completing his family's present that year. But they didn't mind. He made up for it the next year by building a patio for the house. In fact, every year now Joe builds something for his family for Christmas. To Joe and his family, these gifts are a double symbol— a holiday treat and a reminder that Joe was cured of cancer.

Joe and Marie also learned some important lessons from their experience with cancer. Joe decided not to take any more chances and gave up smoking, which may have caused his mouth cancer in the first place. He had a long talk with his sons about not taking up cigarettes, and they have since become active in school no-smoking programs. And once Marie's cancer consciousness was raised, she began to take advantage of some of the tools of early cancer detection. Now, she examines her breasts every month, gets a Pap smear for cervical cancer every six months and never misses a thorough annual checkup.

"I was lucky," Joe says. "When I heard the word cancer, I was

6

sure I was a goner. In fact, I almost put off the surgery because I figured this would be my last Christmas and I should at least spend it at home. Then the doctor talked to Marie and told her there was a good chance that my cancer was curable, but that delaying treatment could make the difference between life and death. So she wouldn't let me wait. I guess I never realized before that cancer can often be cured."

Joe's former fatalistic attitude about cancer is still common today. Few words fill people with more terror and sense of inevitability than does a diagnosis of cancer. Cancer is widely feared and, although it is one of the most common serious diseases of modern man, it is generally misunderstood. Sometimes the fear of cancer can become a self-fulfilling prophecy, leading people to disregard preventive measures and ignore cancer's early warning signs, thus increasing their chances of an untimely death. On the other hand, knowledge and action based on that knowledge can be surprisingly effective weapons in defeating cancer before it defeats you.

Statistically, the incidence of cancer is formidable. Nearly one in five deaths in the United States is due to cancer. Some 1,000 Americans die of cancer each day—about one person every minute and a half. Nearly twice that number are diagnosed as having cancer. Deaths from cancer have become increasingly common during the twentieth century, but this is not because medical science is getting further and further behind in the battle against cancer. In large part, the increase in cancer deaths reflects a victory over other, once more common causes of death. At the turn of the century, tuberculosis was the leading cause of death in the United States, and cancer was only the eighth most common killer. Then, with the conquest of most life-threatening infectious diseases and the extension of life expectancy to around age 70, the so-called chronic ills of man took over as the main causes of mortality in modern countries. Today, cancer is the second leading cause of death—after heart disease—among American men and women, white and nonwhite. Between 1950 and 1970, the cancer death rate among Americans increased six times faster than the death rate from heart disease.

Much of this increase was due to the cancer-causing effects of cigarette smoking, which has produced, among other things, an epidemic of lung cancer among American men. Lung cancer is the most common type of life-threatening cancer and the leading cause of cancer deaths among American men, and is the third leading cancer killer (soon to become second) among American women. The incidence of lung cancer—that is, the number of new cases diagnosed each year per 100,000 people in the population—has increased twenty-fold in the last forty years, and since 1960 it has been increasing at a faster rate in women than in men. Since lung cancer is currently curable in fewer than 10 percent of cases, the soaring incidence of this disease has contributed significantly to the increase in the cancer death rate.

Other cancers have also become more common over the years, including cancer of the colon, pancreas, breast, prostate, and, in males, cancer of the bladder. At the same time, however, certain cancers are occurring less often, including cancer of the stomach, uterine cervix, rectum, esophagus, and, in females, cancer of the bladder.

Though cancer can be a frightening, painful, and fatal disease, it is by no means an automatic death sentence, and most types of cancer do not warrant an attitude of resignation and hopelessness. As noted in Chapter 1, one third of those who develop cancer will be cured of the disease, but one half of all patients could be cured if all took advantage of current methods of early detection and treatment. More than three million Americans are alive today who have been treated for cancer. More than half of them have been "cured" of their disease; that is, they have been free of any sign of cancer for at least five years after completion of therapy (although for some cancers, such as breast cancer, patients must remain free of cancer for longer than five years before they can be considered cured). By the end of the next five years, more than a million new patients will have been cured of cancer. None of these figures includes the nearly always curable cases of superficial skin cancers, which afflict between 300,000 and 600,000 persons a year, or pre-cancer of the cervix, diagnosed in more than 40,000 women each year.

Overall, the chances of surviving most forms of cancer have increased over the last thirty years. By "survival" is meant the likelihood of being alive five years after a diagnosis of cancer, with the figures adjusted for normal life expectancy, since a cancer patient may die of something other than cancer during the five-year period. Five-year survival does not mean the person is likely to die after the five years are up. It simply indicates his chances of living *at least* five years after diagnosis. Significantly better survival chances now accompany cancer of the prostate, uterus, thyroid, kidney, bladder, larynx, melanoma, Hodgkin's disease, chronic leukemia, and a number of childhood cancers.

In some cases, these changes in survival expectations reflect improvements in treatment, such as the widening use of new and better anticancer drugs; in other cases, improved survival rates

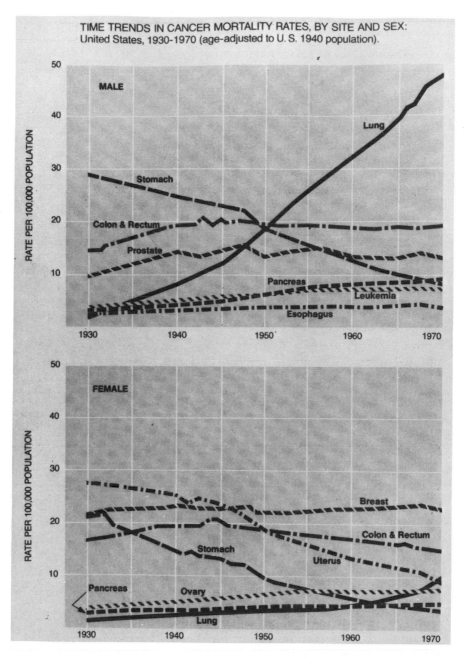

TIME TRENDS IN CANCER MORTALITY RATES, BY SITE AND SEX:
United States, 1930-1970 (age-adjusted to U. S. 1940 population).

The relative contribution of various types of cancer to total cancer deaths in the United States has changed with such factors as increasing or decreasing exposure to cancer-causing agents (such as cigarette smoke), wider use of early detection methods (such as the Pap smear for uterine cancer) and improvements in treatment. But many mysteries remain, such as the reason for the steady drop in cases and deaths from stomach cancer.

PERSONS ALIVE IN 1971 WITH HISTORY OF CANCER: UNITED STATES

Breast	677,000
Colon/Rectum	495,000
Total Uterus	387,000
Prostate	201,000
Lung & Bronchus	85,000
Lymphomas	45,000
Stomach	39,000
Leukemias	37,000
Pancreas	5,000
Esophagus	4,000
All Sites	2,922,000

Note: This table, compiled by the National Cancer Institute, excludes millions of persons who have been cured of superficial skin cancers or in situ cancer of the cervix or elsewhere.

have resulted mainly from many more cases being detected early while the cancer was still localized.

Some critics of the nation's cancer research program have pointed out that most of the dramatic improvements in survival have been achieved for the relatively infrequent forms of cancer, such as acute leukemia (a blood cancer) in children and Hodgkin's disease, a cancer of the lymph system that most commonly attacks young adults. Ten years ago, claims that leukemia or Hodgkin's disease could be cured were greeted with extreme skepticism. But today, half the children with leukemia and 80 percent of those who get Hodgkin's disease can look forward to cure if they receive the most up-to-date therapies.

Is this a small achievement because these are uncommon cancers? Hardly, if you look at them in terms of the years of potential life that are saved. A child cured of leukemia can look forward to six decades or more of productive life, whereas a person who gets a more common cancer against which little progress has been made but which mainly strikes the elderly may have only a few years left to live in any case, even if he did not have cancer.

For two of the most common cancers—breast cancer and cancer of the colon and rectum—there has been little improvement in survival rates in the last few decades. However, recent advances in techniques of early detection of these cancers and postoperative drug therapy for apparently advanced cases promise to send death rates on a downward course in this decade.

But while survival rates have not decreased for any cancer site in the last quarter century, they remain dismally low for certain cancers, including cancer of the lung, esophagus, stomach, liver and pancreas. The survival rate is still less than 10 percent for these cancers. Here, further reasearch on ways to prevent, detect, and effectively treat cancer are necessary to improve the survival rate for the more than nine in ten patients who currently succumb to these cancers.

The secret of preventing deaths from cancer lies in understanding the nature of the disease and its causes. Although "cancer" is one word, it actually represents at least one hundred different diseases, most of which share certain properties. The common properties of cancers are that they can continue to grow, heedless of the rules that govern and limit the growth of normal tissues; they can invade surrounding tissues, and they can dispatch small groups of cells to set up colonies of cancer in distant parts of the body.

Cancer is described in the American Cancer Society's publication, "Cancer Facts and Figures":

Most cancers originate on the surface of some tissues such as the skin, the surface of the uterus, the lining of the mouth, stomach, intestines, bladder or a bronchial tube, or the lining of a duct in the breast, prostate gland or elsewhere. For a time, such cancers typically remain in the lining or on the surface at the site of origin ("in situ") and are visible only under a microscope.

After a while, some of the cancer cells penetrate beyond the surface and "invade" the underlying tissues. This is "invasive cancer." After invading, the cancer continues to grow. . . . For a time, the cancer cells may remain as an intact mass which may be visible to the naked eye. As long as all the living cancer cells remain where the disease started, it is said to be "localized."

The more dangerous phases of cancer are the later ones. Some of the cancer cells eventually become detached and are carried through the lymph channels or blood vessels to other parts of the body. This process is known as "metastasis" (muh-TASS-ta-sis). But the body has a protective mechanism. The detached cancer cells may be trapped in a lymph node in the region of the original organ. This retards the spread for a time. This stage of the disease is known as "regional involvement."

If left untreated the cancer cells eventually spread to other parts of the body. This is "advanced cancer." Death is almost inevitable.

In most cases of cancer, it is the metastases that actually kill the patient by invading vital body organs. Completely localized cancers can nearly always be cured through surgery, radiation therapy, or drug therapy, used alone or in combination with one another. That is why cancer specialists put so much emphasis on early

1976 ESTIMATES

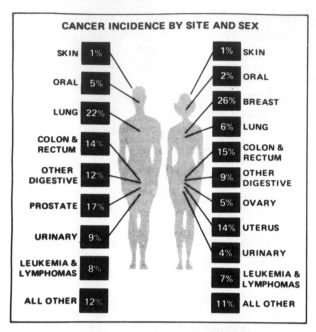

CANCER INCIDENCE BY SITE AND SEX

	Male		Female	
SKIN	1%		1%	SKIN
ORAL	5%		2%	ORAL
			26%	BREAST
LUNG	22%		6%	LUNG
COLON & RECTUM	14%		15%	COLON & RECTUM
OTHER DIGESTIVE	12%		9%	OTHER DIGESTIVE
PROSTATE	17%		5%	OVARY
			14%	UTERUS
URINARY	9%		4%	URINARY
LEUKEMIA & LYMPHOMAS	8%		7%	LEUKEMIA & LYMPHOMAS
ALL OTHER	12%		11%	ALL OTHER

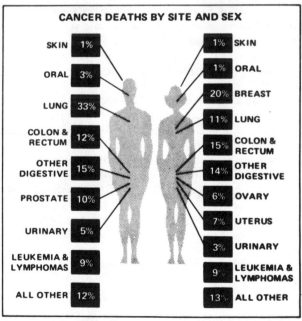

CANCER DEATHS BY SITE AND SEX

	Male		Female	
SKIN	1%		1%	SKIN
ORAL	3%		1%	ORAL
			20%	BREAST
LUNG	33%		11%	LUNG
COLON & RECTUM	12%		15%	COLON & RECTUM
OTHER DIGESTIVE	15%		14%	OTHER DIGESTIVE
PROSTATE	10%		6%	OVARY
			7%	UTERUS
URINARY	5%		3%	URINARY
LEUKEMIA & LYMPHOMAS	9%		9%	LEUKEMIA & LYMPHOMAS
ALL OTHER	12%		13%	ALL OTHER

These charts, based on data gathered in the National Cancer Institute's Third National Cancer Survey, do not include the 300,000 to 600,000 cases of superficial skin cancer and the more than 40,000 cases of in situ cancer of the cervix that are diagnosed annually.

detection—finding and then treating the cancer while it is still confined to its original site.

The name used for a particular cancer depends on where in the body the cancer started—for example, in the breast or prostate gland—and the type of cells it is composed of—muscle, skin, blood, bone, and so forth. Thus, a cancer that began in the breast is called breast cancer, and even after the cancerous breast has been removed, should the cancer spread to some other part of the body, it is still called breast cancer (metastatic breast cancer) because it is composed of breast cancer cells. Cancers arising from connective or supporting tissues, such as the bone and muscle, are called sarcomas. Cancers of the blood-forming tissues are called leukemias, those of the lymphatic system are called lymphomas, and those arising from the body's glandular and lining (epithelial) cells are called carcinomas.

It is important to know where in the body a cancer originated (this is referred to medically as the "primary site") and what type it is because these factors often determine what treatment is likely to be most effective, as well as the patient's chances of cure. Some cancers are more responsive to certain drugs or to radiation therapy than are other cancers. Some cancers are rapidly fatal despite all modern attempts at treatment; others are readily controlled and even totally eradicated by one or a combination of therapies. But because cancer is so many different diseases, it seems doubtful that any one method—a single test, vaccine, drug or other therapy —will ever be found that can detect, prevent, or eradicate all cancers.

While your chances of getting cancer increase with age, cancer is also an important life-threatening disease in children and young adults. Since we all have to die of something sometime, most people accept cancer in an elderly person with relative equanimity (although it is a form of death few people would choose if they had their druthers). But cancer in a child or young parent is often a devastating tragedy that disrupts families and breaks hearts.

Cancer is also a costly disease that can wreck a family financially. But it is much cheaper to treat and cure an early case of cancer than it is to care for a person with advanced cancer who ultimately succumbs to his disease. Initial treatment of cancer costs an average of $2,000, but it may cost $20,000 or more to care for a patient with advanced cancer. Thus, for every cancer that is detected early enough for cure, the difference—$18,000, in addition to the life— is saved.

The "cheapest" way to deal with cancer—both financially and emotionally—is to prevent it from occurring in the first place. Success in preventing cancer depends on understanding what can cause cancer and then avoiding exposure to those causes. The causes of all cancers are by no means understood, but a great deal has been learned about the various substances that can start a cancer and factors that may predispose different persons to develop cancer.

- Gordon had worked for two years during World War II in a shipyard insulating Naval ships with asbestos. In 1972, Gordon, who had been suffering from a lingering cough and shortness of breath for two months, was found to have a fatal form of cancer called mesothelioma (mez-o-theel-ee-O-ma), which involves the lining of the chest cavity. Mesotheliomas have been linked in nearly all cases to exposure to asbestos fibers decades earlier.
- Marcia comes from a Midwestern family in which nearly half of her dead close relatives died of cancer of the colon. Marcia herself has had several small tumors (polyps) removed from her colon, one of which proved to harbor the beginnings of cancer. She has frequent checkups to see whether more polyps are developing.
- Sarah is a first generation Japanese-American. She lost both her maternal grandfather and paternal grandmother to stomach cancer, the most common cancer killer in Japan. Now her father, who migrated to Hawaii when he was a teenager, also has the disease, which is believed to be initiated by something in the diet early in life. But Sarah and her two brothers have been eating primarily a Western-style diet all their lives and they are far less likely than their ancestors were to ever develop stomach cancer.
- As an infant, Jonathan had an enlarged thymus, a gland in the upper chest that shrinks during childhood. As was a common practice mainly in the 1930s and 1940s. Jonathan's oversized gland was "treated" with X-rays. Twenty-five years later, Jonathan was found to have thyroid cancer as a result of the radiation treatments during his first year of life.
- Susan was also the victim of a once-common but now abandoned medical practice. During the early months of pregnancy, her mother was given a hormone-like medication called diethylstilbestrol (DES), to prevent threatened miscarriage. The miscarriage did not occur (but not necessarily because the drug was effective in preventing it), and Susan arrived as a healthy, full-term baby. Just before her seventeenth birthday, Susan was found to have vaginal cancer, an extremely rare disease that is now known to be caused by exposure of the fetus to DES.

● You could probably write your own true story of a person whose cancer was caused by years of cigarette smoking, for this is the most common single cause of serious cancer in the United States today and there are few of us who have not known or heard about one of its victims. Ironically, cigarette smoking is also an entirely preventable cause of cancer, yet for all the government and public action that has been taken against other *suspected* cancer-causing agents in our modern environment, relatively little in the way of direct government regulation protects the American public against this major *proven* cause of cancer in man. Cigarettes can cause far more than cancer of the lung, although this is the cancer that cigarette smoking is most commonly associated with. Other smoking-related cancers include cancer of the larynx (voice box), oral cavity, esophagus, bladder, kidney, stomach, prostate, and pancreas.

As the above examples illustrate, your chances of getting cancer are influenced by a wide range of factors—diet, heredity, where you live, what you do to earn a living, your personal medical history, your habits, and a variety of other circumstances that may expose or predispose you to one or another cancer-causing factor.

The list of known cancer-causing agents—carcinogens (car-SIN-o-gens)—includes physical things like ultraviolet light, X-rays, and radioactive elements; inorganic substances like asbestos, arsenic, and nickel; organic chemicals like benzidine, tobacco products, and dyes derived from coal tars; natural body substances like estrogens; and poisons like aflatoxin, which is produced by a mold.

Hardly a week goes by without a news report that scientists have discovered yet another cause of cancer. To date, some 1,000 different chemicals have been shown to produce cancer in animals (about three dozen of them in man), and many times that number are suspected of causing cancer.

The average person in modern societies lives in a veritable sea of carcinogens. The air we breathe, the food we eat, the drugs we take, the water we drink, the clothing we wear, all may contain substances that have been shown to cause cancer in animals or man. We are exposed to carcinogens through the habits we develop and the jobs we hold. Even the natural radiation from sky and earth, as well as the ultraviolet rays of life-giving sunlight, probably contribute to the human burden of cancer. As many as 85 percent of all human cancers may be caused by environmental agents, according to estimates prepared by the World Health Organization.

But this doesn't mean you have to be a defeatist or that you can throw up your hands and say, "What's the use? Everything causes cancer. There's no escaping. I might as well accept the inevitable." Exposure to many of these carcinogens, such as cigarette smoke or asbestos fibers, can be largely or entirely avoided and the cancers they cause can thus be prevented. While it is true that some carcinogens may be difficult, impossible, too valuable, or too costly to eliminate from the general environment, many could be readily controlled if society (or individuals) chose to do so. There is little doubt that prevention is currently our most effective weapon against cancer, and as researchers identify more and more cancer-causing agents, the possibility of preventing the disease comes closer to reality.

Moreover, exposure to cancer-causing agents does not mean you are doomed to get the disease. Despite the widespread presence of carcinogens, relatively few of the people exposed to them actually get cancer. For example, only one in ten cigarette smokers eventually develops lung cancer, although a smoker's chances of getting this disease are ten times higher than they would be if he did not smoke. While many smokers die of other smoking-caused diseases before they have a chance to develop lung cancer, a few people seem to smoke heavily for decades and live to a ripe old age without getting cancer, giving some smokers the illusion of immortality. Thus, there must be something inherent in some individuals that makes them prone—or resistant—to the effects of certain cancer-causing substances. The differences between cancer-prone and cancer-resistant individuals may involve an inherited lack of certain enzymes, defects in their body's natural immunological defense system, exposure to certain viruses, an inherited condition that predisposes to cancer, changes in hormone patterns, and possibly their psychological state and personality patterns.

Further information on what is known about the various proven and suspected causes of cancer and who is most susceptible to the various types of cancer are elaborated on in Part II: Preventing Cancer Deaths, and again in Part IV: Understanding Cancer.

Part II
PREVENTING CANCER DEATHS

3. Preventing Cancer

John, a talented photographer and 39-year-old father of three, smokes nearly two packs of cigarettes a day. His wife and children have been after him to quit, but John is fatalistic. "My father and two uncles died of cancer," John says, "and if I don't get hit by a car first, I'm bound to go that way too. So what difference does my smoking make?"

Grace is a fair-skinned brunette who was convinced, like millions of other Americans, that a suntan made her look young and beautiful. She baked in the blazing summer sun year after year and returned from every vacation deeply tanned—that is, until one day she noticed a scaly patch on her nose that simply would not go away no matter how much lotion she applied.

Grace's doctor diagnosed it as the beginnings of a potential skin cancer, removed it, and warned her about further prolonged exposure to the sun's damaging rays. "Now I stay a paleface," Grace reports. "I wear a big beautiful hat in the sun, sit under an umbrella on the beach, and use gobs of sun-blocking lotion." And she looks none the less beautiful for it all.

Maryann went to her gynecologist for a routine checkup and was very distressed when a few days after her visit, the doctor's nurse called to tell her that the laboratory had reported abnormality on her Pap smear—a sampling of cells shed by the uterine cervix, the mouth of the womb. The doctor had Maryann return for a repeat test, which confirmed the first result and indicated that Maryann might one day develop cervical cancer. He urged her to come back for treatment and then for Pap tests once every three months so that should the beginnings of cancer appear, he could treat it properly.

But Maryann was scared—scared that if she followed the doctor's advice, she might discover she had cancer. So she delayed going back and ignored the doctor's reminder notices. But, of course, she could not ignore her nagging fears.

John, Grace, and Maryann are all dealing with preventable cancers—cancers that probably would never occur if they each followed simple, health-saving measures. But, as you can see, their attitudes differ. While Grace's scare convinced her to adopt a more sensible approach to the sun, Maryann's scare provoked an inhibiting fear that could eventually threaten her life. And because of John's fatalistic attitude which he uses to justify his continued heavy smoking, he is, in effect, greatly increasing his chances of getting cancer and getting it at a relatively early age.

Few people realize just how much of the cancer problem we currently face is actually preventable. Through wise application of current knowledge, more than a quarter—and perhaps more than half—of the life-threatening cancers that strike Americans each year need not occur in the first place.

Many of the clues to cancer prevention are obvious once the causes of cancer are recognized. Some, like the effects of sunlight and tobacco, are generally well-known, but there seems to be an enormous gap between knowing about a cancer risk and taking the steps necessary to greatly reduce or entirely eliminate that risk.

Other preventable cancers—such as those that might result from excessive exposure to radiation or from carcinogens encountered on the job—are not always in the hands of individuals and may require concerted action to control. But if government agencies, unions, or other groups insist on reducing or eliminating exposure to such cancer-inducing agents, many thousands of cancers could be prevented each year.

Still other cancers can be prevented by diagnosing and treating precancerous conditions, such as abnormalities of the cervix, precancerous patches in the mouth and on the skin, and certain benign polyps in the large intestine. But failing to notice the presence or realize the significance of the precancer, as well as fear of finding out that "it might be cancer," often stands in the way of proper treatment and results in many thousands of avoidable cancer deaths each year.

SMOKING

People are often shocked when they are told that one simple step requiring no government intervention or complex control measure could prevent about 30 percent of the cancer deaths among men in the United States and increasing thousands of cancer deaths among women. That step is *avoiding or stopping cigarette smoking*.

Cigarette smoking is directly responsible for an estimated 70,000 (about 75 percent) of the cases of lung cancer that occur among Americans each year. Lung cancer is the most lethal of the common cancers—it claims the lives of 90 percent of its victims—and this disease alone accounts for one-quarter of all cancer deaths in this country.

The average male smoker is ten times more likely and the average female smoker is five times more likely to develop lung cancer than nonsmokers, and the risk for men who smoke heavily is increased by as much as thirty-fold. In addition, cigarette smokers are more likely than nonsmokers to die of cancer of the larynx, mouth, esophagus, bladder, kidney, stomach, prostate, and pancreas (as well as heart disease and emphysema).

Considering the frequency of these established cancer deaths in man and the relative apathy about controlling their cause, it is hard to understand the excitement generated by the findings that some chemicals, such as the artificial sweetener cyclamate, may cause cancer in animals. While it is certainly wise to be vigilant about potential cancer-causing substances that creep into the human environment, it would make more sense to focus cancer prevention efforts on agents known to cause human cancers—especially agents with so widespread an effect as cigarettes have.

If, for example, oral contraceptives were shown (which they have not been) to cause even 10 percent of the 89,000 cases of breast cancer that strike American women each year (not to mention 75 percent, as is the case with lung cancer caused by smoking), there is little doubt that an enormous public uproar would result, probably ending with a marketing ban on the pill. Yet, considering the benefit–cost ratio—that is, the value of the pill as a contraceptive to the women who take it, compared to the hazard they might face if it increased their breast cancer risk slightly—it would be far easier to justify continued use of the pill than continued sale of cigarettes.

Why has the battle against cigarettes been so long and hard and still so far from resolution? For one thing, agricultural interests in tobacco (it is a cash crop in sixteen states and dominates the agricultural economy of several) have blocked all efforts to reduce or eliminate its production. In fact, the U.S. Department of Agriculture still subsidizes the growing of tobacco to the tune of $60 million a year. Since 1933, when tobacco price supports began, the government has lent more than $3 billion to tobacco farmers.

A second factor is the tax revenue governments glean from tobacco sales. But in an important way, these taxes—amounting to nearly $6 billion a year for local, state, and federal governments—are equivalent to borrowing from Peter to pay Paul, because an equal or greater amount of money is spent or lost by governments because of the health consequences of smoking. Hundreds of millions are spent for medical care of those individuals who develop smoking-caused illnesses. Millions are lost in income taxes and millions more are paid out as Social Security and other benefits to the families of those who succumb to smoking-caused diseases. And who can put a measure on the personal costs of the lives lost?

A further reason for the continued popularity of cigarettes is the more than $300 million spent each year by the tobacco industry to advertise its product. The persuasive power of advertising is well-established, particularly when it appeals to the desire to be sexier, more "with it," and happier, as does cigarette advertising.

The ban on advertising of tobacco products on radio and television that took effect in January 1971 merely resulted in the expenditure of an equivalent amount of advertising money in the printed media, on billboards, and through sponsorship of leading sports events. Now, one can hardly pick up a magazine without being bombarded with page after page of cigarette ads.

Even in the heyday of cigarette advertising on television, when a 1967 Federal Communications Commission ruling required stations that accepted cigarette advertising to donate time to anti-smoking messages, health professionals could raise only a tiny portion of the advertising money spent by commercial interests. And once radio and television advertising of tobacco products was ended, virtually every station also stopped broadcasting antismoking messages. Now the only health message to counter the powerful commercial advertising is a small boxed warning on all ads and cigarette packages stating: "Warning: The Surgeon General has determined that cigarette smoking is dangerous to your health." Tobacco companies have been sued for failing to display even this warning adequately.

Undoubtedly the greatest obstacle to controlling the health hazards that cigarettes create is the psychological and physical pleasure that millions of Americans feel cigarettes bring them. Surveys have shown that well over 90 percent of Americans are aware of the health hazards of smoking, and two-thirds of current smokers say they have tried to quit smoking on one or more occasions. So it must be an extraordinarily strong force that stands in the way of the would-be quitter.

Physicians and psychologists are only now beginning to understand the nature and strength of the cigarette habit and some are finally coming to view the heavy smoker as an addict not unlike persons addicted to heroin or other drugs. The main difference is that addiction to tobacco is still socially acceptable and relatively inexpensive, whereas other forms of addiction are antisocial, costly, and in some cases illegal. Just like other drug addicts, the cigarette addict exhibits such traits as confidence at the start of smoking that he will not become "hooked" and increasing dependence on the effects of smoking, reinforced with each cigarette, to the point where stopping produces a distinct distress syndrome that is only relieved by the drug (in this case, cigarettes).

Yet, even heavily addicted smokers can sever their dependence on cigarettes. It is not easy, and it often takes more than one attempt to finally quit smoking for good, but millions of Americans have proved that it can be done.

For Linda and Arnold L., quitting smoking was a hard-won battle but one which they are convinced was more than worth the agony. Each had made some feeble attempts to give up cigarettes several times in the past, but success was limited to a few weeks or months at best. Then, after Linda had suffered with a lingering cough following a cold for four weeks, the L.'s made a pact to quit together once and for all.

"I was depressed for months, and Arnold was so crabby you had to measure every word before speaking to him," Linda recalls. "We noticed these effects on our personalities for up to a year after our last cigarettes, but we stuck to our decision. Neither of us has had one cigarette since we agreed to quit, and that was ten years ago."

Stopping smoking not only relieved the L.'s of worry about the possible effects of smoking on their health, it also meant that "we were through with the expense, the smell, the messy ashtrays, the bad breath, the annoying cough, stained fingers, and the frantic search for more cigarettes when the pack was suddenly empty," Linda said with a shudder of recalled disgust. "Our son and daughter were very proud of us and having seen what we went through to break the cigarette habit, they are determined never to become smokers themselves."

In 1964 when the Surgeon General's first report on Smoking and Health was issued naming cigarettes as the main cause of lung cancer and chronic lung disease and the probable cause of other cancers and heart disease, cigarette smoking was at an all-time high. At that time 46 percent of adult Americans smoked—53 percent of men and 34 percent of women aged 21 and over. By 1975, the percentage of adult smokers had dropped to 33.8, with 39.3 percent of men and 28.9 percent of women smoking. In 1976, an estimated total of 52 million Americans continue to smoke, but nearly 30 million have given up cigarettes. With each year of not smoking, the ex-smoker's risk of lung cancer diminishes, and ten years after quitting cigarettes, the risk of lung cancer is nearly as

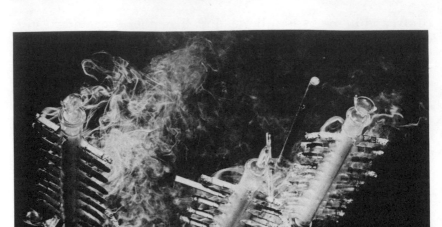

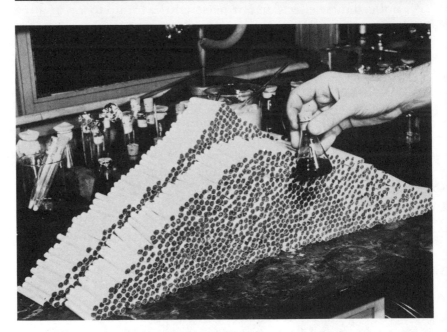

A "smoking robot," developed under a grant from the American Cancer Society, automatically puffs on cigarettes and collects the smoke residue they would deposit in a smoker's respiratory tract. The pile of 2,000 cigarettes—the amount a pack-a-day smoker would consume in 100 days—yielded the tobacco "tar" shown in the flask.

low as that of persons who have never smoked. See chapter 4 for a guide to quitting.

If you find you are simply unable or unwilling to give up cigarettes, there are ways to reduce your risk of cancer. One is to eliminate all those cigarettes that you feel you can do without. In other words, reduce the number of cigarettes smoked each day. Another is to smoke only half of each cigarette, since the last third contains half the total tar and nicotine. You can also take fewer puffs on each cigarette and reduce the depth and frequency of inhaling. But most important is to choose a cigarette that has low tar content, the factor that is believed to determine the cigarette's cancer-causing ability. The tar content of the average cigarette today is 50 percent lower than it was thirty years ago and 30 percent lower than it was ten years ago, and some brands are far below the current average.

Eighty-five percent of cigarettes currently sold have filter tips that screen out much of the tobacco tars before the smoker inhales, and many cigarettes contain considerable synthetic material mixed with the tobacco which reduces the tar content. But brands vary by as much as fifteen-fold in tar content. Tobacco companies now state tar-nicotine content on all cigarette advertisements (some brands also state the contents on the pack). The Federal Trade Commission periodically releases a brand-by-brand analysis of tar and nicotine. The latest list can be obtained free from the Commission (Pennsylvania Avenue at Sixth Street N.W., Washington, D.C. 20580) or from your local American Cancer Society chapter.

No matter how low in tar a cigarette is, if you smoke you must realize that there is no such thing as a "safe" cigarette. All cigarettes increase a person's chances of developing smoking-caused illnesses, especially lung cancer.

Some cigarette smokers have switched to pipes and cigars, which are usually not inhaled and thus present considerably less of a disease risk. But neither is harmless. Both have been associated with greater than normal chances of developing cancer of the mouth, lips, throat, larynx, stomach, kidneys, and lungs. And a recent study of cigarette smokers who switched to cigars indicated that they were so used to inhaling tobacco smoke that they continued to inhale even when they smoked cigars. Since cigar smoke contains more tars than most cigarettes, these persons could actually be increasing their chances of developing a smoking-related cancer.

The American Cancer Society has played an extremely active role in trying to prevent smoking-caused cancers. Its activities have ranged from supporting studies that helped to define the precise risks of cigarettes to preparing antismoking messages and establishing stop-smoking clinics. More than 1,500 society-sponsored clinics to help smokers quit were held in 1975. In addition, the Society is seeking a stronger warning on cigarette labels, taxation based on tar and nicotine content, the elimination of direct cigarette advertising in all media and indirect advertising through sponsorship of sports events, and increased restrictions on smoking in public places. The organization is also expanding its antismoking educational efforts for schools and is extending the involvement of health professionals in educational and stop-smoking programs.

If there is ever to be a substantial and lasting reduction of smoking-caused cancers, it will depend largely on our ability to keep young persons from taking up the cigarette habit. But while the rate at which teen-age boys take up smoking has remained fairly stable for the last decade (one in three 18-year-olds is a smoker), today many more teen-age girls are becoming smokers than formerly. In another decade or so, there will probably be as many female as male smokers among adult Americans. Thus, the current generation of teen-age girls is likely to face the same risk of lung cancer as the boys. Lung cancer deaths among women are already rising rapidly as a result of their smoking habits. Since there is a strong tendency for youngsters to emulate the habits of their parents, reducing smoking among the next generation of adult Americans will depend to some extent on the determination of the current generation of adults to stop smoking.

The increasing insistence of nonsmokers on their right to breathe air unpolluted with tobacco smoke is also expected to discourage cigarette smoking by ostracizing the smoker and making him socially less acceptable. More and more, smokers are being segregated in public places and told that they cannot light up except in designated smoking areas, where the air often gets so thick with smoke that even smokers are annoyed by it. Some families do not allow smoking in their homes, and many individuals do not hesitate to ask a smoker—whether friend or stranger—to refrain because they find the smoke bothersome.

SUNSHINE

The life-giving rays that stream through our atmosphere from the sun are also the principal cause of skin cancer, which afflicts hundreds of thousands of Americans each year. The relationship of sunshine to skin cancer is a graphic example of "too much of a good thing." The sun is the source of radiant energy on which life on earth depends: it is the means by which plants manufacture the foods for animal life to grow, the heat source that recycles water and keeps us all from freezing, the rays that stimulate the production of life-essential vitamin D in our skin. For most of us, sunshine warms our bodies, cheers our souls, and makes us feel at one with the universe. Small wonder, then, that so many people love to bask under its soothing rays.

But sunshine—too much sunshine—can also be harmful. The sun's energy spectrum contains rays that damage the skin and destroy its elastic fibers, causing wrinkling, permanent brown patches, scaling, and—well-known to nearly everyone—sunburn. Doctors who practice in the warmer sections of the United States are very familiar with the "wrinkled prune" look of prematurely aged skin in chronic sunbathers. Frequently, the parts of a person's skin that are continually exposed to the sun (on the face, arms, and neck) will appear twenty to forty years older than skin that is usually protected from sun damage (for example, on the buttocks).

The most serious damage associated with overexposure to the sun is skin cancer, caused by the sun's ultraviolet rays. Between 300,000 and 600,000 persons are treated for skin cancer in this country each year. By far the most common form of skin cancer— referred to as superficial cancer—is curable in 95 percent of cases because it rarely spreads beyond the site where it arises. In fact, since it is so common, so readily cured, and so often treated in doctors' offices rather than in hospitals, this form of cancer is not even counted in the statistics gathered by the National Cancer Institute and the American Cancer Society.

However, about 1 percent of sunlight-induced superficial skin cancers do eventually kill their victims, and overexposure to sun now is believed to increase the chances of developing a far more serious form of skin cancer called malignant melanoma, which spreads quickly to other parts of the body. About 5,000 Americans die of skin cancer each year, mainly the victims of melanoma.

A cooperative study by four medical centers has revealed that the incidence of malignant melanoma is increasing rapidly among light-skinned persons on areas of the body that are now commonly exposed to sunlight, such as the legs of women. Until the last three decades, women wore opaque stockings or long dresses, protecting their legs from sunlight. Now 90 percent of the cases of malignant melanomas that appear between the knee and the ankle involve women. Both men and women are most commonly affected on the face and neck, and in men, the disease often occurs on the shoulders and back. For skin cancers in general, the parts of the body most frequently exposed to the sun—the face, neck, forearms, and backs of the hands—are the areas where the disease is most likely to arise.

As with other cancer-causing agents, sun has a cumulative effect. You don't get skin cancer from one long exposure to the sun, but rather from years of repeated exposure. Thus, skin cancer almost never occurs in children, but is common in older people whose skin has been overly exposed to the sun, perhaps thousands of times.

The amount of natural pigmentation in your skin determines how vulnerable you may be to the damaging effects of sunlight. The skin pigment, melanin, absorbs the sun's ultraviolet rays and partially prevents this radiation from reaching the cell layers where skin cancers arise. Thus, blacks are far less likely to develop sun-caused skin cancers than light-skinned persons. Persons of Northern European ancestry—especially the Irish, Scots, and Scandinavians—are the most susceptible to skin cancer. In general, persons with fair, ruddy, or sandy complexions are the sun's most likely victims, but anyone who chronically overdoes exposure to sunlight is liable to get skin cancer.

This does not mean that you are endangering your health by acquiring a light tan in the summer. If you control your exposure to the sun—especially by limiting the initial exposures to about 15 minutes and slowly building up to longer periods—the melanin that forms in your skin as you tan can help protect the underlying cell layers during future exposures. It is important, though, to avoid excessive exposure, no matter how darkly you may tan.

Preventing skin cancer is relatively easy once you understand how it arises and learn to exercise some common sense in the sun. Basically, the sun is most likely to produce cancerous changes under the same circumstances that it is most likely to cause sunburn. Thus, the fairer one's skin, the closer to the equator one lives, and the more directly overhead the sun's rays, the greater the risk. In the northern hemisphere, the sun is closest to the earth and its rays strike at the most direct angle at the summer solstice on June 21 (you are more likely to get burned on May 3 than on August 27), and during the course of a day, the sun strikes the earth most directly between the hours of 10 A.M. and 3 P.M. If you are fair-skinned, you are advised to try to restrict outdoor summer activity to the early morning or late afternoon hours.

One dermatologist, who has practiced in both Southern California and New York State, reports that skin cancer occurs three to four times more often among residents of sunny Los Angeles than among those living under the cold, grey skies of Buffalo, New York. Also, the higher one goes above sea level, the greater the ultraviolet exposure—for each 1,000 feet increase in altitude, there is a 5 percent increase in utraviolet rays that reach the skin.

Window glass screens out the burning ultraviolet rays, which is why you don't get sunburned driving a car with the windows closed. But you can get burned when overexposed on a day of light cloud cover (70 to 80 percent of the sun's ultraviolet rays penetrate an overcast sky) or when sitting on the beach under an umbrella. The latter happens because the ultraviolet rays can be reflected back from the sand. Dry sand reflects about 17 percent of the sun's burning rays, whereas grass reflects only 2.5 percent. Even city pavement reflects the sun and, as skiers know, snow is an excellent reflector—fresh snow throws back 85 percent of the sun's rays.

For those who choose to or who must be out for long periods when the sun is high in the sky (like farmers and construction workers), there are ways to protect against overexposure to ultraviolet radiation. An obvious one is to wear protective clothing—wide-brimmed hats and long-sleeved shirts. Another is to apply to exposed skin any one of several effective agents that block out ultraviolet light. Unfortunately, if you try to select such an agent you are likely to face a bewildering assortment of creams, lotions, oils, sprays, and what-have-you, most of which are valueless in screening out the damaging rays. Such popular "tanning agents" as baby oil, mineral oil, and olive oil lubricate the skin but offer no protection whatsoever against the sun's burning rays. Most other commercial suntan lotions, creams, and sprays allow ultraviolet rays to reach the skin (or else you would not tan at all) and thus are inadequate protection against skin cancer.

The best protection is obtained through the use of agents called "sunscreens." There are two kinds: physical and chemical blocking agents. Physical blockers are usually opaque substances such as zinc oxide, red veterinary petrolatum, and titanium dioxide; they are best used on small areas that are especially vulnerable to sunburn like the nose and lips. Chemical sunscreens are more acceptable to most people because they form a clear film on the skin. They work by "absorbing" most of the ultraviolet light before it reaches the skin and thus prevent burning or tanning. The best of these sunscreens contain a chemical called para-aminobenzoic acid (PABA) or the esters of PABA. Somewhat less effective sunscreens contain benzophenones (also called diphenylketones). To choose an effective sunscreen, you must ignore advertising claims and read the label to see if it contains one of the protective ingredients. Also, regardless of what the manufacturer says, dermatologists recommend reapplying the sunscreen after swimming or heavy sweating. The agents are said to work best if first applied an hour before going out into the sunlight.

Even after sun damage has already occurred, skin cancer can be prevented in many cases by proper treatment of what are generally regarded as precancerous or potentially malignant skin changes. By far the most common of these is senile or actinic keratosis, a scaly thickening that resembles "onion skin." Keratoses can be treated by a freeze technique called cryotherapy or by using a topical drug called 5-fluorouracil (5-FU). About one-quarter of those with many keratosis lesions eventually develop skin cancer.

Another premalignant lesion that can affect surface cells is a white scaly patch called leukoplakia, which usually develops on the lip, the tongue, or in the mouth. It is frequently associated with heavy pipe-smoking or the use of chewing tobacco. Sometimes leukoplakia develops at a point where jagged teeth or ill-fitting dentures constantly irritate the delicate mucous membrane that lines the mouth. When you go to your dentist for a checkup, he should examine your entire mouth carefully and any suspicious patches should be promptly seen and evaluated by a surgeon.

Mouth cancers can be prevented by avoiding or correcting the conditions that may cause them. The American Cancer Society recommends the following: make sure your lips are covered with a protective cream in strong sunlight; avoid irritating tobacco habits; have your dentist correct irritating dental structures; eat a balanced diet (dietary deficiencies render mucous membranes especially susceptible to cancer); avoid repeated consumption of very hot foods or drinks since these irritate living tissue; and keep your mouth clean by frequently brushing your teeth.

RADIATION

The sun's dangerous rays do not penetrate any further than the top layers of the skin, but man-made radiation—X-rays, fallout from nuclear weapons, radioactive elements used in industry and medicine—all emit high-energy radiation capable of penetrating and causing cancer in tissues deep in the body many years later. The damaging effects of such radiation are cumulative, so that theoretically it doesn't matter whether you get a large dose all at one time (as did the survivors of the atomic bombings of Hiroshima and Nagasaki) or many smaller doses over a period of time, because they eventually add up to one large dose.

The most common source of radiation exposure is through medical X-rays for diagnosis or treatment. About 90 percent of people's exposure to penetrating radiation is through medicine, 5 percent from nuclear fallout, and currently less than 1 percent from the use of nuclear power. The unfortunate legacy of cancer that resulted from the unwitting misuse of X-ray therapy for minor medical problems, such as acne, ringworm and inflamed tonsils, is described in Part IV. Because cancer can sometimes result from X-ray therapy does not mean, of course, that such treatments should never be used. It only means that radiation therapy should be reserved for the treatment of very serious, potentially life-threatening conditions for which no other equally effective, safer treatment is available. As in dealing with all other useful but dangerous agents, the expected benefits must be weighed against the possible risks. It must also be remembered that the risk involved in radiation therapy is only a possibility, not a probability. Everyone—in fact, the overwhelming majority of persons—exposed to a given amount of radiation will not get cancer as a result. So, while the benefits of radiation therapy theoretically would accrue to all who received it, the risks are faced by only a relative few. In each instance where radiation therapy is considered, the doctor must decide whether the treatment is potentially so valuable that it is worth the chance. Thus, in treating a life-threatening cancer, radiation therapy would be used even though it may minimally increase the patient's chances of developing a second cancer years later. The important thing is to destroy the existing cancer now.

Similarly, benefits versus risks should be considered in deciding when and how often to use diagnostic X-rays. Diagnostic X-rays use far lower doses of radiation than are used in X-ray therapy, but since even very small doses add up with time, diagnostic X-rays should also be used with discretion and with respect for their possible harmful effects. Is the X-ray being taken because the patient insists on it, or because the doctor wants to protect himself against a possible future malpractice suit by ordering unnecessary tests? Is it a routine procedure that is likely to yield little of diagnostic usefulness, or can the patient really be expected to benefit from the information the X-ray reveals?

In 1970 national statistics revealed that 129 million Americans (two-thirds of the population) received 210 million medical and dental X-ray examinations involving a total of 650 million X-ray films. Between 1964 and 1970 the rate of medical X-ray examinations increased from 50 to 56 per 100 persons a year, and the rate of dental X-ray visits increased from 27 to 34 per 100. While many of these X-rays are important to the patient's welfare and may even be life-saving, according to the United States Bureau of

Radiological Health, at least 30 percent of them do not contribute any useful information.

Experts on the hazards of radiation advise the patient to consider these questions before an X-ray is taken: Is this X-ray clearly necessary to my well-being? What useful information might it reveal? Are there previous X-rays available or might other tests be taken that would serve the purpose? If the X-ray is necessary, is everything being done to be sure I receive the lowest radiation dose?

This last question involves the quality of the X-ray equipment used and the competence of the technician or physician who takes the X-ray. You are least likely to be subjected to an unnecessary X-ray or one that involves an unnecessarily high radiation dose if the X-ray is done by a specialist in radiology. Dr. Karl Z. Morgan, who for 30 years was director of health services at the Atomic Energy Commission's Oak Ridge National Laboratories, reports that because of poor technique (mainly overexposed and underdeveloped X-rays), patients sometimes receive ten times the radiation dose really needed to obtain a useful X-ray. Dr. Morgan says that too many diagnostic X-rays are taken by untrained persons using outmoded equipment. Only five states require that radiation technicians be properly trained and certified. Only 1 percent of dentists use the most modern X-ray equipment which delivers the lowest radiation dose.

In many states, X-ray equipment is not inspected each year to be sure it is delivering the amount of radiation it was intended to deliver. In fact, in many cases, X-ray equipment is inspected no more often than once in four or five years. In 1973 one in five of the X-ray units inspected throughout the country was delivering excessive and illegal amounts of radiation because the equipment was faulty. Dr. Morgan suggests that before submitting to an X-ray, the patient should check the certificate posted near the machine to see when it was last inspected, and if it was more than a few years ago, ask to have the X-ray done elsewhere.

Dr. Morgan estimates that with relatively little effort, medical radiation exposure could be reduced to less than one-tenth its present level without any reduction in medical benefits—and with improved results in many cases. Techniques to reduce radiation exposure during X-ray examinations include the use of fast films (they are more sensitive, and therefore less radiation is needed to get a good image) and proper collimation of the X-ray beam. A collimator (which can be as simple as a lead washer) narrows the X-ray beam to the size of the film, whereas without collimation the beam may be four times larger than necessary. More than half of the diagnostic X-ray examinations in 1973 exposed people to unnecessary radiation because the beam was larger than it needed to be.

Dr. Morgan also urges the replacement of old X-ray and fluoroscopy equipment with modern X-ray machines that deliver 100 times less radiation. In modern machines the X-ray beam is delivered through a lead-lined open-ended cylinder about 8 inches long. If the X-ray machine your dentist uses has a short, pointed cone, that is a clue to its age and the higher radiation dose it delivers.

Lead sheets should be used to shield the body parts not intended for the X-ray film. A lead shield should always be used (unless it interferes directly with the area to be X-rayed) to protect the sex organs of men and women from X-ray scatter, since radiation can damage the genetic material of eggs and sperm and result in birth defects in future offspring. Since exposure of unborn children to X-rays increases the children's later chances of developing cancer, X-rays during pregnancy should be avoided wherever possible. Dr. Morgan and others recommend that except in emergency situations, X-rays of women who are in their childbearing years should be restricted to the first ten days after the start of the menstrual period, when pregnancy is unlikely. If X-rays must be taken during pregnancy, a lead shield should be used to protect the woman's abdomen, if that will not interfere with the information needed on the X-ray.

CANCER ON THE JOB

Cancer can also be prevented by controlling the exposure of workers to cancer-causing agents that they encounter on the job. The problem of occupational cancer is discussed at length in Part IV, but in the table below you will find an extensive list of known or suspected carcinogens that are potential hazards for millions of American workers. Each day, scores of workers die of cancers that were caused by on-the-job exposure to hazardous substances. They have, in many instances, needlessly traded their lives for their paychecks.

Prevention of occupational cancers may entail such measures as substituting a safer substance for the known carcinogen, dealing with the carcinogen only in closed systems that effectively prevent worker exposure, and instituting protective measures—such as wearing special clothing or breathing through respirators that filter the air—to reduce as much as practicable the amount of the carcinogen that reaches the worker. In extreme cases, there may be

CAUSES OF OCCUPATIONAL CANCERS

Agent	Affected Organ	Incubation Period (years)	Occupation
A. Organic agents			
Coal soot Coal tar Other products of coal combustion	Lung, larynx, skin, scrotum, urinary bladder	9–23	Gashouse workers, stokers, and producers; asphalt, coal tar, and pitch workers; coke-oven workers; miners; still cleaners; chimney sweeps
Petroleum Petroleum coke Wax Creosote Anthracene Paraffin Shale Mineral oils	Nasal cavity, larynx, lung, skin, scrotum	12–30	Contact with lubricating, cooling, paraffin or wax fuel oils, or coke; rubber fillers; retortmen; textile weavers; diesel jet testers
Benzene	Bone marrow (leukemia)	6–14	Explosives, benzene, or rubber cement workers; distillers; dye users; painters; shoemakers
Auramine Benzidine α-naphthylamine β-naphthylamine Magenta 4-aminodiphenyl 4-nitrodiphenyl	Urinary bladder	13–30	Dyestuffs manufacturers and users; rubber workers (pressmen, filtermen, laborers); textile dyers; paint manufacturers
Mustard Gas	Larynx, lung, trachea, bronchi	10–25	Mustard gas workers
Isopropyl oil	Nasal cavity	10+	Producers
Vinyl chloride	Liver (angiosarcoma), brain	20–30	Plastic workers
Bis(chloromethyl) ether Chloromethyl methyl ether	Lung (oat cell carcinoma)	5+	Chemical workers
B. Inorganic agents			
1. Metals Arsenic	Skin, lung. liver	10+	Miners; smelters; insecticide makers and sprayers; tanners; chemical workers; oil refiners; vintners

Agent	Affected Organ	Incubation Period (years)	Occupation
Chromium	Nasal cavity and sinuses, lung, larynx	15–25	Producers, processors, and users; acetylene and aniline workers; bleachers; glass, pottery and linoleum workers; battery makers
Iron oxide	Lung, larynx	—	Iron ore (hematite) miners; metal grinders and polishers; silver finishers; iron foundry workers
Nickel	Nasal sinuses, lung	3–30	Nickel smelters, mixers, and roasters; electrolysis workers
2. Fibers			
Asbestos	Lung, pleural and peritoneal mesothelioma, gastrointestinal tract	4–50	Miners; millers; textile, insulation, and shipyard workers
3. Dusts			
Wood	Nasal cavity and sinuses	30–40	Woodworkers
Leather	Nasal cavity and sinuses, urinary bladder	40–50	Leather and shoe workers
C. Physical agents			
1. Nonionizing radiation			
Ultraviolet rays	Skin	varies with skin pigment and texture	Farmers; sailors
2. Ionizing radiation			
X-rays	Skin, bone marrow (leukemia)	10–25	Radiologists; medical personnel
Uranium Radon Radium Mesothorium	Skin, lung, bone, bone marrow (leukemia)	10–15	Radiologists; miners; radium dial painters; radium chemists
3. Other			
Hypoxia	Bone		Caisson workers

Source: Dr. Philip Cole, Harvard Medical School

no alternative but to put an end to the industrial process involved because no safe and economical way can be found to carry it out.

Whatever the solution, if you look at this list and find that your job exposes you to a known or suspected cancer-causing agent, you should take measures to protect yourself. You might discuss the situation with your union leader or your employer. If no action results or you are self-employed, you might contact the National Institute for Occupational Safety and Health (5600 Fishers Lane, Rockville, Maryland 20852) or the Occupational Safety and Health Administration (Department of Labor, Third Street and Constitution Avenue, N.W., Washington, D.C. 20210). These organizations are charged with the responsibility of assessing hazards to workers and establishing and regulating protective measures. In any case, don't wait until an occupational cancer strikes among your coworkers. By then it may be too late to protect the others.

PREVENTING UTERINE CANCER

Cindy and Paul had been married for nearly three years when they decided that it was time to start a family. Cindy thought it would be a good idea to get a thorough health checkup before becoming pregnant, although she felt perfectly fine and fully expected to be given a clean bill of health.

Cindy was not too worried at first when the doctor called her back to repeat the Pap smear. The repeat examination confirmed the results of the first—Cindy had a severe abnormality of the cervical cells that had a good chance of developing into cancer. The doctor advised prompt treatment, which in Cindy's case involved relatively minor surgery that did not impair her ability to bear children. The doctor assured her that the treatment would effectively prevent the development of cervical cancer. He also told Cindy and Paul that they could start their family any time they wanted, but he cautioned Cindy to return every three months for another Pap smear to be sure the cervical abnormality did not recur.

Prior to Cindy's experience, she had not thought of the Pap test as a means of preventing cancer. She, like many others, thought it only showed the presence of cancer once it had already developed. In fact, if every woman has a Pap smear at least once a year, followed by the proper treatment if a potentially malignant abnormality is found, most cases of actual cervical cancer can be prevented. The increasingly widespread use of the Pap smear is credited with contributing significantly to the dramatic decline in deaths from cervical cancer—a 50 or 60 percent drop in the last 30 years—that has occurred in the United States.

At the same time, an increasing number of so-called in situ carcinomas (surface noninvasive cancers) are being found and treated before invasive cancer develops. For example, in a city-wide study in London, Ontario, where nearly all adult women received a Pap smear between 1968 and 1972, the incidence of invasive cervical cancer dropped 72 percent—from 1.6 per 1,000 women tested in 1968 to 0.44 per 1,000 in 1972, and the incidence of preinvasive cancer was cut in half.

More than 40,000 cases of carcinoma in situ of the cervix were discovered through the Pap smear in American women in 1975 and by treating them potentially fatal cancers were prevented. But in the same year, another 19,000 women were found to have invasive cervical cancer and 7,800 women died of the disease.

A Gallup survey sponsored by the American Cancer Society in 1974 revealed that in the previous decade there had been a 60 percent increase in the proportion of American women who have had Pap smears. In that year, more than three-fourths of adult women said they had had at least one Pap smear at some time during their lives. But only about one-quarter of those women have the test repeated annually, which is the minimum recommended frequency if abnormalities are to be detected and treated before they become cancer. As Cindy's case illustrates, in some situations doctors recommend a Pap smear two to four times a year. It is a harmless and painless procedure.

The Pap test is named for the late Dr. George N. Papanicolaou who in 1928 first reported that long before any symptoms of cancer appeared, one could sometimes find cancer cells by studying under a microscope the cells found in the vaginal fluid. Just like the skin, the lining of a uterus continually sheds cells. It is these sloughed-off cells that are studied in the Pap test.

Dr. Papanicolaou had a hard time convincing his fellow physicians of the potential value of such an examination and it was not until the early 1950s that the Pap test began to catch on. The American Cancer Society, which supported much of Dr. Papanicolaou's research, was largely responsible for promoting widespread use of the test. The Society informed physicians of the test's value through professional materials. In addition, through articles in newspapers and general magazines, the Society convinced many American women of the importance of the test and these women in turn began demanding that their doctors perform it. Right now the American Cancer Society is working toward a goal of a Pap test

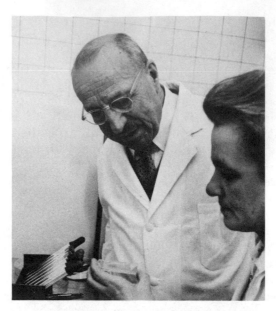

Dr. George N. Papanicolaou developed the simple test known as the Pap smear which can be used both to prevent and to detect cancer of the uterine cervix. His test has been credited with saving the lives of hundreds of thousands of women.

for every adult woman in the United States, and by the end of 1975, 85 percent of American women had had at least one Pap smear. The National Cancer Institute, through grants to state health departments, has begun an extensive program to bring the test to the low-income women who are currently least likely to get a Pap smear. By mid-1975, thirty-four states and two territories were conducting free screening programs for low-income women, with follow-up care when needed.

From the woman's standpoint, the test could not be more simple. In the course of a routine pelvic examination, the doctor takes a swab of the cervix and vaginal fluids and smears it on a glass slide. The sampling is completely painless and at most may cause slight spotting for a day. The test can be done at any time during the menstrual cycle.

The cells on the slide are stained with a special dye and then examined under a microscope in a laboratory. A trained technician determines whether the cells appear normal or abnormal, and if abnormal, to what degree. Abnormal smears are evaluated by a pathologist and the final report is sent to the patient's physician. The National Cancer Institute reports that the Pap test can detect abnormal changes (called dysplasia) in cervical cells five to ten years before symptoms of cancer appear. Studies indicate that the Pap test is approximately 90 percent effective in detecting the early warning signs of cervical cancer. It can also detect about 60 percent of cases of cancer of the body of the uterus, which more commonly occur in women past the menopause.

Experts recommend that every woman have an annual Pap test from the time she first becomes sexually active, at whatever age that may be. Even though cervical cancer is relatively infrequent in women below the age of 40, a study in Houston of more than 10,000 teen-age girls showed that significant cervical abnormalities can and do occur even before the age of 20. The researchers were "quite surprised" to find seriously abnormal Pap tests in as many as 23 of every 1,000 girls between the ages of 13 and 19 who had attended a hospital gynecology clinic. Some of the girls had already developed carcinoma in situ. In recent screening programs, up to 30 percent of the abnormal Pap tests were found among women under the age of 35.

Abnormal conditions of the lining of the uterus (endometrium) that may develop into cancer can also be detected by a recently developed device called an endometrial aspirator. The device consists of a disposable tube connected to a syringe. The doctor inserts the tube through the cervix into the uterus and a piece of tissue is scraped from the uterine lining. This tissue is sucked back through the tube into a cylinder. The tissue specimen is then sent to a laboratory for analysis. If the analysis reveals an overgrowth of lining cells (a condition called endometrial hyperplasia), the woman is advised to have a D and C (dilitation and curettage) which will correct the problem and prevent the later development of cancer.

The examination can be performed in a doctor's office without anesthesia. It should be done at least once, usually around the time of menopause, in women who face a higher than usual risk of developing endometrial cancer: those who are obese, who have diabetes or high blood pressure, or who have been on estrogen replacement therapy.

PREVENTING COLON CANCER

The most common life-threatening cancer among American men and women can be prevented in the majority of cases by detecting and removing benign polyps in the rectum and colon (the large intestine). Polyps are variously shaped projections from the lining of the colon. Most polyps remain benign indefinitely, but certain polyps may eventually become malignant, and proctologists and cancer detection specialists generally believe that to be on the safe side, all polyps should be removed when they are discovered.

Polyps are found during examination of the large intestine with an instrument called the proctosigmoidoscope, a lighted tube which when inserted through the rectum permits the doctor to see directly inside the rectum and the lower part of the large bowel, where about 70 percent of colon and rectal cancers arise. The examination is commonly referred to as a "procto."

Dr. Victor A. Gilbertsen, Director of the Cancer Detection Center at the University of Minnesota, reports that when patients are examined via the proctosigmoidoscope once a year, and all polyps that are found are removed, more than three-quarters of the colon cancers that would be expected to develop in those patients never occur. Those cancers that do develop in spite of this preventive measure are generally early, easily treated, and curable cancers, Dr. Gilbertsen reports. He has based this conclusion on a 25-year study of 18,000 patients, who had more than 85,000 repeated proctoscopic examinations over the years. Usually, any polyps found were removed through the scope at the time of the examination in the doctor's office.

Dr. Gilbertsen's conclusion is that most cases of colon-rectal cancer—which is second only to skin cancer in the number of Americans it strikes and second only to lung cancer in the number it kills—can be prevented by removing polyps found during an annual procto. He recommends that the procto be included as part of the routine physical for all persons aged 40 or older, because most colon-rectal cancers occur after the fifth decade of life.

Other researchers have obtained similar results with periodic procto examinations and support Dr. Gilbertsen's recommendations. In a study at the Kaiser Permanente Medical Care Program in California, death rates from colon-rectal cancer were 400 percent lower among patients who received an annual procto.

The procto will be discussed further in the section on early cancer detection (see Chapter 5) as will a newer instrument—the fiberoptic colonoscope—which permits the doctor to examine the entire 6-foot length of the large intestine and to remove any polyps that are found.

Annual proctos and removal of polyps and other suspicious lesions found during the exam is considered vital for persons whose close blood relatives have had colon cancer, because there is a tendency for this disease to be hereditary. For the relatively rare in-

dividual who has inherited a condition known as familial polyposis, removal of the entire colon is recommended as the most
effective cancer preventive, since all patients with that condition
eventually develop colon cancer.

PREVENTING BREAST CANCER

Other methods of cancer prevention have their strong advocates
but are the subject of intense controversy. One is the finding of
noninvasive cancer in the breast—carcinoma in situ. These may be
accidentally detected in the course of a biopsy of breast tissue for
some other problem or they may show up as tiny, suspicious areas
on a mammogram, a special X-ray of the breasts that is currently
being widely used to examine women for hidden breast cancers.

A certain percentage of patients with these cancers in situ eventually will go on to develop invasive cancer; others never do. But
since patients with one in situ breast cancer usually have similar
lesions elsewhere in the breast, most doctors recommend that the
safest approach is removal of the breast (simple or total mastectomy) at the outset, which, in effect, prevents the development of
an invasive cancer in that breast.

Among the latter group of physicians is Dr. Jerome A. Urban,
the breast cancer surgeon at Memorial Hospital in New York who
operated on Margaretta (Happy) Rockefeller shortly before her husband was confirmed as Vice President. Mrs. Rockefeller was found
to have a cancer in her left breast, which Dr. Urban removed along
with many of the lymph nodes that surround the breast. These
nodes could harbor cancer cells that might later spread to the rest
of the body. At the same time, Dr. Urban took a biopsy of Mrs.
Rockefeller's right breast at the mirror image site of the cancer in
the left breast. He did this because his studies have shown that 16
percent of women with cancer in one breast eventually develop a
cancer in the opposite breast, most often in the mirror-image location. The biopsy indicated that Mrs. Rockefeller's right breast
harbored a tiny cancer in situ, and Dr. Urban then removed that
breast as well. According to Mr. Rockefeller, his wife decided she
would prefer the mastectomy to worrying about the possibility
that the in situ cancer would develop into a full-blown invasive—
and less curable—cancer at some later date.

Some breast cancer specialists now recommend an operation
that is far less disfiguring than total mastectomy to prevent breast
cancer in women who are considered high-risk individuals, women
with certain benign breast abnormalities, as well as women whose

mothers and sisters had breast cancer. In some cases, a strong family history of breast cancer can increase a woman's chance of getting the disease by 47 times. (The relationship between heredity and breast cancer is described at length in Part IV.)

Surgery to prevent breast cancer in such cases generally involves removal of the breast tissue beneath the skin, leaving a sac consisting of the outer skin and nipples alone and replacing the removed tissue with a plastic implant. The woman awakens after surgery with two breasts that look very much like the ones she had before. Her muscles and lymph nodes have not been removed, and she experiences no impairment of her normal functions. Sometimes this operation is done in two stages—first the subcutaneous mastectomy and then the implant. Doctors who do preventive—or prophylactic—breast surgery report that for those patients who accept the operation, it often gives them great peace of mind. Until the surgery many of these women fretted for weeks before each breast examination and lived with a constant fear of developing breast cancer. However, such women still need to be examined periodically, because they retain some breast tissue in which a cancer could arise.

Preventing cancer is clearly the surest way to prevent deaths from cancer. Many of the tools of cancer prevention are already available and need only be applied to their full life-saving potential.

As doctors gain a better understanding about how cancers develop, they are discovering new ways of detecting cell changes that precede the actual development of invasive, and therefore potentially fatal, cancers. Studies are underway of Pap-type tests for cancer in such organs as the lungs, bladder, esophagus, and stomach. It is not yet certain whether examinations of cells shed by these organs can consistently reveal the precancerous state—and even if they do whether it will be possible to locate and remove the suspicious lesion before it has a chance to become invasive cancer—but there is no doubt that the tests have the potential, at least, of becoming a valuable weapon in the battle to prevent cancer.

As more is understood about cancer's causes, reducing cancer deaths will focus increasingly on preventing cancer from starting in the first place by avoiding exposure to those agents that cause it. But right now, in many ways, preventing cancer is up to you. It is up to you to control known causes of cancer like smoking and excessive sun exposure. It is up to you to get regular examinations, including such cancer-prevention tests as the Pap and the procto. It is up to you to find out the nature of the substances you work with and, through your union or joint action with fellow workers, insist that your employer protect you from exposure to agents that can cause cancer or otherwise damage your health. It is even up to you to protect yourself and your children from excessive exposure to penetrating radiation by questioning the need for medical and dental X-rays that are ordered, by checking to be sure up-to-date equipment and lead shielding are used, and by not insisting on an X-ray if the doctor thinks it is unnecessary.

Such measures will undoubtedly always be important to cancer prevention, because it now seems highly unlikely that the coming years will yield anything like a "vaccine" or other simplistic preventive tool that will protect people from developing cancer.

4. How to Stop Smoking

Anyone who wants to can give up cigarettes. Does that sound like a rash statement? Not to the experts who have carefully studied the reasons people smoke and who have helped thousands to quit smoking. The secret, they say, is in the wanting. Giving up smoking must be a personal decision. If you make that decision and commitment, you can quit.

It is this commitment that can overcome the fear some smokers have of being unable to function without cigarettes, of being so miserable they can't stand themselves. It is this commitment that can carry the quitter over the temporary discomfort and feelings of loss that often mark the first days or weeks after stopping smoking. It is this commitment that helps you find the way that will enable you to quit.

Cigarette smoking is a learned behavior—a habit, not an instinct or reflex one is born with. Like all other learned behaviors, it can be unlearned or a new behavior can be learned in its place. For some people, cigarette smoking is a habit that has been reinforced forty times a day for thirty years (the two-packs-a-day smokers). But no matter how strong the habit, it can be broken and a new habit —the habit of nonsmoking—can replace it.

For some people, breaking the smoking habit is relatively easy. One man who smoked four packs a day was dating a woman who objected to his incessant smoking. When he asked her to marry him, she said "yes" but only if he gave up cigarettes. "What will I do," he asked, "when I want to smoke?" She replied, "Take a deep breath." The man tried it and it worked.

Another man was leaving the house one Sunday evening to get a pack of cigarettes. His wife asked him to pick up some milk for the children's breakfast. When he got to the store, he realized he didn't have enough money for both items. The mere fact that he debated about which one to buy suddenly struck him as so "sick" that he gave up smoking on the spot.

But if quitting cigarettes were that simple for most people, there would be far more than 30 million former smokers by now, since two-thirds of the 52 million people currently smoking have tried to quit at least once.

Countless schemes and gadgets have been devised to aid those smokers who cannot quit by making a decision to do so. A number of these techniques are highly successful; others, less so. They include cigarette counting devices, special filters, nicotine substitutes, plastic cigarettes, hypnosis, behavioral reconditioning, sleep learning, and a variety of free and paying stop-smoking clinics and group sessions. Since each person is different and smokes for his own set of reasons, different methods help different people to quit. In a sense, you need to tailor-make your own stop-smoking plan.

Dr. Donald T. Fredrickson, director of the Inter-Society Commission for Heart Disease Resources and former director of New York City's Smoking Research Project, believes that only a relative handful of smokers actually need professional help to give up cigarettes. Given the right circumstances, he says, most people can do it on their own. These circumstances, or "basic ingredients" of a stop-smoking program, are:

- *Motivation:* Finding the right incentive to quit smoking is a must. Your reasons must be strong and important, because success depends on your willingness and determination to carry through.
- *Insight:* Understanding what you get out of cigarettes will help you to find substitutes and learn to do without smoking. The United States Public Health Service has prepared a "Smoker's Self-Testing Kit" to help you understand your smoking behavior.
- *Practice:* You've had a lot of practice at smoking. Now you must be willing to practice *not* smoking.
- *Attitude:* If you think of quitting smoking as giving something up, a loss, your outlook will not help support your determination to stick with it. Rather, stopping should be considered a plus, a building into your personality of a new and exciting dimension of self-control.

Dr. Daniel Horn, former head of the National Clearinghouse for Smoking and Health and the psychologist who developed the Smoker's Self-Testing Kit, says the first step toward quitting is to start thinking about your smoking instead of just drifting along, smoking mindlessly. Part One of the kit examines what you know about smoking and how you feel about it, "Do You Want to Change Your Smoking Habits?" It will help you to assess the relative importance to you of such matters as your concern about health, the example you set for others, the esthetics of smoking, and self-mastery over cigarettes.

Part Two of the self-test helps you determine what you think the effects of smoking on your health might be. How important are these effects, are they likely to affect you, will you benefit from quitting, do you think you can quit? Smokers often try to justify their habit by saying, "I want to enjoy life, and smoking is part of enjoying life. I'd rather live a few years less and enjoy the life I have." What these people forget is that the health effect of smoking is rarely sudden, painless death. More likely, smoking will cause a chronic, limiting illness—such as emphysema—which is hardly compatible with enjoyment of life. Emphysema can strike in the thirties and forties and turn an active person into a respiratory cripple who is constantly short of breath. Similarly, heart disease can be a crippler as well as an instant killer. And lung cancer—or any smoking-caused cancer—is hardly a pleasant illness or a painless way to die.

Some smokers try to rationalize that other things cause cancer, so why pick on smoking? Some convince themselves that "It's not going to happen to me." They rationalize: "I heard you have to smoke forty cigarettes a day for twenty years to have a harmful effect, and I only smoke thirty-nine," or "I don't smoke on Sundays so that gives my lungs a chance to clear out the poisons." But once you realize that the hazards of smoking apply to you as much as to "the other guy," you are more likely to make the commitment to quit.

Part Three of the self-test examines why you smoke. Psychological research has shown that cigarettes are commonly used for one or more of six reasons. The same person is likely to put different cigarettes he smokes during the day to different purposes. The reasons, as itemized by Dr. Silvan Tomkins of the City College of New York, are as follows:

- *Stimulation:* Stimulation smokers use cigarettes to get themselves going, to increase their energy and focus their sense of purpose. They frequently are heavy morning smokers, sometimes having their first cigarette the moment they step out of bed.
- *Handling:* Cigarettes give smokers something to do with their hands (and mouths), the satisfaction of manipulating objects: taking out the cigarette, lighting up, watching the smoke, playing with the ashes and butt.
- *Pleasurable Relaxation:* About 15 percent of smokers use cigar-

ettes to enhance good feelings and help them relax, after meals
or after making love, or when they have finished a task.
- *Crutch or Tension Reduction:* For nearly a third of smokers
cigarettes are a means of relieving tension, reducing anxiety,
coping with anger, disappointment, fear, depression, and other
bad feelings. They light up more often when the going gets
rough.
- *Psychological Addiction:* About one in four smokers really
craves cigarettes—feels "hooked" by them. The craving for the
next cigarette begins to grow the moment the last one is stubbed
out.
- *Habit:* Some smokers reach for their cigarettes unconsciously,
in an automatic response. They are not even aware of the fact
that they are smoking, and they often light a new cigarette while
one is still burning in the ashtray.

Part Four of the self-testing kit concerns the world around you
and how easy or difficult this environment will make it for you to
change your cigarette habit. How supportive are the key people in
your life, your colleagues at work and family at home? Are you
influenced by doctors, advertising, the general climate?

Dr. Horn emphasizes that this self-testing kit is designed to help
you focus on why you smoke, your motivations for quitting, and
the kind of support you are likely to get if you do quit. But the
decision to quit is up to you. Without that decision, no technique
will be successful.

Dr. Fredrickson has outlined a four-week program for stopping
smoking. His approach can be applied on your own or in a group.
The same program can be condensed into a two-week or even
shorter period. It is designed to prepare you for quitting, which
you may not actually do until the end of the program. It is basically a shortened version of the program used in Helping Smokers
Quit clinics sponsored by local units of the American Cancer Society and several other groups. This is the basic program:

- *First Week:* 1. Develop a list of reasons for wanting to give up
smoking, concentrating on the positive benefits. Read the list
daily and add to it. Then focus on the two or three most important reasons.

  2. Complete the Self-Testing Kit.

  3. Wrap your cigarette pack in an 8½-by-11-inch piece of paper
and secure it with two rubber bands. You may smoke whenever
you wish, but before you light up you must unwrap the pack

and write down the time, what you were doing, how you were feeling and how important (on a scale of one to five, where one is most important and five least important) that particular cigarette is to you. Then rewrap the pack.

This procedure, which should be repeated each time you want to smoke, is designed to make you aware of when and how you use cigarettes and make the act of lighting up a more conscious one. "The wrapping technique makes it virtually impossible to smoke automatically," Dr. Fredrickson says. You begin to see that smoking is a habit you have taught yourself by associating cigarettes with different emotions and activities. With this understanding, you can start to reverse what you learned—you can retrain yourself into a new habit of nonsmoking. For instance, with the wrap technique, one smoker discovered that half of his cigarettes were smoked when he drank coffee. By reducing his coffee consumption, he was able to cut down on his smoking.

● *Second Week:* 1. Review your reasons for wanting to stop smoking.

2. Continue wrapping your cigarettes and keeping a detailed smoking record.

3. Never carry matches or a lighter.

4. Do not carry cigarettes on your person. At home, keep them far from reach, in the basement or mailbox; at work, lock them in a desk or give them to a secretary. Whatever you do, never have your wrapped pack within arm's reach.

5. Begin a gradual program of smoking reduction: make a pledge each morning of the number of cigarettes you think you can manage on that day and see how close you come. Start eliminating some cigarettes systematically—start either with those that are least important to you or those that are most important, whichever way works best for you. Try to smoke fewer cigarettes each day than you smoked the day before. Many people find it helpful to try to delay their first cigarette one-half hour longer each day.

● *Third Week:* 1. Continue all the previous instructions.

2. Do not buy a fresh pack until you have finished your last cigarette, and never buy a carton.

3. Change brands twice during the week, and with each change choose a brand that is lower in tar and nicotine content than the previous one. Do not return to your old brand.

4. Select a period that is likely to be easiest for you and try to go 48 hours without smoking at all. When you succeed with your first 48 hours (and if you don't make it on the first try, try

again), ask yourself whether you are ready to stop altogether at that point.

● *Fourth Week:* 1. Increase your physical activity. This helps to reduce tension and nervousness.

2. Temporarily avoid the activities you most powerfully associate with cigarettes. If, for example, you normally smoke after meals, don't linger when you've finished eating. Get up and do something, especially something that distracts your attention or makes it difficult for you to smoke at the same time.

3. Find a temporary cigarette substitute—gum, celery or carrot sticks, headless matches, flavored toothpicks, a plastic cigarette. One woman found it helped to suck on two small stones.

4. Whenever you feel the urge to smoke, try a deep-breathing exercise. Let yourself go limp. Inhale slowly and deeply, holding your breath, and count to five. Then slowly exhale. This is similar to a meditation exercise which cured one inveterate smoker after all else had failed, including an attempt at hypnosis.

5. Have a plan of action ready when temptation comes, an activity that will keep your hands busy. One woman took up knitting and in one year had completed a magnificent bedspread.

It is important, Dr. Horn maintains, to tailor your stop-smoking program to your own needs and lifestyle and in accordance with how you use cigarettes. For example, the stimulation smoker will do best to substitute other activities that help him get going, such as a cold shower, brisk walk, deep breathing, or a new hobby. For the "handler," finding something else to manipulate may be vital. The crutch smoker has to try deliberately facing difficult situations without cigarettes. This may seem forbidding when you think about it, but many people find it is not as hard as they had anticipated.

The addicted smoker is one who must quit cold turkey, Dr. Horn reports. He never gets unhooked simply by cutting down, because each cigarette he smokes reinforces the addiction. But once an addicted smoker quits, he's unlikely to resume because he remembers what a hard time he had quitting and doesn't ever want to have to go through it again.

The important thing to remember, no matter what kind of smoker you are and how wedded you think you are to cigarettes, is you *can* give them up if you are really motivated to do so and you adopt a plan of action personalized to suit your needs and smoking pattern. It is also important to realize that many—probably most—smokers are not successful at quitting for good the first time they try. Backsliding is common, and it should not be taken as a sign that you can't give up cigarettes. *If you don't succeed at first, try again and again and again, if necessary, because eventually you can make it if you really want to.*

Each smoker who has gone the route has his own answer to how to quit. For one, it was establishing strict rules as to when, where, and under what circumstances he was allowed to smoke. For another, carrying one cigarette with him as a security blanket kept him from panicking and enabled him to resist the temptation to smoke. Some men switched temporarily—or permanently—to a pipe. One man carried a thermos filled with a very peppery soup which he drank whenever he felt the urge to smoke. Some find it helpful to chew gum. Others use a nicotine substitute like lobeline for a while. Many make announcements to everyone they know that they are giving up cigarettes and feel strengthened by this public commitment. Others don't want to be noticed—they prefer to be sure they are successful before they tell a soul.

Dr. Horn points out that most how-to-stop-smoking books are not particularly helpful because they contain generalized hints for quitting that do not take into account individual differences in the reasons for smoking and the need for individualized substitutes. For example, some recommend taking a cold shower whenever you feel an irresistible urge to smoke. If you smoke for stimulation, the shower might help, but it is hardly an adequate substitute for someone who smokes for the enjoyment of handling a cigarette.

There are at least two books, however, that do take individual needs into account and can help you tailor your personal stop-smoking program. One is *The Thinking Man's Guide To Quitting Cigarettes* by Eliot Tozer (an Award Books paperback, $1.25), based on the nationwide television series "Why You Smoke," which was produced under a grant from the American Cancer Society. Another is *You Can Quit Smoking in 14 Days* by Walter S. Ross (Reader's Digest Press, hardcover $6.95). Mr. Ross has written on smoking and health for 15 years for the Reader's Digest and the American Cancer Society. Both books contain the four short tests included in the Smoker's Self-Testing Kit. In addition, individual copies of the self-testing kit can be obtained free from the Center for Disease Control (Bureau of Health Education, National Clearinghouse for Smoking and Health, Atlanta, Georgia 30333). (It is also available for 40 cents from the U.S. Government Printing Office, Washington, D.C. 20402.)

If you feel you can't quit smoking on your own, there are groups and clinics throughout the country where you can get guidance and group support. Virtually all these groups are run by former smokers who have been specially trained to be "facilitators" in quit-smoking programs. To find out if there is a free clinic in your area, check with the local affiliate of the American Cancer Society, the American Heart Association, or the American Lung Association. In 1975, the Cancer Society alone sponsored more than 1,500 such clinics around the country.

Your community's health department or the local hospital's department of community health or preventive medicine may also know of or operate such programs. The Seventh-day Adventists also conduct nondenominational five-day quit smoking clinics in communities throughout the United States. Some of these programs charge a small fee to cover operating costs, such as room rental, but most also offer the course free to those who are unable to pay.

Other programs run by commercial (profit-making) organizations charge larger sums. For some smokers, paying a sizable amount for a stop-smoking program gives them an added incentive to stay off cigarettes. As John M., who completed a ten-week SmokEnders program a year ago remarked, "I figure that first cigarette I smoke will cost me $150, and that helps to keep me from smoking it." SmokEnders, the oldest and largest commercial organization of its kind, conducts stop-smoking seminars in twenty states, Washington D.C., and Canada. Its national headquarters are at Memorial Parkway (at Prospect Street), Phillipsburg, New Jersey 18865 (201-454-4444).

5. Early Detection

Consider these odds:

When breast cancer is detected and treated in its early stages, there is a more than eight-in-ten chance that the patient will be alive five years later. But if the cancer has already spread to the nearby lymph nodes (glands), the five-year survival chances are closer to one in two.

When cancer of the uterus is detected early while it is still confined to its original site, the five-year survival rate is also better than 80 percent. But the rate is only half that if the cancer has already spread regionally by the time it is detected and treated.

Similarly, for cancer of the larynx, 79 percent of patients survive five or more years in early cases, but only 38 percent of more advanced cases live that long. And for cancer of the colon and rectum, 71 percent in early cases, 43 percent in later ones. Bladder cancer, also 71 percent for early cases, but only 21 percent when the cancer is already advanced at the time of diagnosis. And so on and so forth.

If these were the odds in a race, it wouldn't be hard to guess which way the betting would go. Little wonder, then, that cancer specialists place so much emphasis on early detection. Not all serious cancers can be prevented—at this point at least. But in many instances where prevention of the cancer itself is impossible or unsuccessful, death from cancer can still be avoided by detecting and treating the disease early, before it has spread beyond the site of origin.

Cancers remain confined that way for varying periods of time—some for years, even decades, others for only months. Although a few kinds of cancer—for example, cancer of the pancreas—do not produce readily detectable signs or symptoms until the disease is well advanced, most of the common cancers can be found early, long before the patient himself has any clue that he or she may be ill.

It stands to reason biologically that if a cancer is found and treated while it is still localized, the treatment has the best chance

FIVE YEAR CANCER SURVIVAL RATES*
FOR SELECTED SITES

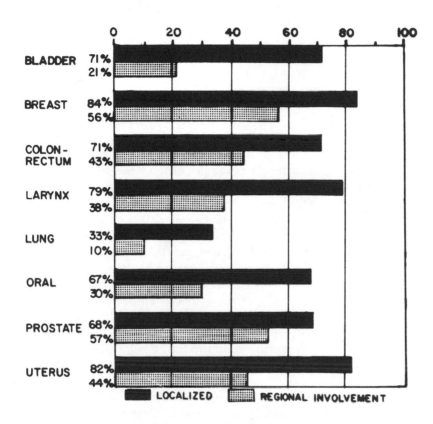

*ADJUSTED FOR NORMAL LIFE EXPECTANCY
SOURCE: END RESULTS GROUP, NATIONAL CANCER INSTITUTE 1965-69

The cure rate for cancers that are treated before they have started to spread beyond the site in which they arose (that is, localized cancer) is usually considerably higher than when there is regional involvement, or spread of the cancer to nearby lymph nodes. This demonstrates the life-saving value of early detection.

of totally eradicating the cancer. But if some cancer cells have already escaped to other parts of the body when the cancer is first treated, it is far more difficult to wipe out every last cancer cell and the patient is much more likely to suffer a recurrence and to die of his disease.

As indicated earlier, for many of the more common types of

cancer—including cancers of the breast, colon, uterus, bladder, and prostate—more than two-thirds of patients can be cured if the cancer is detected and adequately treated while still localized. In recent decades increasing percentages of patients with these cancers have been saved because more and more cases are being diagnosed in their early stages.

Although we are still a long way from a single test to detect all or even most cancers, a host of excellent diagnostic tools are currently available and doctors and the public are learning to take advantage of them. But further improvements can be made. Experts estimate that if the methods we already have for early cancer detection were universally applied, there could be a doubling or tripling of survival rates for all patients with these cancers. It is up to you to take advantage wherever possible of the life-saving tools already in hand.

Unlike most of the diseases with which we are all familiar, cancer in its early stages almost never causes pain or clear-cut feeling of sickness. Because of the absence of these traditional warning signs, detecting early, curable cancer means searching for clues to the possible existence of cancer in otherwise healthy people.

Too often Americans feel embarrassed to go to a doctor or medical clinic when they feel perfectly okay—embarrassed and a bit guilty about taking up the time and energy of health professionals when other, obviously sick people may need them. But those who avail themselves of the tools medicine has developed for early cancer detection and who periodically check their own bodies for possible signs of cancer are actually saving medicine a great deal of time, effort, and expense in the long run. It is far simpler (and less costly), as well as life-saving, to find and treat an early localized cancer than to wage a long, hard war against a cancer that did not come to medical attention until it had spread beyond its original site and caused undeniable symptoms of illness.

Biologically speaking, the importance of early detection in symptomless people is evident from the following fact: on the average, half of cancers (excluding cancers of the blood-forming organs) develop metastases during their "hidden" life before they produce symptoms that would prompt the average person to visit a doctor.

This is not to say, however, that cancer never gives any clues to its presence until it is well on its way to claiming the lives of its victims. Even early cancers sometimes produce noticeable warning signals, but many people who develop these cautionary signs tend to ignore them or shrug them off as "nothing important." The American Cancer Society has been working for decades to publicize what it calls the "seven warning signals" of cancer—the "seven signals that can save your life . . . if you see your doctor." The Society's seven signals are: *a change in bowel or bladder habits; a sore that does not heal; unusual bleeding or discharge from the genital, urinary, or digestive tract; a thickening or lump in a breast or elsewhere; indigestion or difficulty in swallowing; an obvious change in a wart or mole; and a nagging cough or hoarseness.* These signals and their potential significance will be discussed more fully later in this section.

Early cancers may also produce warning signals that are not apparent to the individual with the disease, but are detectable through special tests. Two of these were described in the previous section on preventing cancer: the Pap test, which detects the beginnings of cancer of the cervix, and the procto, which enables the physician to spot precancer of the colon or rectum. These tests can also reveal more advanced but still frequently curable stages of these cancers. There are many other such tests for picking up early, symptomless, and usually curable cancers, and their wider use among persons who are at risk of developing one or another form of cancer, followed by prompt treatment of any cancer discovered, could save many lives that are currently being lost.

But no single, general test has yet been developed that can detect all kinds of cancers. Rather, there are a variety of specific tests that can be used to detect specific cancers in their early, most curable stages. The tools for early cancer detection most commonly used include the following:

● Physical examination in which a physician or trained medical assistant is able to feel for abnormalities in various parts of the body. Manual examination of the breast, thyroid, ovaries, uterus, and prostate may discover a lump, a change in shape, or other findings that warrant further investigation.
● Examinations of sloughed-off cells, such as from the cervix, to detect early malignant changes in cells. Such "cytology" examinations, as they are called, are being used to detect early cancers of the lung and bladder in addition to the uterine cervix (in a Pap smear) and may be applicable to some other organs as well.
● X-ray examinations of organs, such as the breasts and colon, to pinpoint suspicious areas that might harbor a cancer. Breast X-rays, called mammograms or xeroradiograms, use special film or paper and as little radiation as is needed to produce an adequate image. Colon X-rays, known as barium enemas, use a contrast dye to highlight abnormal areas of the large intestine.
● Lighted instruments, such as the proctosigmoidoscope, which

allow the physician to view directly an otherwise hidden part of the body. The proctosigmoidoscope is used to detect colon-rectal cancers and the bronchoscope is used to locate early lung cancers which may first show up in sputum cytology and may be too small to be seen on an X-ray of the chest.

- Thermography, a heat-sensitive picture made with infra-red rays, is used to detect "hot spots" in tissue that might mean cancer, because cancers as well as some other abnormalities tend to produce a higher temperature than normal tissues. Thus far, thermography for cancer detection has been used mainly for examining the breasts.

- Ultrasound, which uses very high frequency sound waves as a "radar" system to explore tissues inside the body, is being used more and more experimentally as a possible cancer detection device. Its advantages are that it is thought to do no harm to the person being examined, it gives immediate results, and, since it involves no radiation, it can be repeated often apparently with-out hazard.

- Laboratory tests of samples of stool and urine for the presence of blood. The finding of blood in body excretions requires closer examination for hidden cancers of the colon, rectum, kidney, or bladder.

- Various blood tests, such as the CEA (carcinoembryonic anti-gen) test, detect changes in the immunological status of the body that often accompany cancers. Thus far, however, these blood tests are not sufficiently accurate to be used to screen large numbers of ostensibly healthy people for the possible presence of very early cancer. The tests may come out positive when no cancer is present and sometimes come out negative even if the person is known to have cancer. Currently, therefore, these blood tests are used only as an adjunct to other cancer detection examinations.

Some cancers do not lend themselves to early detection with any of the currently available tools. Cancer of the pancreas, for exam-ple, has thus far defied all efforts to find it early. Leukemia, a blood cancer, and Hodgkin's disease, a cancer of the lymph sys-tem, are nonlocalized by definition, no matter when they are diagnosed. With leukemia the chances for cure do not seem to be much affected by how early the disease is diagnosed, although if an individual is extremely ill and deteriorated at the time of diag-nosis, the powerful drugs and radiation used to treat leukemia may be more than the patient can withstand. For Hodgkin's disease, however, the earlier in the course of the disease it is diagnosed and treated, the greater are the chances for cure.

Once an area that may harbor a cancer has been detected, the next step is to confirm the diagnosis by directly examining a small sample of tissue removed from the area. This is called a biopsy. It involves making laboratory slides of the removed tissue and studying the slides under a microscope. For the breast, four out of five biopsies turn out to show no cancer. Sometimes, when the organ suspected of harboring a cancer is not readily accessible, such as the pancreas, or when X-ray examination indicates with a fair degree of certainty that the abnormality seen suggests cancer, a diagnosis must be made during exploratory surgery.

Thanks to early cancer detection, Mrs. Betty P. of Williston, North Dakota, says she has thus far had "ten good years which I might not otherwise have enjoyed." At the age of 54 following the funeral of a relative who had died of cancer, Betty decided to go to her doctor for a routine physical examination. "In examining my breasts, the doctor found a tiny tumor. It was so small I couldn't even feel it myself. The biopsy indicated it was cancerous and I had my breast removed. I've been fine ever since. I should say I was lucky."

Harry L., a vigorous 77-year-old, also knows well the value of early cancer detection. Twenty-five years ago, in mid-career as a labor leader in Minneapolis, Harry decided to go for a checkup at the University of Minnesota's Cancer Detection Center.

"I felt fit as a fiddle," Harry recalls, "but the doctors found something suspicious—polyps in my bowel." The polyps were removed and one polyp proved to harbor the beginnings of a cancer of the colon. "That examination probably saved my life," Harry says. "My mother had colon cancer, but she didn't get hers diagnosed until she had symptoms of intestinal obstruction and her disease was pretty far advanced. She lived only a year after her surgery."

Harry says he goes back to the Minnesota detection center for a complete checkup every year, and he has encouraged hundreds of others among his colleagues and friends to do the same. He even periodically shows a film on cancer detection to his union members. "There are about half a dozen very grateful people in my union, because when they went for their exam, a cancer was found and found early. A thorough annual checkup is the best health bargain you can get," the labor leader says.

To be effective in detecting a hidden cancer, a complete checkup should include, among other things, blood and urine tests; a digital rectal exam; a procto; a pelvic exam as well as a Pap test for women; a chest X-ray; a manual examination of the abdomen, thyroid gland, and of prostate gland in men and the breasts in women; a thorough scrutiny of all skin areas and the mouth using a mirror that allows the examiner to see into the throat and larynx; a look into the back of the eyes with a lighted scope; a careful medical history; and a listing and checking out of any suspicious symptoms that the person may have noticed. And if the doctor is really doing a thorough job, he will take this opportunity to advise his patient on cancer prevention.

Unfortunately, relatively few Americans get anything like the yearly examination Harry receives at the University of Minnesota, although there is nothing involved in that examination that any physician could not do. It is not necessary to go to a special cancer detection clinic to get a proper physical that could ferret out an early cancer (as well as other health problems). The American Cancer Society conducts numerous educational programs for family and other physicians to keep them up to date on the latest techniques of cancer detection that could be applied to their patients.

Sometimes, however, the patient must be forthright in insisting that the doctor perform certain tests that he might otherwise skip. Far too often a male doctor is reluctant to examine the breasts or pelvic region of his female patients, although these are among the most common areas in which cancer develops in women. Only a small percentage of doctors include the procto as part of a routine physical for men and women past the age of 40, although this test can detect while still curable the most common life-threatening cancer in the nation today. You can usually tell if your doctor is planning to do a procto because he will ask that you follow a special diet and take an enema or laxative the day before your examination is scheduled. If he has not done so, ask him before your visit if he intends to do a procto.

Examination of the prostate gland (by inserting a gloved finger into the rectum) is also often skipped in a routine physical, even though prostate cancer is the third largest cancer killer in men. Thus, it is the patient's job to see to it that a routine physical includes the complete list of dectection procedures. It is also the patient's responsibility to do self-examination, heed possible warning signs of cancer that might be noticed, and see the doctor promptly for a proper workup if anything suspicious is found, rather than wait for the next annual exam.

Although a thorough annual physical is probably the surest way to pick up early, curable cancers (as well as early stages of other diseases), such a checkup for every adult American is currently not practical or even possible. Even if everyone wanted a complete annual physical and could afford it, there would not be adequate medical facilities and personnel to perform all the examinations. Therefore, specialists have worked out approaches that help doctors pick out for more thorough examination those people who are at greatest risk of developing one of another form of cancer. In most cases, this amounts to restricting certain tests to patients in the age groups when the various cancers are most likely to develop. It may also mean that people who face a higher than usual risk of cancer—for example, because of their family or personal medical histories, their habits, or their occupational exposures— are singled out for more frequent examinations starting at much younger ages than would otherwise be recommended. The National Cancer Institute is now attempting to develop a cancer screening system that will identify at least 75 percent of individuals with cancer at a time when the disease is still localized in at least 90 percent of them.

DETECTING BREAST CANCER

Lillian F., a 45-year-old mother of two teen-age sons, is very proud of the fact that she discovered her own breast cancer and in doing so saved her life. An avid tennis player and swimmer (she became a senior life saver after her mastectomy), she is living proof that ritualistic adherence to a simple monthly procedure called breast self-examination (BSE) can be life-saving. Ten years ago while performing the monthly examination her doctor had taught her, Mrs. F. discovered a tiny lump in her right breast. She immediately visited the doctor, who said he could feel the lump too and referred her to a specialist for an X-ray and possible biopsy. The lump proved to be a tiny cancer—less than one centimeter in diameter—and after an examination of the tissue removed during surgery, the doctor told Mrs. F. that the disease seemed to be confined to her breast. With that removed, the doctor said, Mrs. F. could expect to see her sons graduate from high school and college and she could look forward to the day when she would be a grandmother. The surgeon said her prompt action after discovering the lump was wise indeed. To this day Mrs. F. wonders what might have happened to her without BSE, since she was not due for her next medical checkup for another six months.

Mrs. F. still does BSE each month, in addition to being checked twice a year by her doctor. After all, she has another breast, and having once had breast cancer, her chance of developing cancer in the remaining breast is somewhat greater than if she had not had the disease.

Breast self-examination involves just a few minutes of your life once each month but could mean twenty or more years added to your life. Yet a Gallup survey sponsored by the American Cancer Society in 1973 revealed that while three-fourths of American women know about BSE, only one in five women practice it monthly, and three in ten who are aware of BSE have never done it at all. The survey showed that most of those women who regularly do BSE had learned the technique from their physicians but only one-fourth of all women had ever received such instruction from a doctor. Another reason for failing to do BSE regularly, the survey indicated, was the fear of many women that checking their breasts each month would cause them to worry unnecessarily. Few were aware of the fact that eight out of ten lumps found in the breast are not cancerous.

While breast cancer is the most common serious cancer among American women—striking approximately one in thirteen—it is also a fact that the vast majority of women—twelve out of thirteen, to be exact—never get it. And since the early, more curable breast cancers are likely to be discovered through a monthly examination, it is really the women who neglect to do BSE who should be worrying.

Recently, the widely publicized discovery that both the wife of the President and the wife of the Vice President (then Vice President designate) had breast cancer inspired countless women—temporarily, at least—to do BSE. Betty Ford underwent a mastectomy, in September 1974, for a cancer found by her physician during a routine examination, and Margaretta (Happy) Rockefeller had her left breast removed less than three weeks later for a cancer she discovered while performing breast self-examination. Mrs. Rockefeller said she had been stimulated to do BSE by Mrs. Ford's experience with breast cancer. Since Mrs. Rockefeller had an annual checkup seven months earlier, her discovery through BSE of the cancer five months before she was due for her next routine physical could well have meant the difference between the small, localized cancer she actually had and more extensive, less curable disease.

The best time to do BSE is right after the menstrual period, when the breasts are least swollen and tender. For women who are past the menopause, pick a date—the beginning of the month or the date of your birthday is usually easiest to remember—and do it at approximately the same time each month. Women who have had a hysterectomy should consult their doctors about the best time for them to do BSE.

Start BSE while in the shower or bathtub. With wet (even soapy) fingers, held flat and together, massage gently and in a circular motion every area of each breast from the chest bone to the armpit. Check for any lump, hard knot, or thickening. When examining the right breast, use the fingers of the left hand and place the right hand behind your head. Repeat the procedure on the left breast, this time using your right hand to massage and placing your left hand behind your head.

After bathing, stand in front of a mirror with your arms raised over your head. Look for any changes in the shape of each breast, or any swelling, dimpling of the skin, or changes in the nipples. Then place your hands firmly on your hips, tensing your muscles by pushing inward. Again, look for dimpling or changes in shape. Chances are your left and right breast will not match exactly—few women's do—but by examining them regularly, you will be able to notice readily if the shape of one breast changes.

For the final part of BSE, lie down flat on your back. To examine your right breast, place a pillow under your right shoulder and fold your right arm under your head. Using your left hand (with fingers together and flat) and thinking of your breast as the face of a clock, feel gently with a small circular motion at each hour of the clock. Begin at the outermost portion of your breast at the 12 o'clock position, then move to 1 o'clock, 2 o'clock, and so on.

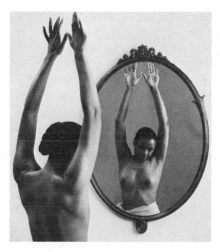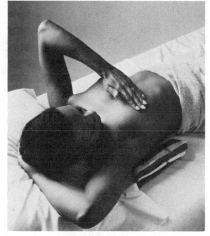

A model demonstrates Steps 2 and 3 of breast self-examination.

When the first circle is completed, move your hand one inch inward toward the nipple and repeat the process until the entire breast has been examined, including the nipple. While your arm is raised, be sure to check for swellings in the armpit. Reverse the process for your left breast. Pay attention to how your breast tissue feels. That way, if a change occurs, you will be able to notice it right away.

Finally, squeeze the nipple of each breast gently between the thumb and index finger, looking for discharge. A discharge is not a reason to panic, but it should be reported to your doctor. Any unusual findings discovered during BSE or at any other time should be reported immediately to your physician. Remember, only one in five breast abnormalities turns out to be cancer, but if it should be cancer, delay in reporting it to your doctor could make the difference between life and death.

The best time to start doing BSE is in your doctor's office. Have him show you how and tell you what is normal for you.

Who should do BSE? According to the American Cancer Society, every woman should from the time her breasts develop. Although breast cancer is relatively rare in young women, approximately 9,000 cases a year (10 percent of the total) are diagnosed in women aged 35 or younger, and the earlier in life the BSE habit is established, the more likely it will be used monthly—and knowledgeably—for life.

Currently more than 90 percent of breast cancers are first discovered by the women themselves (occasionally by their husbands). By the time these cancers are first brought to medical attention, 50 to 60 percent have already spread to the lymph nodes adjacent to the breast, indicating the possibility that the disease has metastasized to other parts of the body. When the lymph nodes in the armpit contain cancer cells, the five-year survival rate free of recurrence is only 45 percent.

However, few of the cancers that women currently find by themselves are discovered through the ritualistic practice of BSE, but rather are noticed "accidentally," usually when the lump is already quite large or obvious. The American Cancer Society believes that through monthly BSE, breast cancer can be detected by women at a much earlier stage in the disease, with the result that more women will be saved.

More widespread and consistent use of BSE is not the only way to improve the breast cancer survival statistics. In addition to BSE, every woman should have her breasts examined manually by a physician at least once a year. (In fact, the best time to start doing BSE is right after a doctor has examined your breasts and

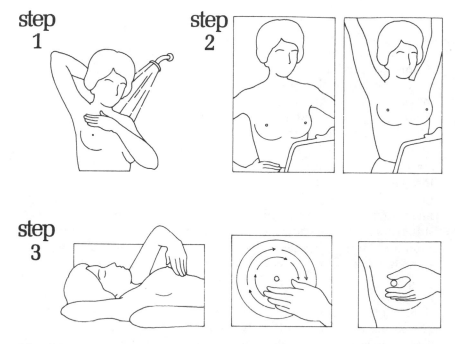

step
1

step
2

step
3

Monthly breast self-examination—BSE—is best done right after the menstrual period. Start (Step 1) in the shower or bath, and with wet fingers held flat and together, massage gently in a circular motion every area of each breast from the chest bone to the armpit. Check for any lump, hard knot or thickening. To examine the right breast, place your right hand behind your head and use the left hand to massage the breast. Reverse the procedure for the left breast. After bathing (Step 2) stand in front of a mirror and look at your breasts while your hands are on your hips and your muscles are tensed by pushing inward. Then raise your arms above your head. Check your breasts for any dimpling or changes in shape. In the final part (Step 3) of BSE, lie on your back with a pillow under your right shoulder and your right hand behind your head. Using your left hand and thinking of your breast as the face of a clock, feel gently with a circular motion at each hour of the clock. Begin at the outermost portion of your breast, and when the first circle is completed, start again one inch inward toward the nipple. Repeat until the entire breast has been covered. Then reverse the procedure for the left breast. Finally, squeeze each nipple gently and look for discharge.

told you they feel normal. Getting to "know" your breasts when they are normal will help you to recognize an abnormality should one develop.)

Besides the manual examination by a physician or trained

nurse, there are now available screening techniques that can detect breast cancers long before they are apparent to the touch. These include thermography, a heat-sensitive picture of the breast, and mammography, an X-ray image of the breast tissue. The thermogram works on the principle that the vast majority of breast cancers have a slightly higher temperature than surrounding normal tissue. The mammogram is a special X-ray of soft tissue that uses far less radiation than is ordinarily needed for an X-ray image of internal organs. A newer version of mammography, called xeroradiography, reproduces the X-ray on selenium-coated paper instead of film. Mammograms today are done using very little radiation and, for women over 50, the benefits of repeated mammograms are expected to far outweigh the risks that may result from the radiation exposure. During the last several years, thousands upon thousands of American women age 35 and over have been flocking to any of 27 special breast cancer detection projects for examinations that include a manual exam by a physician, a thermogram, and a mammogram (for women 50 and over). The women are supposed to be free of any known suspicious breast symptoms at the time of the screening. They are asked to return each year for at least 5 years to undergo a similar exam. If an abnormality is found, the women are referred back to their own physician for further examination or asked to return for a repeat exam in a few months. The 27 projects are part of a $9-million-a-year nationwide demonstration project initiated by the American Cancer Society and now supported jointly by the Society and the National Cancer Institute. Before the project is completed, at least 270,000 women will have been screened for each of five years and then followed for another five years. These projects are designed to determine whether annual screening of women in this age group in which 90 percent of breast cancers occur can turn around the currently dismal breast cancer death rate, which hasn't changed substantially for four decades. The accumulated data should also help to identify those groups of women who would be most likely to benefit from annual screening (since there are inadequate facilities currently to examine all women over 35 each year), to determine how often such screening should be done (once every two years or longer may be enough for some women), and select the most effective screening tools for detecting early, curable cancers.

In their early months of operation, the projects uncovered two and a half times the expected number of cancers among the women screened. The unusual number of cases largely reflected the fact that many of the women's cancers were discovered much earlier than they would otherwise have been, thus greatly increasing their chances for cure. In only 23 percent of the women whose cancers were revealed had the cancer spread to the nodes adjacent to the breast. This is less than half the percentage of women usually found to have cancer that has spread beyond the breast at the time of surgery.

To put these statistics another way, four out of five women whose breast cancers were detected through the screening project were found to have an early, localized cancer with a very high chance of cure. This is twice the percentage of breast cancer patients who are ordinarily found at the time of surgery to have highly curable cancers.

Women with only localized disease have between an 85 and 99 percent chance of being alive and well five years after breast cancer surgery, compared to a 45 percent five-year survival rate free of apparent cancer for women whose tumor had already spread to nearby nodes when their cancers were first diagnosed. At ten years, the difference in survival chances remains 74 percent for women with localized breast cancer compared to 38 percent for those with cancer in the nodes. Thus, it already appears that early breast cancer detection through the screening program will ultimately save significant numbers of lives.

The potential value of such a program was initially suggested by the impressive findings of a study conducted by the Health Insurance Plan of Greater New York under a contract from the National Cancer Institute. In the study, 31,000 presumed healthy women between the ages of 40 and 64 were screened annually by manual examination and mammography (thermography was added later), and their breast cancer experience was compared to a similar group of 31,000 women who did not go through the special detection program. Of the women in both groups who developed breast cancer, the death rate in the screened group was one-third lower than among those women whose cancers were discovered through the ordinary course of events. This meant that screening was picking up cancers at earlier, more curable stages. The study showed that an annual manual exam and mammography could pick up approximately 95 percent of cancers that develop among screened women and can often do so at a stage when the cure rate approaches 100 percent.

In 1968, while the HIP study was still in progress, one of its researchers, Dr. Philip Strax, a New York radiologist, established a prototype screening center for breast cancer—the Guttman Institute. Currently, each day at the clinic nearly 300 women receive a complete breast exam, including an interview, manual exam, mammography and thermography, and each woman is taught

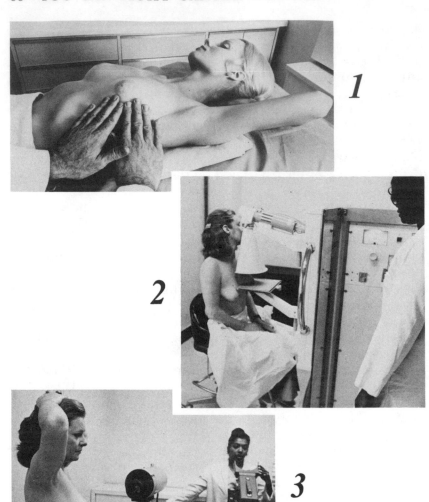

A complete medical examination to check for possible breast cancer takes only about 15 minutes. The three-step procedure involves 1) a manual examination by a physician or specially trained nurse, 2) a mammogram, or special low-dose X-ray of each breast and 3) a thermogram to check for "hot spots" in the breast. Preliminary results of a national breast cancer detection study suggest that this type of examination done regularly on women with no outward signs of breast cancer can greatly increase the percentage of cases that are detected early enough for cure.

breast self-examination. Two-thirds of the cancers found through the annual clinic examination or through BSE between annual exams turn out to be early cases with very high potential for cure.

The Guttman Institute is one of the 27 centers in the National Breast Cancer Detection Demonstration Project and was the model around which the remaining 26 programs were built.

A long-term study conducted at the University of Minnesota's Cancer Detection Center suggested that even without mammography, annual breast examinations by a physician plus monthly BSE can practically eliminate deaths from breast cancer. Women whose breast cancers were discovered through manual examination by a physician once a year had a five-year survival rate identical to that of women the same age who did not have breast cancer. In other words, survival among the breast cancer patients was 100 percent the expected rate, and this apparent cure rate did not change even fifteen years after treatment. In addition to the cancers discovered by examining physicians, some were found between annual examinations by the women themselves. When all cases were considered, the survival rate fifteen years after surgery was 92 percent—double that in the general population of breast cancer patients. The National Breast Cancer Detection Demonstration Project is expected to show how applicable the Minnesota findings may be to American women generally.

A long-standing problem such cancer detection programs face has been figuring out how to get people to take advantage of them. The publicity surrounding the breast cancer surgery undergone by Mrs. Ford and Mrs. Rockefeller awakened many thousands of American women to their opportunity for early breast cancer detection and resulted not only in many doing BSE for the first time, but also in the filling of clinic appointment books to overflowing. The problem now is how to sustain women's interest in these potentially life-saving health measures.

Monthly BSE and a manual breast examination by a physician at least once a year are recommended for women of all ages. Thermography, since it involves no radiation, can be used as a screening tool at any age as frequently as a woman's doctor suggests, although currently thermograms are being done routinely at breast cancer detection clinics starting with women age 35. But since mammography (both ordinary breast X-ray and xeroradiography) involves exposure to some radiation, albeit very small amounts, routine annual use of this technique is currently restricted to women aged 50 and older when the chance of picking up an early, curable breast cancer justifies any possible risk involved. Of course, a mammogram may also be recommended for younger women who are considered high risk for breast cancer or who develop suspicious breast symptoms.

For certain women who face a higher than average risk of developing breast cancer, more frequent physical examinations starting at a younger age may be recommended. Thus, if your mother or sister had breast cancer, the doctor may suggest a manual examination two or more times a year starting at age 30. Other high-risk groups for whom more frequent examinations may be recommended include women with fibrocystic disease of the breast and women who have already been treated for cancer in one breast.

DETECTING COLON AND RECTAL CANCER

"Don't be embarrassed to death," the American Cancer Society says in one of its public service advertisements about the most common internal cancer among American men and women, cancer of the colon and rectum. Often called "the cancer nobody talks about," this disease was diagnosed in 99,000 Americans in 1975 and it claimed the lives of 49,000 that year—second only to lung cancer as a cause of cancer deaths.

For more than sixty years, medicine has had the means to detect early cancer of the colon and rectum, but as of 1973 a Cancer Society-sponsored survey showed that only 24 percent of adult Americans had ever taken advantage of the technique and far fewer used it regularly. The technique is direct examination of the last twelve inches of the large bowel by an instrument called the proctosigmoidoscope.

The procto, as the examination is usually called, was described earlier as a means of preventing colon-rectal cancer, because it enables the physician to detect and remove most precancerous lesions in the lower bowel, where 70 percent of the colon-rectal cancers arise. Through the procto the doctor can also detect most lower bowel cancers while they are still localized. Early discovery may allow less extensive surgery to produce a cure. Yet the vast majority of physicians do not include the procto as part of a routine physical, and it is the rare patient who asks his doctor to do one.

The procto invades an area that most of us—including physicians—have been conditioned to think of as private, unmentionable, and unclean. Even when we notice abnormalities in the lower digestive tract, such as rectal bleeding, chronic diarrhea, or difficult, painful bowel movements, many of us are reluctant to mention these symptoms to a doctor. When our concern with toilet privacy is carried to the extreme of failing to detect and treat an early bowel cancer, the modesty is false indeed.

The fault does not always lie with the patient, however. Monica W. had been telling her doctor for at least three years that she had been bothered by frequent persistent diarrhea, a condition she had never had before the age of 63. But the doctor brushed off the complaint as "nervousness" and never checked into it. Finally, just before her 66th birthday, Monica started bleeding profusely from the rectum and was rushed to the hospital, where she underwent emergency surgery for what turned out to be a massive cancer of the colon. She was dead a year later, and her two sisters, Ida and Myra, blame the doctor who had long ignored Monica's symptoms for her painful death.

The sisters had learned a bitter lesson; following Monica's surgery both went for proctos. Myra was found to have unsuspected colon cancer as well, but surgery showed it had not yet spread beyond the polyp in which it arose, and she is alive and well now five years later. Ida, like Myra, goes for a procto each year without fail and has had numerous polyps removed, some of which had harbored precancerous cells. Ida says, "The procto may not be the most pleasant experience I've had, but it's certainly worth the momentary discomfort once a year to know that I am protecting myself from the awful experience my sister Monica suffered through." As another American Cancer Society ad proclaims, "Maybe a procto isn't exactly a pleasure. Neither is cancer."

Preparing for a procto usually begins the day before your scheduled exam with a diet that contains no roughage, an enema, and sometimes a laxative. The morning of the exam, the enema is repeated until the bowel is cleaned out. The better prepared a patient is, the better able the doctor is to spot an abnormality in the bowel wall. (Sometimes, preparation for the procto is done at the doctor's office on the day of the examination.) The exam may take as little as ten minutes, and the more relaxed the patient is, the less discomfort he is likely to feel and the quicker the exam will be over.

To do the procto, the doctor uses a well-lubricated hollow instrument about twelve inches in length, with a light at one end. With the instrument gently inserted into the rectum, the doctor can see the lining of the lower portion of the large intestine and the rectum. Abnormalities seen during the procto may alert the physician to the need for a barium enema X-ray, which enables him to see indirectly the rest of the large intestine, where the remaining 30 percent of bowel cancers arise.

If the doctor finds something suspicious during the procto, he can usually take a biopsy or remove any polyps through the scope at the same time, right in his office. When cancer of the colon is found early in a polyp, major surgery (that is, removal of a portion of the colon) is rarely necessary. The American Cancer Society points out that "since the vast majority of procto exams reveal no cancer, and many of those which are found can so easily be cured, a procto exam once a year gives real peace of mind."

Annual proctos are usually recommended for all persons without symptoms aged 40 and over. The examination should always be done for any patient with symptoms related to the colon and rectum, except those who have severe diverticulitis, an inflammation of the bowel wall. For patients without symptoms, an annual procto is the best insurance against this prevalent life-threatening cancer.

A recent advance in techniques for examining the bowel has been the development of the fiberoptic colonoscope, a narrow, lighted, flexible tube that can be threaded through the entire six-foot length of the large intestine. Light-transmitting glass fibers inside the rod show the bowel wall to the examining physician. The light actually "bends" around corners and curves. The patient is given a mild sedative (but no anesthetic) before the examination, which is most often done in an outpatient clinic in a hospital. At the time of the initial examination, polyps can be removed, biopsies taken, and cell washings obtained for cytology directly through the instrument. Although relatively few physicians are currently trained to use this instrument, it promises to become an important tool in the diagnosis and treatment of bowel diseases, especially cancer, that are beyond the range of the foot-long rigid proctosigmoidoscope.

The usefulness of colonoscopy is evident from cases like Mr. P., who had a procto and barium enema X-ray after he had experienced some rectal bleeding. The procto showed nothing, and the X-ray revealed a benign-looking polyp. Colonoscopy was done, which confirmed that the polyp was benign, but a short distance away a small, early cancer that had not appeared on the X-ray was found. Mr. P. was treated surgically and has been fine since.

Cancer of the colon and rectum tends to grow slowly and silently for years, remaining localized and therefore curable for a long time. Usually, by the time symptoms are noticeable, the disease is more advanced, but there may still be an excellent chance for cure if the situation is promptly attended to. The warning signals of bowel cancer may include any of the following: blood in the stool, constipation or diarrhea lasting more than a few weeks or returning intermittently, and chronic "gassy pains" in the lower abdomen. The problem with all these symptoms is that they are extremely common, although rarely prolonged beyond two weeks, and readily attributed to some other, relatively innocent cause, such as hemorrhoids that bleed. All too often, patients have monkeyed around for months with over-the-counter "pile cures" only to discover when they finally visited a doctor that they really had cancer.

In November 1974, a lady from Evanston, Illinois, wrote to thank *Woman's Day* magazine for an article it published called "How to Protect Your Family From Cancer," in which the procto was described. Mrs. W. said, "I'm sure that without having read it, I would have put up with vague discomfort until . . . ?" Instead, halfway through reading the article, she called her doctor for an appointment, and—after a procto and barium enema X-ray indicated trouble—two weeks later underwent surgery for colon cancer. "Even though over two feet of colon was removed," Mrs. W. wrote, "I have been given nothing but good news for the future. No lymph nodes were involved [indicating that the disease was still confined to the site in which it arose] and all seems to be well."

Recently, another simple test for uncovering unsuspected colon cancer has been developed: a means of testing for "occult"— hidden—blood in the stool. Although it is usually the more advanced cancers that bleed noticeably, very early colon cancers often lose tiny "invisible" amounts of blood that can be detected by smearing a very small sample of stool on a specially prepared test slide. For four days the patient is asked to adhere strictly to a special diet containing a lot of roughage, such as fruits, vegetables, and bran, but no meat. Starting on the second day of the diet, two samples are taken from each of the next three stools passed, and each sample is smeared on a labeled slide. The six slides are then sent to the doctor or clinic for evaluation. If any of the slides indicates there was blood in the stool, the patient is called in for further examination—usually a procto and a barium enema X-ray.

In a study by one physician among patients in his private practice, five persons in 556 tested were found to have "silent" colon cancers that would have been missed by procto because they were higher in the colon than the instrument reaches. Three of the cancers were in an early, curable stage. In another community-wide study sponsored by the Mercer County, New Jersey, unit of the American Cancer Society, again five persons were found to have unsuspected colon cancers, three of whom were considered surgically cured.

One person who was glad he showed up for the screening exam

was a 45-year-old man who had hemorrhoids and whose mother had had colon cancer. One of his test slides indicated blood in the stool and he was given an X-ray and procto. The X-ray was negative, but the procto revealed a polyp which was removed through the scope. Microscopic examination of the polyp showed it harbored the beginnings of cancer. The man also had his hemorrhoids removed and he has been fine ever since.

Doctors who use the occult blood test emphasize that it is not a substitute for, but rather a supplement to, the procto. Experts also point out that a digital rectal exam alone (a gloved finger inserted into the rectum) is not adequate to detect all colon or rectal cancer. Seven out of eight cancers detectable through the procto are missed by a digital exam. The digital rectal exam, however, *is* important for cancer detection and in the examination of the prostate gland in men.

Proctoscopy and a test of the stool for occult blood are recommended for all persons over age 40. But for certain people, regular bowel exams are especially important because they face a higher than normal risk of developing colon or rectal cancer. Included are people whose close blood relatives have had the disease, persons with ulcerative colitis, and people with various hereditary bowel diseases that result in repeated formation of polyps in the colon.

DETECTING UTERINE CANCER

Sharon K., a strikingly attractive journalist and mother of two girls, was about to remarry four years after the tragic death of her husband in an automobile accident. A few months before the wedding Sharon decided to see her doctor for a complete checkup, something she had been neglecting because of "lack of time." She was shocked and not a little frightened when her doctor called her back to his office to tell her that the Pap smear he took indicated she had cancer of the cervix. A biopsy confirmed his suspicion, and Sharon had a hysterectomy. Fortunately, the cancer was localized and Sharon has been healthy for the last eight years. But she no longer misses her annual checkup. "I took one gamble with my life and I was lucky. I won't do that again," she says. "And I'm going to see to it that my daughters don't neglect their health, either. My 22-year-old is about to get married, and I made sure she had a thorough checkup, including a Pap smear."

The usefulness of the Pap smear in preventing cervical cancer was described in the previous section, and actually, if a Pap is done every six to twelve months, the vast majority of cervical cancers would never occur, since precancerous conditions can be readily detected and treated with simple surgery that does not impair fertility.

That 20,000 cases of cervical cancer were diagnosed in 1976 and 7,700 women died of the disease that year is testimony to the fact that many women do not get a Pap smear done regularly. A survey for the American Cancer Society in 1973 revealed that only 52 percent of adult women had had a Pap smear during the previous year (although this was an encouraging increase from 23 percent a decade earlier).

The Pap smear is said to be 90 percent effective in detecting cervical cancer at the time when the disease is virtually 100 percent curable. Cancer of the body of the uterus, usually called endometrial cancer, is also readily cured if detected early, but the Pap smear is not quite as effective in ferreting out this disease as it is in finding early cervical cancer. About 60 percent of endometrial cancers are detected through the Pap smear.

A gynecologist at the University of Alabama, Dr. Leland Clark Gravelee, Jr., has devised a "jet washer" that can safely and painlessly flush out from the uterus tiny samples of tissue for laboratory analysis. In a study of 1,084 women who had symptoms of uterine disorders, the jet washer indicated that 53 had endometrial cancer, later confirmed by a surgical scrape (D and C) of the uterine lining. Thirty-five of the 53 women had had a Pap smear as well, but the Pap picked up only nine of the endometrial cancer cases. In another study of 101 women with no uterine symptoms, the jet washer suggested the possibility of cancer in two, one of whom was found subsequently to have the disease.

The Gravelee test, which must be done by a physician, involves inserting the tip of what resembles an oversized hypodermic needle into the uterine cavity. A plunger squirts a mild salt solution into the cavity and the fluid and washings from the uterine wall are then sucked back into the device. A plug of tissue can then be prepared from the washings and analyzed for the presence of cancer cells in the same way as any other tissue specimen. The endometrial aspirator, which was described earlier as a means for preventing endometrial cancer, can also be used to detect cancer of the uterine lining.

Endometrial cancer most commonly occurs at the time of or after menopause. Unlike most other cancers, symptoms of endometrial cancer often occur early in the disease, when it is still readily curable. The symptoms may include bleeding between periods, a prolonged or heavier than normal menstrual flow, or resumption of bleeding after menopause. While most often these symptoms *do not* indicate cancer, if a woman experiences any one of them she should bring it to a doctor's attention immediately. Some women face a higher than usual risk of developing endometrial cancer, and for them, periodic testing with the jet washer could be especially valuable. They include women with a history of obesity, diabetes, high blood pressure, infertility, irregular menstrual periods, or failure to ovulate. Such women are advised to have an aspiration biopsy around the time of menopause. Endometrial cancer is also more common among women who were treated with estrogens for several years during or after their menopause.

DETECTING LUNG CANCER

Early detection of lung cancer is in the vanguard of efforts to reduce deaths from this disease, which is currently the nation's leading cancer killer. Under present circumstances, fewer than 10 percent of lung cancer patients can expect to be cured. By the time the vast majority of lung cancers produce clear-cut symptoms —chest pain or blood-tinged sputum—the cancer is already well advanced, with only a 7 percent chance of cure. Very early lung cancers are generally not visible on a chest X-ray. In fact, only 30 to 40 percent of lung cancer patients have operable disease when it is first discovered. In the remainder, the cancer is too widespread to be removed surgically. Other forms of treatment, such as radiation therapy and drugs, may temporarily slow or stop the malignant growth, but thus far at least, they usually do not cure the patient.

While prevention is clearly the most effective means of substantially reducing the lung cancer death rate, some 52 million Americans currently smoke cigarettes and thousands of teen-agers take up the habit each day. Therefore, the lung cancer death rate is expected to continue its steady climb for some time to come. It takes about 15 years of exposure to cigarette smoke to get a lung cancer started, but once established, the disease often develops to a lethal state within a few months. Therefore annual screening with a chest X-ray is not adequate to detect early, curable disease in most patients.

Most lung cancers start in the bronchial tubes, the passageways that carry inhaled air from the windpipe to the lungs and collect air to be exhaled from the lungs. Recent studies have shown that cells shed by early lung cancers can often be found in coughed-up sputum. A sputum test for detecting early lung cancers is currently under investigation at four medical centers—the Mayo Clinic in Rochester, Minnesota, Johns Hopkins Hospital in Baltimore, and in New York, at the Preventive Medicine Institute-Strang Clinic and Memorial Sloan-Kettering Cancer Center—working under grants from the National Cancer Institute. The first five years of the ten-year study will cost an estimated total of $13 million. Preliminary results from the Mayo Clinic and Johns Hopkins indicate that the sputum test, done every four months, is capable of detecting lung cancers when there is a good chance for cure. This does not mean, however, that the test can pick up all lung cancers at such an early curable stage, but its regular use among persons with a high risk of developing lung cancer may increase the five-year survival rate from 10 to 40 percent. At Mayo, study participants also get a chest X-ray (which involves a very low radiation dose) every four months, because the X-ray seems able to detect early curable cancers that originate in the periphery of the lungs, where cells are not likely to be shed into the sputum.

Some 30,000 smokers are expected to participate in the study sponsored by the National Cancer Institute. The participants are all men over 45 years of age who smoke at least one pack of cigarettes a day. From past experience, doctors anticipate that every year, between three and five lung cancers will be found among each 1,000 men screened. At the outset, the participants all complete a detailed questionnaire, receive a chest X-ray, and are taught how to produce a sputum specimen by inhaling deeply and coughing. The men are asked to collect the phlegm they cough up every morning for three days. The sputum specimens are then analyzed for the presence of cancer or otherwise abnormal cells. Among the first 500 persons tentatively accepted in the Mayo Clinic study, seven persons could not be enrolled in the study because they were found to have cancer at the outset and another eleven persons had suspicious findings on a chest X-ray. Two of the cancers were found only through the sputum test.

Every four months for five years, the men are asked to obtain a repeat examination. After the five-year-study, the men will be followed for an additional five years to determine whether any get lung cancer. If the sputum test proves capable of detecting a large percentage of lung cancers when they are still localized and potentially curable, the test is likely to be made widely available to persons who face a high risk of developing the disease.

Someone who has smoked two packs of cigarettes a day for ten years or more faces a one in ten chance of developing lung cancer. In addition to smokers, certain occupational groups, including workers who were exposed to asbestos, arsenic, chromates, uranium, and bischloromethyl ether, are especially prone to developing lung cancer. A screening exam like the sputum test done several times a year could prove life-saving to those who unfortunately "earned" lung cancer along with their pay checks.

For example, in Tyler, Texas, the home of a now-defunct asbestos factory, 878 former employes at the factory are being examined every six months to see if the early signs of lung cancer and other asbestos-related diseases can be picked up in time for cure. The Tyler plant was opened in 1954 after a similar plant owned by the same company was closed in Paterson, New Jersey. Studies of 1,560 former Paterson workers have shown that they are six times more likely than the general population to die of lung cancer, the legacy of their exposure to asbestos fibers in the factory. Since the same equipment and processing procedures were used in Tyler, the Texas workers are thought to face a similar risk. The project, which is being supported by the National Cancer Institute at a cost of nearly half a million dollars for the first two years, involves a two-hour battery of tests, including a physical examination, chest X-ray, and sputum test.

Once cancer cells are found in a sputum sample, the next trick is to locate their source in the respiratory tract. This is especially difficult in cases where the cancer is still too small to show up on an X-ray. The fiberoptic bronchoscope, an instrument similar in design to the flexible colonoscope described earlier, has proven useful in locating many of these early hidden cancers. The flexible lighted instrument enables the doctor to examine most of the bronchial tree where lung cancer usually arises.

DETECTING ORAL CANCER

"Open wide," says a big-mouthed hippopotamus in an American Cancer Society brochure, "and keep it open long enough for your dentist or physician to examine it for oral cancer." Eighty-five percent of cancers in the mouth region can be seen by the examiner either directly or indirectly with a mirror, and 11 percent of those not visible can be felt.

Yet fewer patients survive oral cancer than cancer in such relatively "hidden" regions as the colon, breast, and bladder, and the death rate from oral cancer has not decreased since 1950. This is because examination of the mouth is rarely included in a routine physical and even dentists, who have frequent opportunity to check this area for possible cancer signs, often fail to look beyond

cavities and gum disease when examining their patients. As a result, only two-thirds of patients with oral cancers have their disease
diagnosed while it is still confined to the original site. Yet in one
study, the five-year survival rate increased more than 45 percent
when oral cancer was diagnosed before it had spread to other parts
of the body.

Because sores in the mouth are so common, many people delay
far too long before bringing them to the attention of a physician
or dentist. Any mouth irritation that persists beyond a week or
two should be examined professionally. Other warning signals of
oral cancer include a swelling, lump, or growth anywhere in or
around the mouth or neck; white, scaly patches (leukoplakia)
inside the mouth (a precancerous condition that is readily treated
to prevent progression to cancer); difficulty in chewing or swallowing food; numbness or pain anywhere in the mouth area; and
repeated bleeding in the mouth without an established cause. The
existence of any of these signs does not necessarily mean cancer—
bleeding in the mouth, for example, is most often caused by gum
disease—but their presence should be a signal to see your doctor or
dentist immediately.

Mouth cancers are usually painless, so don't wait until it hurts
to see the doctor. Symptoms of oral cancer may also appear outside
the mouth, as a lump around the ear or in the upper neck. Any
such symptoms should be reported promptly to a physician. You
can help further in the early detection of oral cancer by asking
your dentist or doctor to examine your mouth carefully at each
regular visit. The medical examination should include the use of a
mirror to look down into your throat and voice box (larynx).

Although traditionally the mouth examination has focused on
white patches, oral surgeons at the East Orange Veterans Administration Hospital in New Jersey say that the examination should
include a search for velvety red areas with or without white spots
that are especially common in persons over the age of 40. The
painless lesions occur mainly on the floor of the mouth, on the
side, under the tongue, and on the soft palate. The East Orange
surgeons report that the vast majority of early cancers they have
found were mostly red, and that treatment of these lesions has
yielded a 5-year survival rate of over 90 percent.

DETECTING PROSTATE CANCER

The survival rate for cancer of the prostate could also be significantly increased if all men over the age of 40 had an annual digital

examination of this gland, followed by surgical removal of the prostate when cancer is found. At the University of Minnesota, this approach has yielded a survival rate of 100 percent—that is, the men lived out their lives as if they never had had this often fatal disease. In the military services, where regular physicals—including prostate examinations—are compulsory, the death rate from prostate cancer is much lower than in the general population of the same age.

The prostate is normally a chestnut-sized gland that produces the seminal fluid that is part of the male ejaculate. It is located just below the bladder and surrounds the beginning of the urethra, the tube that carries urine from the bladder. To examine the prostate, the doctor inserts a gloved finger into the rectum, which enables him to feel for any irregularities or abnormally firm areas in the gland. Any doctor can and should do this exam, but it is often skipped in the general physical. Since early prostate cancer often produces no symptoms, a routine rectal examination is the most effective way to uncover early, curable disease. Presently, however, in the general population only 10 percent of prostate cancers are discovered before the disease has spread to other organs. Generalized enlargement of the prostate gland is extremely common in older men and is most often benign. Only a doctor can tell whether cancer may be present. Symptoms of prostate enlargement, which afflicts more than half of the men in the United States over the age of 50, include a weak or interrupted flow of urine, inability to urinate, or difficulty in starting urination; the need to urinate frequently, especially at night; occasional blood in the urine; a urine flow that is not easily stopped; and painful or burning urination. These symptoms may occur whether the enlargement is malignant or benign, so any of them should be brought promptly to medical attention. In addition to urinary symptoms, continuing pain in the lower back, pelvis, or upper thighs may be the first or major sign of prostate cancer that has spread. There is no good evidence to indicate that benign prostatic enlargement increases a man's chances of developing prostate cancer.

Prostate cancer is very common and is generally a slow-growing disease. As many as 15 or 20 percent of men over the age of 50 may unknowingly have prostate cancer, but in only a small percentage does the disease progress and cause death. At autopsy many men are found to have harbored prostate cancers that apparently remained dormant and localized for years. Because of this fact, some doctors are reluctant to operate on older men when a localized prostate cancer is discovered. However, for men with an otherwise reasonably long life expectancy, surgery offers the best chance that the cancer will not spread.

Recently, doctors at Columbia-Presbyterian Medical Center in New York discovered that the wives of men who had prostate cancer were far more likely than other women their age to develop cancers of the breast and genital organs, suggesting the possibility that these cancers may be caused by a common factor. The wives' cancers, which were diagnosed at least a year after their husbands' cancers had been discovered, occurred eleven times more frequently than expected. Based on these findings, the doctors recommend that women whose husbands have prostate cancer should have breast and pelvic exams three times a year in the hope of catching any cancers that may develop while they are still curable.

EARLY WARNING SYSTEMS

As medical research further defines what factors increase a person's risk of developing one type of cancer or another, early detection programs will focus more and more on those people who face an unusually high risk of getting particular cancers. A program similar to the one among the Tyler, Texas, asbestos workers might be established for uranium miners and other workers who also face a high risk of lung cancer. Chemical dye workers who were exposed to aromatic amines might be screened regularly for bladder cancer, and those exposed to arsenic might be examined periodically for evidence of skin cancers.

Indentification and examination of at least one high-risk group —young women who had been exposed while still in their mother's womb to a synthetic hormone called DES (diethylstilbestrol) —has clearly demonstrated the life-saving rewards of this approach to early cancer detection. These women, whose mothers took DES during pregnancy to prevent a threatened miscarriage, are prone to developing an otherwise rare form of cancer, clear-cell adenocarcinoma of the vagina and cervix. The disease can be detected by a thorough pelvic examination in which the doctor looks directly into the vaginal canal.

The Harvard Medical School investigators who uncovered the relationship between DES and adenocarcinoma in 1971 have also found that the disease can be cured when it is discovered before the young victims develop obvious symptoms (a lower but still sizable percentage of cases are also apparently cured even after symptoms develop). Thus, they say, it is vitally important that the hundreds of thousands of young women at risk of developing this disease be examined regularly, although overall fewer than one in 1,000 women exposed to DES before birth seem to develop this special kind of cancer.

Periodic screening for early signs of cancer should also be focused on those persons with a family history of certain cancers, such as cancer of the breast and large bowel and on persons who have benign conditions that predispose them to developing cancer, as well as on those individuals who are "high risk" simply because of their age. Ideally, all persons should have some sort of periodic checkup to detect possible cancers. Therefore, more and more, experts in preventive medicine are looking to specially trained nurses and physicians' assistants to carry out the task of screening apparently healthy people for possible signs of disease.

One such center is CANSCREEN, with clinics now operating in New York, Philadelphia, and Omaha, where the screening is done by nurses trained in cancer detection. Dr. Daniel G. Miller, medical director of the Preventive Medicine Institute–Strang Clinic, reports that in a test of the nurses' effectiveness in examining patients when compared to the findings of doctors who examined the same patients, "there was not a single lesion suspicious for cancer or other serious disease that the nurse missed. The nurses took 30 percent more time than the doctors to do the same examination . . . and patient satisfaction was high."

CANSCREEN is an experiment to determine the practicality and life-saving value of periodically examining persons who are believed to face a higher than usual risk of developing cancer and of educating such persons about ways to reduce their cancer risk. The clinics are operated entirely by paramedical personnel. The patients are selected on the basis of such factors as family history of cancer and personal medical history of precancerous conditions, as well as exposure to known cancer-causing substances. But all the early warning systems that might be established for detecting cancers while they are still curable are useless unless people take advantage of them and get any suspicious finding attended to promptly.

A study at a major Boston hospital in 1973 revealed that two-thirds of patients waited longer than a month, 39 percent delayed more than three months, and 15 percent let a year go by before seeing a doctor after they first noticed a possible cancer symptom. The average delay in getting cancer diagnosed was four months. Fear, denial, and fatalism seemed to prevail, causing many of the patients to in effect seal their own fate. Those who after diagnosis readily acknowledged that they had "cancer" were faster in seeking medical help than those who called their disease "a tumor."

Those with a history of cancer in their families and those who worried a lot about cancer were likely to delay *longer* than most. And the last patients to come in were those with pain as their principal symptom. The study's most encouraging finding was that when cancer was discovered in the course of a routine examination, treatment was instituted with relatively little delay. Thus, more widespread detection programs would help to bring more cancer patients to treatment early in the course of their disease.

It is not only the patient who may be reluctant to recognize the significance of an early cancer symptom. Doctors, too, sometimes deny or ignore the possibility of cancer in their patients and thus fail to do the proper examinations. While this is not usually the case, it is in part the patient's responsibility to be sure his symptoms get properly checked out. Dr. Henry T. Lynch, preventive medicine specialist at Creighton University School of Medicine in Omaha, tells of Mrs. J., a middle-aged woman with diabetes, who developed a pain in her right shoulder which moved down into her arm and elbow. Aspirin gave her some relief and her physician, assuming she had arthritis, prescribed a pain killer. Whenever she mentioned the shoulder pain to her doctor, he reassured her and told her to continue with the pain killers. A year and a half after she first told her doctor of the pain, a medical student she encountered at a hospital clinic decided to investigate further.

It didn't take him long to find a large cancer in her right breast and three large lymph nodes under her right arm. Little wonder she was in pain! But by that time, her cancer was inoperable and Mrs. J. died four months after the medical student made the diagnosis that should have been made eighteen months earlier, at a time when effective therapy might have been instituted.

Mrs. J. conceded that she had considered the possiblity of cancer, but because her doctor didn't mention it, she put the thought out of her mind even though the doctor had done no examination to rule out cancer. While Mrs. J.'s physician was clearly at fault in his offhand approach to her persistent symptom, as a patient Mrs. J. also fell down on her job. She forgot that doctors are human beings subject to the same failings as the rest of us, and that patients must assume some responsibility for their own care. Sometimes patients are reluctant to report symptoms of ill health to their doctors lest the physician think they are hypochondriacs. But when it comes to your health, there is no time to be timid or to leave everything to the doctor. You have the right, in fact the obligation, to participate in your care—to ask your doctor questions and to be sure he does the kind of examination necessary to preserve your health.

As often as not, cancer is a curable disease. But it is up to you and your doctor to see to it that if cancer develops, it is detected early and treated promptly enough for cure.

Since 1956 the National Cancer Institute has been conducting what it calls the "End Results Evaluation Program" in which statistics are gathered on several hundred thousand patients treated for cancer at more than 100 hospitals across the country. The program measures the survival of patients with regard to the kind of cancer, the stage at which it is diagnosed, and the type of treatment received. The program helps to define the types of therapy that are most likely to lead to cure of particular types of cancer. The data collected have demonstrated unequivocally that the best chance of surviving cancer—regardless of the type of treatment received—follows diagnosis of the disease while it is still localized. While progress is continuously being made in developing improved cancer treatments, most cancer specialists are convinced that the greatest dent can be made in the cancer death rate—and in the shortest time—through more widespread use of early detection methods.

6. Treatment and Advances in Therapy

It was 1962 and Michael Finamore was a normal, active 12-year-old boy attending junior high school in New Jersey. One day, while taking a shower, Michael noticed a lump on his chest. His mother promptly took him to a local doctor who said it was probably a sprained rib and told him to come back in three weeks. Michael's mother was doubtful, however, and that same day she took him to another physician who did a blood test and X-ray and found that the boy's chest housed a tumor the size of two grapefruits and that his blood contained twenty times the normal number of white blood cells. Suspecting leukemia, that very night the physician sent Michael to Memorial Sloan-Kettering Cancer Center in New York where doctors were experimenting with potent drugs that could kill off leukemic cells. There, the diagnosis of acute lymphocytic leukemia was confirmed and Michael's prospects were outlined. Untreated, the doctors said, Michael might have only a few weeks—perhaps months—to live. There was no known cure for leukemia, they continued, but they did have a small battery of experimental drugs that could destroy leukemic cells and in some cases suppress the disease for long periods. These drugs, however, also damaged normal cells and could cause highly unpleasant and sometimes life-threatening reactions.

For Michael's parents, the decision was easy. If there was even a small chance that the rapidly growing tumor could be halted by the drugs, they were willing to take it. The alternative amounted to a death sentence for their young son. The doctors used radiation therapy to shrink the massive tumor in Michael's chest and periodically pumped two potent drugs into his veins to kill off the millions of leukemic cells that his bone marrow was manufacturing and steadily pouring into his bloodstream. Michael, who had

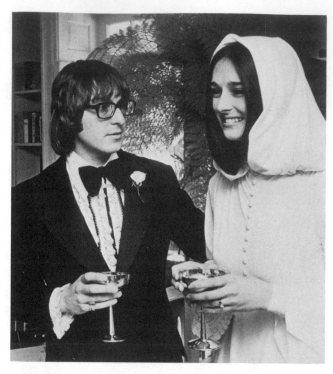

Michael Finamore at his marriage in 1974 to Ann Murdach, more than 11 years after he began treatment for acute lymphocytic leukemia. At one time this disease claimed the lives of 99 percent of its victims. Now, thanks to modern chemotherapy, more than half of young leukemia patients can look forward to being alive and well at least five years after diagnosis.

felt fine before his cancer was diagnosed, now was very sick as a result of the treatment. But in a few months, all traces of leukemia were gone and for about 2 years, Michael went to school and did all the things teen-age boys do. Then the leukemia came back.

By that time, however, the doctors had another half-dozen anti-leukemic drugs they could try. Michael was placed on more intensive drug therapy that made him feel even sicker. His hair fell out, he was nauseated much of the time, he lost weight and had to be tutored through two years of high school. But the leukemic cells once again disappeared from his blood and bone marrow. This time they stayed away.

Michael Finamore is now 26. He got married to Ann Murdach in 1974, and a year before the wedding, he stopped the small doses of antileukemic drugs that he had taken for five years in the hope of wiping out any new leukemic cells that might arise. Today, Michael looks, acts, and feels like any normal young man trying to establish a life for himself. He works as a plumbing and heating contractor. In his spare time he enjoys water-skiing, scuba diving, snow skiing, tennis, and baseball and does volunteer work for the American Cancer Society.

Michael is one of cancer therapy's success stories. There are perhaps two million other people like him in the United States, people who have had cancer and are considered cured. Most cancer treatment stories are not nearly as dramatic as Michael's, but they are nonetheless significant to the patients and their families.

In recent years, cancer specialists have demonstrated that most cancers are far from hopeless and that many, once thought hopeless, are now curable. After decades of shying away from publicity lest it give people false hopes, these specialists are now loudly proclaiming the good news about new cancer treatments. They have seen that fear, pessimism, and resignation to inevitable death from cancer are self-fulfilling prophecies. These attitudes cause patients to delay going to a doctor when they first suspect cancer. Many doctors themselves in fact, still hold such attitudes, and their mistaken belief that cancer is hopeless prevents them from trying the very therapies that might wipe out their patients' cancers or at least give the patients years of meaningful life. Through professional meetings and literature, the American Cancer Society is continually working to keep physicians who are not cancer specialists up to date on the prospects of modern therapy.

But cancer specialists also realize that educating the public is one of the fastest ways of getting new information about cancer therapies to the practicing physician, whose initial decision about how to treat a patient's cancer could well make the difference between life and death.

The best chance for curing most cancers results from early detection, while the cancer is still confined to the site where it began and before any cancer cells have escaped to other parts of the body. But now with refinements in therapy, even some advanced cancers can be cured. And a number of cancers which until recently have been considered hopeless, such as Michael Finamore's leukemia, are now being effectively treated with modern therapies in a large percentage of cases.

Other once almost hopeless cancers in which significant numbers of patients are now being cured include Hodgkin's disease (many advanced as well as the vast majority of early cases), testicular cancer, choriocarcinoma which involves the uterus of young women, and such childhood cancers as Wilms's tumor (a kidney cancer), rhabdomyosarcoma (involving the muscle tissue), and Ewing's sarcoma (a bone cancer). Improved chances of cure now also prevail for some of the more common cancers, including cancer of the prostate, bladder, and ovary, through the use of modern radiation therapy as well as surgery. In addition, aggressive treatment with anticancer drugs can in many cases prevent recurrence or produce shrinkage of the cancer and longer survival among victims of advanced breast and ovarian cancer, colon cancer, the lymphomas, osteogenic sarcoma (the most common form of bone cancer), multiple myeloma (a cancer originating in the bone marrow), chronic leukemia, and acute myelocytic leukemia. It is still too early, however, to say if any of these patients are permanently cured.

There are three main approaches to cancer therapy—surgery, radiation therapy, and chemo (or drug) therapy. In addition, a fourth, still-experimental approach, immunotherapy, in which the body is stimulated to reject the cancer as if it were a foreign organ, has shown considerable promise in recent studies and may soon become standard for certain kinds of cancers. Today, these various approaches are often used in combination to eradicate a cancer where one approach alone would not effectively do the job.

Behind the recent improvements in therapy is the recognition that cancer is a relentless disease that demands aggressive action, often involving a combination of anticancer weapons. Dr. Audrey Evans, director of pediatric cancer at the Children's Hospital in Philadelphia, says, "Instead of going to one doctor—say, a surgeon —who does his thing, then hands the patient to someone else—the radiologist or chemotherapist—when things go wrong, the current approach for many cancers is to use all the anticancer weapons at the same time." The surgeon removes the lump, the radiation therapist wipes out any cancer cells remaining in the area of the lump, and the chemotherapist kills off any tiny, as yet invisible, groups of cancer cells that may already have escaped to other parts of the body. This approach allows the therapist to get the jump on cancer before untreatable metastases become well-established.

Dr. Ralph E. Johnson, radiation therapist at the National Cancer Institute, points out that the old approach to cancer treatment, where secondary therapies were not used until metastases were obvious, large, and widespread, "might be compared to asking the little boy, once successful in plugging the hole in the dike with his finger, to stop the ocean following collapse of the dike." In the new treatment approaches, cancer specialists are concentrating on "plugging the holes"—stopping metastases while they are still small, even invisible—instead of trying to stop the "ocean" of wide-spread metastases.

SURGERY

Surgery, the most common method of cancer treatment, offers the best chance of cure for most solid tumors—cancers that form growths in places where they can be removed. For sugery alone to be able to cure a cancer, the disease must be treated while it is still confined to a site that can be encompassed and removed by the surgeon's tools. Surgeons usually try to remove not only the visible cancer tissue, but also some of the surrounding seemingly normal tissue in case it might be harboring hidden cancer cells that could lead to recurrent disease.

Many improvements, not only in surgical technique but also in supportive care during and after surgery, have made it possible to perform some cancer operations that previously would have been too life-threatening. Surgery in general and cancer surgery in particular is far safer today than it was two or three decades ago, because doctors are now able to control infection with antibiotics and build up the patient's blood supply with transfusions. Anesthesia is also much safer and can be used for longer periods, making extensive, complicated surgery possible.

Today it is possible to surgically remove large numbers of lymph nodes that may be harboring cancer cells or to remove an entire lung, the larynx, stomach, part of the liver, and part or all of the large bowel or the urinary bladder. And the use of modern plastic surgery and various rehabilitation techniques and devices make it possible for many patients who have undergone extensive cancer surgery to lead relatively normal lives.

Surgery is the primary method of treating a wide range of cancers, including cancers of the skin, breast, ovary, uterus, lung, stomach, pancreas, large bowel (colon), rectum, thyroid gland, head and neck, bladder, kidney, testis, prostate, bone and connective tissue, brain, spinal cord, and outlying nervous system. Even when the cancer has already apparently spread beyond the initial site, surgery can reduce the amount of cancerous tissue present and increase the effectiveness of other modes of therapy that might subsequently be used to try to eradicate the remaining cancer cells.

Sometimes, even in cases where the cancer cannot be cured, palliative surgery is extremely effective in relieving a cancer patient's discomfort and in giving the patient several more years of useful life. For example, in about a third of patients with advanced breast cancer, removal of hormone-producing glands, such as the ovaries, adrenal glands, or pituitary can lead to a disappearance of the cancer sometimes lasting for several years.

One of the most crucial aspects of cancer surgery is the choice of surgeon. Since each type of cancer has its own peculiar "natural history," growing and spreading in certain characteristic ways, it is extremely important that the surgeon know how your cancer might spread so that he can do the kind of operation that is most likely to get rid of the disease. Also, the increasing use of combinations of treatments—such as surgery plus radiation (either before or after the operation) or surgery plus chemotherapy—means that it is in your best interest if your surgeon is part of a team that is well-informed about the treatment of cancer. Further information on how to find the best cancer treatment will be presented later.

RADIATION THERAPY

Radiation therapy is the second most common approach to treating cancer. About half of all cancer patients receive some radiation treatment. Originally, radiation therapy was primarily used as a postsurgical "mop" to clean up any cancer cells that the surgeon may have left behind. The amount of radiation that could be delivered to the tumor was limited by the fact that radiation also harmed the normal tissues exposed to it and caused damage to the skin and debilitating "radiation sickness."

In the last decade, however, enormous improvements have been made in understanding the radiation sensitivity of cancer cells and normal tissues. New techniques and strategies of radiation therapy and new and more effective sources of radiation have been developed. Now high doses of radiation can be directed at the cancer with minimal exposure of normal tissues. As a result, cancer specialists are now using radiation more and more as a primary form of treatment for some cancers, often effective by itself or in combination with surgery or chemotherapy.

One famous beneficiary of modern radiation therapy is Senator Hubert H. Humphrey of Minnesota. In 1965, during his vice-presidency, a thorough physical examination revealed some wart-like growths in the opening of his bladder. The growths were removed with minor surgery and found to be benign. However, Mr. Humphrey was cautioned to return every six months for a bladder examination to be sure that no cancers had appeared. Occasionally in the succeeding years other benign growths were removed, but in September 1973 his semi annual examination revealed something worrisome: a pinhead-sized tumor that on biopsy appeared to be a potential cancer. Senator Humphrey underwent six weeks of therapy—five minutes each day—with high doses of radiation, which gave him an 80 to 85 percent chance of cure. His cancer disappeared and he remained well for three years until the development of a new, more advanced cancer necessitated surgical removal of his bladder.

Radiation therapy is often effectively used as the primary treatment for cancers of the cervix, head and neck, esophagus, larynx, and prostate, and for Wilms's tumor (a kidney cancer in children), rhabdomyosarcoma (a cancer of the muscle), Ewing's sarcoma (a bone cancer), retinoblastoma (an inherited eye cancer that afflicts children), Hodgkin's disease (a lymph system cancer), and other lymphomas. Radiation therapy can be used in different ways in cancer treatment: it may be used to cure cancers by totally eradicating them, to extend life by temporarily controlling tumor growth, or to make remaining life more pleasant by relieving pain, ulceration, and pressure produced by an advanced cancer. Radiation therapy is especially useful when a cancer is still confined to one region of the body but too advanced to remove completely by surgery. This gives the patient a chance of cure where surgery alone would have failed.

In addition to postsurgical radiation therapy to destroy cancer cells that surgery might have been unable to remove, radiation is now being used in some instances *before* cancer surgery to reduce the size of the cancer, thereby making surgery less complicated, and to diminish the chance that extraneous cancer cells will escape to other parts of the body during the operation. Increased chances of survival have occasionally been reported when radiation therapy is used prior to surgery for some cancers of the breast, colon, and rectum and advanced cancers of the bladder. Sometimes cancers that were initially too large to be removed surgically were rendered operable by the radiation treatment, Dr. John F. Potter, chief of surgery at Georgetown University Hospital, told a scientific conference in 1974.

Still another role for radiation therapy is in controlling and preventing the growth of metastases, which may be present at the time of surgery but not visible to the naked eye. By knowing where a particular type of cancer is most likely to spread, the radiation therapist can, in a sense, head it off at the pass by treating those areas with radiation to clear them of any cancer cells that may be present before they can develop into full-blown metastases.

As with surgery, it is essential that radiation be administered by a specialist in the field—a therapeutic radiologist (more recently called a radiation oncologist). Each kind of tissue, each cancer, and, in fact, each patient has a different sensitivity to the effects of radiation. In addition, there are different kinds of radiation treatments and certain ones work better for some cancers than others. Different cancers grow and spread in different ways. The training and experience of a specialist is needed to plot out an appropriate strategy for radiation therapy in each patient. The therapeutic radiologist is also likely to be part of a cancer treatment team so that radiation therapy can be properly combined with other treatment methods if this is most likely to cure the particular patient.

Therapeutic doses of radiation usually do not kill cells outright. Rather, they work by damaging the cells so that they are unable to reproduce. When a cell harmed by radiation reaches the end of its life, it simply dies without leaving any new cells to carry on its line. The main advantage of radiation therapy in treating cancer is that most cancer cells are more susceptible to—that is, more readily damaged by—the effects of radiation than are normal cells, because cancer cells are more likely to be in an active state of cell division. Thus, a dose of radiation that could mortally wound a cancer cell would allow most normal cells to go on living and reproducing. Certain kinds of cancers, however, are more resistant to the effects of radiation than others. These include melanoma, (a life-threatening form of skin cancer), and glioblastoma, a brain cancer.

Recent years have seen a veritable revolution in the techniques of therapeutic radiology. Previously, the amount of radiation that could be delivered to a cancer was limited by the fact that the highest doses of radiation were received by the skin and the tissues lying between the body surface and the cancer. When the patient began to suffer radiation damage to the skin and radiation sickness, the dose had to be lowered or the treatment discontinued, often before all the cancer had been destroyed. Today, however, new, faster, and more powerful radiation beams are available that deliver the maximum dose to the target tissue—the cancer—with minimum radiation to the skin and organs en route. Treatment strategies have been developed so that radiation beams can be delivered from many different angles of the patient's body, all pointed at the cancer but passing through different normal tissues. That way the cancer, where the beams converge, can receive a very high dose of radiation with relatively little effect on normal tissues.

Radiation sources can also be implanted directly into the cancer where they deliver localized radiation to the cancer cells with very little radiation reaching normal tissues. For instance, "needles" made of such substances as radium, radioactive cobalt, or gold may be inserted directly into the cancer, or hollow, flexible plastic tubes may be placed in the tumor and filled with a radioactive solution. The needles or tubes are removed after the treatment is completed. Extraordinarily precise radiation therapy, essentially limited to the cancer, can be delivered in this way. The technique is especially useful for cancers, for example, certain head and neck tumors, where the tumor is surgically inaccessible or where surgery would be too extensive to permit the patient to go on living a reasonably normal life.

For precision therapy, radiation oncologists can also use radioactive chemicals that have a preference for a particular place in the body. For example, radioactive iodine travels—as does all iodine—to the thyroid gland, and in some cases of thyroid cancer it is possible to use radioactive iodine to destroy the gland and the cancer along with it. Radioactive phosphorus travels to the bone, particularly to actively growing bone, and this chemical can sometimes be used to destroy metastases in the bone.

One who was an eye-witness to the remarkable progress in radiation therapy is Dr. Justin J. Stein, a past president of the American Cancer Society, who himself was cured of a usually fatal cancer —reticulum cell sarcoma, a bone cancer—more than thirty years ago. As a therapeutic radiologist at the University of California, Los Angeles, Dr. Stein saw the introduction of the first cobalt radiation unit in the nation, heralding the era of supervoltage or megavoltage radiation. Compared to the older kilovoltage machines, which delivered radiation doses of thousands of electron volts, megavoltage units, delivering doses of millions of electron volts, can do much more harm to the cancer while sparing the normal tissue. Megavoltage radiation can direct a more precise, intense beam to a tiny target area in the body with less scattering of radiation to surrounding normal tissue and less skin damage. Megavoltage therapy, which is ten to twenty times stronger than the old kilovoltage therapy, has helped to increase greatly the percentage of patients who survive cancers of the cervix, prostate, testis, bladder, ovary, head, and neck. For several cancers, five-year survival has more than doubled with megavoltage radiation.

Perhaps the most dramatic success of modern radiation therapy involves the treatment of Hodgkin's disease, a cancer of the lymphatic system that attacks some 7,000 teen-agers and young adults each year and was considered incurable until the 1960s. Now, in well-equipped centers capable of accurately diagnosing the extent of the disease, the early stages of Hodgkin's disease can be cured in up to 90 percent of cases with expertly administered megavoltage radiation. Many patients are now alive and well ten years after treatment. And even in advanced cases of Hodgkin's disease, combinations of drugs (sometimes with radiation) can cure more than half the patients with two-thirds living at least five years and 58 percent alive ten years later.

At Stanford University where megavoltage treatment of early Hodgkin's disease was pioneered, Dr. Henry Kaplan reports that radiotherapy alone can also cure most patients with early prostate

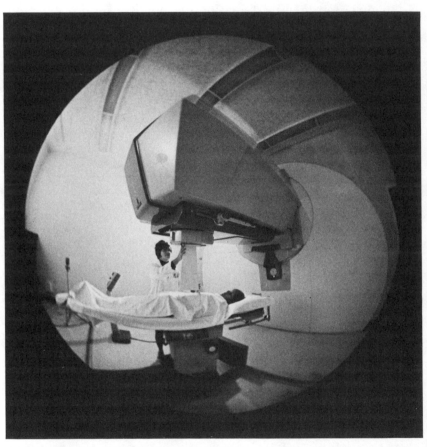

This powerful radiation unit, a betatron installed at the Boston University Medical Center, can deliver 42 million electron volts. Megavoltage units like this can direct a precise, intense beam of lethal radiation to a tiny target of cancer within the body. Megavoltage therapy has greatly increased the percentage of patients who survive several types of common cancers.

cancer, sparing the patients from surgery and the risk of impotence that often follows surgical removal of the prostate gland. Even for advanced prostate cancer, megavoltage radiation can increase survival chances and improve the quality of the patient's life.

In retinoblastoma (a cancer of the eye) megavoltage radiation can cure the cancer in many cases and save the child's eyesight at the same time. An early cancer of the larynx (voice box) can now often be treated effectively with radiation without the patient losing his ability to speak, which necessarily occurs when the larynx is removed surgically. For cancer of the nasopharynx, the part of the throat above the palate, megavoltage radiation offers a 62 percent chance of surviving five years and a 56 percent chance of ten-year survival.

Some cancer centers have begun to irradiate the patient's whole body to treat certain forms of leukemia and lymphoma, which by their very nature are spread throughout the body even in early stages. The National Cancer Institute reports that using whole body irradiation, average survival time is doubled for patients with chronic lymphocytic leukemia, which afflicts 5,580 persons a year. One in three patients so treated has experienced a long-term disappearance of his disease, with some patients living 10 years or more thus far. This approach has also been used effectively against lymphocytic lymphoma (a cancer of the lymph system), which is ordinarily treated with combinations of potent drugs. Since the side effects of radiation are minimal compared to the toxic effects of the drugs, patients prefer it to chemotherapy. It is possible that whole body radiation will be extended to other such cancers in lieu of combination chemotherapy.

The future of radiation therapy for cancer is exciting indeed. Recently, Dr. Herman Suit of Massachusetts General Hospital reported that implants of radium needles can often destroy soft-tissue sarcomas in patients who ordinarily might have required amputation of the cancer-bearing limb. At several centers doctors are exploring the potential of neutron beam radiotherapy. Neutrons—nuclear particles that can be generated for treatment purposes in the $2.5-million cyclotrons originally built for physics studies—are heavier than X-rays and gamma rays and consequently do more damage to the cells they hit. Fast neutrons seem able to attack cancer cells that resist other forms of radiation, including cells that are deficient in oxygen. Such cells are commonly found in large tumors.

Some doctors are studying substances that can increase the radiation-sensitivity of cancer cells. In this way, cancers can be destroyed at a lower dose of radiation.

Perhaps the most promising prospect in radiation therapy for cancer is the development of pi-meson (or pion) beam therapy. Pions, a kind of nuclear "glue" generated by high-energy particle accelerators used in physics research, cause miniature atomic explosions within cells. The beauty of pions as a potential therapeutic tool in cancer is that they have little effect on the tissues they pass through. Their damage is produced only when they stop. When stopped, pions are captured by the nuclei of cells, causing the nuclei to blow apart. This intracellular explosion results in destruction of the cell. Because the stopping region of a beam of pions can be controlled quite precisely by varying the speed of the particles, tissue damage can be confined almost entirely to the area of the cancer, experimenters believe.

Pion therapy is expected to have its greatest usefulness in treating deep-seated and large tumors and may be applicable to as many as 50,000 cancer patients a year. Researchers expect to concentrate their studies of pion therapy on cancers of the head and neck, brain and pancreas, and advanced cancers of the rectum and cervix. Right now, only two centers exist where pion therapy can be used therapeutically. This method of treatment, even if it proves worthwhile, will not be widely available to cancer patients for many years.

CHEMOTHERAPY

Surgery and radiation therapy have been the mainstays of cancer treatment for more than half a century. They work best for cancers that are confined to a certain region of the body. To treat cancer that is established in diverse, inaccessible, and remote regions of the body, systemic therapy—that is, treatment that reaches the entire body—is necessary.

In the last decade or so, systemic therapy with anticancer drugs —referred to generally as chemotherapy—has come into its own. Not long ago, chemotherapy was just a poor relation of surgery and radiation that was used as little more than a last-ditch palliative effort. Give the patient with advanced cancer large doses of potent drugs and maybe, just maybe, they would shrink the tumor, relieve the pain, and prolong life by weeks, months, even a year. But in recent years, specialists called medical oncologists have shown that chemotherapy can cure a number of relatively uncommon but deadly cancers, cancers that without drugs would claim the lives of nearly all their victims within months. In addition, anticancer drugs in combination with surgery or radiation are proving capable of preventing recurrences of a wide variety of common cancers. The main advantage of drugs is that they can reach beyond the surgeon's knife or the radiotherapist's rays to destroy colonies of cancer cells anywhere in the body. More and more, chemotherapy is being used as a front-line weapon in the fight against cancer, and every year several new possibilities for effective use of chemotherapy are discovered.

In fact, progress is being made so rapidly in cancer chemotherapy that it prompted one of the fathers of modern chemotherapy, the late Dr. Sidney Farber of Children's Cancer Research Foundation in Boston, to remark in 1972, "I think the day may come when we won't have to cut off a leg, a breast or a piece of intestine to cure cancer. We will be able to do it with drugs."

Actually, "chemotherapy" has been tried against cancer since ancient times. The Egyptian papyri describe the application of medicine to ulcerating skin tumors. In subsequent years, thousands of chemicals—including snake venom, pokeweed, skunk oil, kerosene, and extracts of scorpions—were tried in an attempt to arrest cancer. Chemotherapy as it is used today is less than four

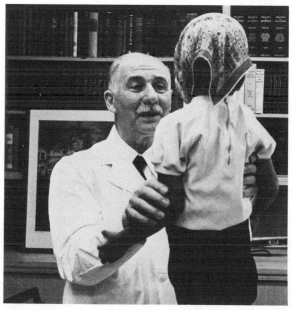

Dr. Sidney Farber greets one of his young cancer patients. The late Dr. Farber, a pioneer in the modern use of drugs to treat cancer, helped to develop the first effective drugs against childhood leukemia. The drugs are now being used effectively against a wide range of deadly cancers.

decades old. It was begun shortly before World War II when Dr. Charles B. Huggins of the University of Chicago showed that the female sex hormone estrogen could arrest the growth of advanced prostate cancer. Dr. Huggins received a Nobel Prize in 1966 for this work.

Then, during the war, the anticancer potential of the nitrogen mustards was inadvertently discovered. A chemical relative of the nitrogen mustards, mustard gas, was used as a poison war gas. When the Liberty ship, the *John E. Harvey*, was sunk on December 3, 1943, it was carrying 100 tons of mustard gas. Victims who survived the sinking died later as a result of mustard gas poisoning. Autopsies revealed that the gas had severely damaged their bone marrow and lymphatic systems, the tissues that form and harbor white blood cells. The potential usefulness of such an agent against cancers that involve a proliferation of white blood cells was recognized, and the nitrogen mustards, some of which are still used today, were developed.

But it was Dr. Farber's discovery that proved most exciting. In 1947 he showed that acute leukemia in children could respond to treatment with a drug called aminopterin. He treated sixteen children, all of whom were seriously ill and had a life expectancy of a few months, with aminopterin. Ten of the sixteen experienced a complete, albeit temporary, disappearance of their leukemia. Aminopterin, and its less toxic relative, methotrexate, which soon replaced it, worked by starving leukemic cells of an essential vitamin, folic acid. The search was now on in earnest for other chemicals that could preferentially attack cancer cells.

Because anticancer drugs were experimental methods of treatment that were often accompanied by severe side effects, these new agents were used primarily in patients for whom all else had failed and who now had widespread cancer and were near death. To friends and relatives—and many physicians—this approach often seemed a cruel hoax. Having grown up in an era of miracle drugs against infectious diseases, they were disappointed when anticancer drugs failed to produce similar results. Sometimes the drug's side effects seemed worse than the cancer. In any event, due to the advanced stage of disease the patient nearly always succumbed to his cancer. Sometimes, however, a new anticancer drug would produce a dramatic response. Patients riddled with cancer and in extreme pain would discard their morphine and return to a semblance of normal life. Occasionally all signs of cancer disappeared. This disappearance, when it occurred, was usually short-lived. The cancer would return and the patient would die. Yet the "experiment" left a life-saving legacy, a clue to the possible effectiveness of a new drug against cancer. Once its effectiveness was known, it could be used in other patients earlier in the course of the disease when it had a better chance of producing a lasting remission.

New anticancer drugs were also tried against such cancers as acute leukemia in children where there was essentially no hope for cure. Since no other effective treatment was known, there was not much to lose. Fortunately for the future of cancer therapy, these were the very cancers against which chemotherapy worked best— the rapidly growing cancers of young people. At last, the glimmers of "wonder drugs" against cancer could be seen. The full extent of this advance is hardly known as yet. Today, as a result of extensive cooperative testing in patients at a dozen or so cancer centers, there are some fifty anticancer drugs established as clinically useful. Hundreds of other chemicals that have shown promise in animal tests are awaiting evaluation in cancer patients. At least half of patients with ten different types of disseminated cancer can now be cured with drugs. These are patients who, without drugs, usually have no chance of overcoming their diseases. These cancers include acute leukemia in children, advanced Hodgkin's disease, histiocytic lymphoma, testicular carcinoma (a cancer of the testicles), embryonal rhabdomyosarcoma (a muscle cancer), Ewing's sarcoma (a bone cancer), Wilms's tumor (a kidney cancer), Burkitt's lymphoma, retinoblastoma (an eye cancer), and choriocarcinoma (a cancer of the uterus). Skin cancer can also be added to this list of cancers that respond to chemotherapy, although this is not among the formerly hopeless cancers and the chemicals are applied locally rather than systemically (throughout the body).

Choriocarcinoma, a rare cancer of the uterus of young women, was once 90 percent fatal within a year but now is 90 percent curable. The difference is the use of two anticancer drugs, methotrexate and actinomycin D, which not only cure this cancer but at the same time preserve the woman's ability to bear children.

Karen D., a 20-year-old Maryland girl, says her high school friends all thought she was a goner when they first heard she had cancer. But when she got to Duke University Medical Center, one of seven regional centers around the country for the treatment of choriocarcinoma, the doctors assured her that although the treatment was "rough," in their experience with drug therapy they had not lost a patient to choriocarcinoma in ten years. Karen suffered all the expected side effects of the drugs plus some that weren't so common: she lost all her hair; she got sores inside her mouth that made it difficult to eat; her weight dropped from 165 to 82 pounds; her skin got blotchy and discolored; and the nerves in her legs became so inflamed that she couldn't walk. But at the same time Karen's cancer completely disappeared, and now, three years later, she is an attractive, healthy young woman. Her leg braces are gone, her hair has grown back, and, she says, "I feel like a million bucks. Like it never happened."

Anticancer drugs work in one of several ways. The so-called alkylating agents, such as the nitrogen mustards, block the replication of DNA, the genetic material in the cell nucleus, a process essential to the cell's ability to reproduce. Antimetabolites, like methotrexate, block the operation of the cell's normal chemical machinery. The vinca alkaloids, derived from the periwinkle plant, stop cell division. L-asparaginase blocks the production of the essential amino acid, l-asparagine, in certain kinds of cancer cells. It is not known exactly how the steroid hormones work, but they are effective in treating certain cancers that need particular hormones to continue growing. In some cases organs that produce certain hormones may be removed surgically, and in others, hormones may be given to suppress the cancer. Some anticancer drugs are antibiotics which interfere with protein synthesis in the cell.

Unfortunately, all drugs that attack cancer cells also damage normal cells, often causing extremely unpleasant, sometimes life-threatening side effects. The normal cells most vulnerable to attack are those that grow and divide rapidly, like most cancer cells. These are the cells that line the gastrointestinal tract, those that form the bone marrow where blood cells are produced, and those in the hair follicles. Accordingly, the most common side effects of anticancer drugs are nausea and vomiting, diarrhea, hair loss (temporary), and a decreased supply of crucial blood cells, causing anemia, reduced clotting ability, and diminished response to infections. Sometimes painful sores develop in the mouth, making it difficult to eat. When on chemotherapy, a patient needs frequent blood tests to be sure his blood cells do not fall to dangerously low levels. In addition, patients are advised to try to avoid infections and to eat protein-rich diets low in roughage and high in iron and vitamins. Sometimes a vitamin-mineral supplement is given.

In a pamphlet called "Understanding Chemotherapy" published by the Franklin County Unit of the American Cancer Society in Columbus, Ohio, Rosalee Bayer, whose own inoperable breast cancer was treated with heavy doses of drugs, advises eating many small meals throughout the day, drinking nutritious "shakes" prepared at home in a blender and high-protein supplements, and using cotton swabs to gently brush your teeth.

To the cancer patient who asks, "At times I feel so depressed, why should I even bother with chemotherapy?", Mrs. Bayer replied, "As a cancer patient, I've experienced some of these thoughts in moments of depression. We all do. But I want to survive, to enjoy as much life as I possibly can. And I know that these drugs may help make this possible. I have been fortunate, for now I feel well nearly all the time and I can maintain a full schedule of activities [which includes the care of a husband and four lively young sons]. . . . Chemotherapy gives you and me the opportunity to choose to try and do something to aid our own survival. The choice is ours. I choose to try."

Mrs. Bayer died a year after this pamphlet was completed. She died, not of her cancer, but of pneumonia which was a complication of intensive chemotherapy. But everyone who knew her said she had courage—the courage to live despite the fact that the odds were against her. During her bout with cancer, she not only cared for her family and wrote this pamphlet (in collaboration with Peggy Krach, a nurse), she also did so much volunteer work that she was named the Outstanding Community Volunteer of 1973 by the *Citizen Journal* in Columbus, Ohio. The job she was most proud of was working at the chemotherapy clinic of University of Ohio Hospital, helping other patients like herself to cope with the trials of chemotherapy. She also helped the nurses with their chores and provided a much-needed sympathetic ear and a vivid example for discouraged patients.

Because of side effects (the severity of which varies from patient to patient, with some having very little and others finding the side effects intolerable), doctors are limited in how much of a given anticancer drug they can administer. Sometimes if enough drug is given to kill the cancer, the complications may kill the patient. Moreover, cancer cells can become resistant to the attack of a particular drug and may no longer be harmed. These facts have spawned a new and exciting era in cancer chemotherapy, an approach that can work where other methods have failed. This is the use of several—two, three, four, and even five—different anticancer drugs at the same time or in close succession. It is called combination chemotherapy, and it is largely responsible for the cures— ranging from 15 to 90 percent of patients—that are now being attained for some susceptible cancers. For example, the nitrogen mustard, mustargen, is active against Hodgkin's disease, but it was the rare patient with advanced Hodgkin's disease (you will recall that radiation therapy is used for early cases) who was permanently cured by mustargen. However, further studies revealed that several other drugs also worked against this disease and that by combining them, as many as 80 percent of patients experienced a long-term disappearance of their cancers and more than half were apparently cured.

The combination therapy is referred to as MOPP—for mustargen (methchlorethamine), Oncovin (vincristine), procarbazine, and prednisone. It was devised by Dr. Vincent T. DeVita and his colleagues at the National Cancer Institute in Bethesda, Maryland. More than half the patients with advanced Hodgkin's disease who are treated with MOPP, sometimes in combination with radiation therapy, live longer than eight years. Dr. DeVita, who is now chief of the division of treatment at the Cancer Institute, says that combination chemotherapy works where single agents fail because the cancer is attacked from many different angles at once and even if the cancer cells become resistant to one drug, they will still be destroyed by the others. The trick in combination chemotherapy is to put together several drugs all of which attack the cancer cells in a different way and have different effects on normal cells. Thus, the maximum anticancer dose of each drug can be given while holding the severity of side effects (damage to normal tissues) to a minimum. The cancer cells, in a sense, get it from all sides and the normal cells are relatively spared.

Another disease where this principle has been put to use with dramatic results is acute lymphocytic leukemia (ALL) in children, which afflicts between 4,000 and 5,000 children a year in the United States. When Dr. Farber discovered the antileukemic effects of aminopterin in 1947, at most 1 percent of children with leukemia recovered permanently and most died within a few months of diagnosis. But in the last decade, a series of coordinated studies in cancer centers around the nation produced steady improvements in the chemical attack on leukemia until today, more than 95 percent of children with ALL who receive the best available combination treatment experience at least a temporary disappearance of their disease and more than half can expect to be alive and well five years later.

At the time these studies began, anyone who spoke of curing leukemia was condemned as a charlatan. Today cure of this disease is a realistic goal, and as improvements continue to be made in the treatment for ALL, more and more children can look forward to permanent recovery.

The essence of modern treatment of leukemia is the use in sequence of four or more drugs, all of which kill leukemic cells but which have differing damaging effects on normal cells. At the same time, steps are taken to prevent recurrence of the cancer. The spread of cancer cells to the central nervous system is prevented by injecting a drug, methotrexate, into the spinal column and by

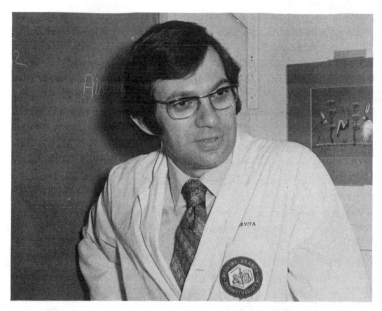

Dr. Vincent DeVita, Jr., now director of cancer treatment at the National Cancer Institute, helped to develop the complex drug schemes that are now curing more than half of the patients with advanced Hodgkin's disease. He is directing and promoting studies of similar drug therapies to prevent recurrence of the more common cancer killers.

irradiating the skull. After the initial large drug doses, smaller amounts of drug therapy are continued for several years to wipe out any new leukemic cells that may start to develop. The side effects of therapy can be drastic. Among other unpleasant effects, the drugs can increase the child's susceptibility to infection and interfere with the ability of his blood to clot. But the treatment offers the possibility of cure, and cure of leukemia is what cancer specialists are now shooting for in every case.

Jean K., now a perfectly healthy, normally developing adolescent, is one of hundreds of children who in all likelihood have been cured by this modern aggressive approach to treating leukemia. Jean was 7 years old when a blood test revealed that instead of the normal white blood count of 5,000 to 8,000, Jean's was 26,000 and the vast majority of the cells were leukemic cells. The diagnosis was confirmed by an examination of her bone marrow, where 90 percent of the cells found were of the primitive leukemic type.

At a hospital that specialized in the treatment of leukemia, Jean was placed on a carefully worked out regimen of potent drugs designed to kill the leukemic cells in her blood and bone marrow and prevent the disease from reestablishing itself. Once a week Jean received an intravenous injection of vincristine, a drug derived from the vinca plant, to stop cell division. At the same time, three times each day she took prednisone, a hormonal drug, to suppress white blood cell formation. The prednisone gave Jean a voracious appetite and made her a little hyperactive, and the vincristine caused some tingling in her fingers and toes, but Jean was able to receive this therapy without spending a single night in the hospital (although many hospitals prefer to keep children hospitalized at least during the first round of treatment). Jean spent a few weeks at home and tried to avoid people with infectious illnesses while the drugs destroyed most of her infection-fighting white blood cells.

By the third week of treatment, Jean was in partial remission—there were no more leukemic cells in her circulating blood and only 7 percent of the cells in her bone marrow were of the leukemic type—and she was able to return to school and keep up with her second-grade classmates. A week later, all the leukemic cells were gone from Jean's bone marrow as well as from her blood, and the team of physicians treating her changed the therapy. Vincristine was stopped and prednisone was tapered off. Instead, once a day for ten days she received an intravenous injection of asparaginase, an enzyme produced by the common intestinal bacterium *E. coli*, to starve leukemic cells by denying them the essential nutrient asparagine. The drug caused some vomiting for a few days, but Jean soon got used to it.

Now Jean was ready to begin the maintenance therapy that she would stay on for five years. Three times a day she swallowed tablets of 6-mercaptopurine, and once a week she took an oral dose of methotrexate. Both drugs block the formation of new cells. The doctors also tapped the fluid in her spine, and once every two weeks for a total of six times they injected methotrexate into the spinal column to prevent the leukemia from reappearing in the central nervous system. The spinal tap gave Jean a headache the first few times. Once a month for six months the maintenance therapy was reinforced with a single injection of vincristine and a week of oral prednisone. After six months the dose of the reinforcement therapy was doubled, but it was given only four times a year. And after five years all of Jean's therapy was stopped. Fifty-eight percent of children with acute lymphocytic leukemia who received the kind of treatment Jean did remain alive and well five or more years after their leukemia was diagnosed, and no child who has been all right for five years has yet experienced a recurrence of the cancer, according to Dr. James F. Holland, chemotherapy expert at Mount Sinai Medical Center in New York.

Of course the drug regimen Jean took does not represent the last word in the treatment of ALL. But while studies go on to try to find ways of permanently halting leukemia in the remaining 40 to 50 percent of victims who still succumb to the disease despite the current best available therapy, cancer specialists are beginning to apply the principles of combination chemotherapy to other forms of cancer, usually in conjunction with surgery or radiotherapy.

One of these is breast cancer, the leading cancer killer of women. Experts estimate that by the time a breast cancer has grown into a detectable lump, there is a 50 percent chance that it already has metastasized. Surgery and radiation, which are local treatments, would be unable to cure these women.

Although it is not yet known how many of the 33,000 lives lost to breast cancer each year might be saved by chemotherapy, studies conducted by the National Cancer Institute among women with advanced breast cancer showed that nearly two-thirds responded at least temporarily to a four-drug combination. Twenty-eight percent experienced a complete disappearance of their metastatic cancer. Sixty percent of those who responded were still alive sixteen months later or longer with or without disease.

The idea now is to use such therapy immediately after initial surgery for breast cancer in those women whose cancer is likely to have spread beyond the breast area by the time it was discovered. Anticancer drugs are much more effective against small, fast-growing tumors than against large, slow-growing ones. Therefore, drug use right after the bulk of tumor is removed may destroy any hidden metastases of the cancer and prevent recurrence.

In one cooperative study, the rate of recurrence of breast cancer was greatly reduced by a single drug called L-PAM used immediately after surgery in women who were found to have cancer in the lymph nodes adjacent to the breast. The lower relapse rate has continued among the treated women for more than 3 years after surgery, but it is not yet known whether survival will also be prolonged.

An even more dramatic reduction in the recurrence rate of breast cancer has been associated with the use after mastectomy of a three-drug combination called CMF—Cytoxan, methotrexate and 5-fluorouracil. In a study done in Italy, after three years the relapse rate among women whose lymph nodes contained cancer was only 13 percent in the drug-treated group compared to 33 percent in

the group that received only surgery. Again, the results are preliminary, since the women will have to be followed for up to ten
years after surgery to determine what effect the drug therapy will
have on their chances for a lasting cure.

Dr. DeVita has begun a similar study of cancer of the ovary. In
1976 this cancer caused 10,800 deaths and was diagnosed in another 17,000 women. Half the women who are thought to have
only localized cancer when their diseased ovary is removed, in fact
already have more cancer elsewhere which can not be seen by the
surgeon. At least one drug, L-PAM, is known to be capable of
curing some 10 percent of patients with advanced ovarian cancer.
If used earlier—at the time of surgery when metastases are small—
drugs that attack ovarian cancer may greatly improve survival, Dr.
DeVita believes. A similar chemotherapy approach is being tested
for cancer of the colon, stomach, pancreas, head and neck, certain
lung cancers, and melanoma.

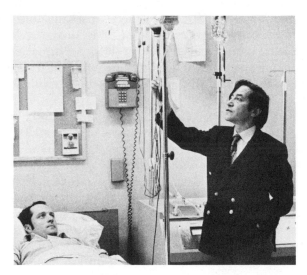

Dr. Isaac Djerassi, director of research hematology at Mercy Catholic
Medical Center in Darby, Pa., adjusts the flow of a transfusion for one
of his patients. Dr. Djerassi was a leader in developing blood cell
fractions to support the lives of cancer patients receiving potent drugs.

During the spring of 1976 Dr. Ralph E. Johnson, head of radiation oncology at the National Cancer Institute, reported that the
combination of radiation therapy and intensive chemotherapy had
dramatically altered the outlook for a small group of patients with
a form of lung cancer that is ordinarily rapidly fatal. The cancer,

called oat cell carcinoma (or undifferentiated small cell carcinoma) of the lung, causes 15,000 deaths a year in this country, half of them within six months of diagnosis. Even with modern treatment methods, only about one in four patients experiences a complete and usually temporary disappearance of his cancer. But the therapy Dr. Johnson devised, which includes three potent drugs that he administers in very high doses over a three-month period, produces complete remission in more than 95 percent of patients. Thus far, of 27 patients so treated, 26 had complete remissions and 21 are alive and free of cancer for up to two years after diagnosis. Dr. Johnson's interest now is two-fold—to modify the therapy so that it will be less toxic and more easily applied, and to use the same principles to derive equally effective therapies for the remaining types of lung cancer, the nation's leading cancer killer.

One cancer that has already yielded largely to postoperative chemotherapy is Wilms's tumor, a kidney cancer of young children. When surgery, radiation therapy, and prompt chemotherapy are used, the five-year survival was doubled to approximately 80 percent of these young patients. At Memorial Sloan-Kettering Cancer Center in New York, the use of a four-drug combination and radiation therapy or surgery to destroy the tumor has drastically reduced recurrences of Ewing's sarcoma, a bone cancer that afflicts children. This combined therapy has thus far led to survival without any evidence of disease in fifteen of nineteen children for an average of thirty-seven months. By contrast, among a group of children who received radiation alone without the drugs, all but one had recurrences within six months. The new approach to treating Ewing's sarcoma is now being used at major cancer centers both here and abroad.

Similarly, at Sloan-Kettering, pediatric oncologists have combined radiation therapy and simultaneous chemotherapy, including treatment to the brain and spinal cord, to reverse completely the prognosis for children with lymphosarcoma. Instead of only 11 percent surviving a year after diagnosis, now 72 percent of 58 children are alive up to three years later, with more than two-thirds of them completely free of recurrence.

But perhaps the most exciting progress in combined therapy has been in the treatment of osteogenic sarcoma, a rare but highly fatal form of bone cancer which kills 80 percent of its young victims within two years, despite amputation of the affected limb. Improvements are being made so rapidly in the treatment of this disease that the therapy described here is likely to be out of date by the time this book is published. But the recent series of innovations in treating osteogenic sarcoma is a vivid example of the kind of progress that is possible in modern cancer therapy and the meaning of that progress to the lives of cancer patients.

The story begins with a drug called methotrexate, a cell-killing substance first used by Dr. Farber in 1947 in children with leukemia. In subsequent years methotrexate was found to be effective against a variety of cancers, but the amount of drug that could be used—and hence its ability to cure them—was limited by its poisonous effects on normal cells. Methotrexate works by tricking cells into thinking it is the essential vitamin, folic acid, and thereby prevents the cells from dividing and multiplying, ultimately killing them. Cells which are undergoing rapid division, such as cancer cells, are most damaged by the drug's effects. However, many normal tissues also contain rapidly dividing cells and this limits how much methotrexate can safely be used.

In the 1960s Dr. Isaac Djerassi of Mercy Catholic Medical Center in Darby, Pennsylvania, among others, began studying the use of extremely large doses of methotrexate—up to 1,000 times the ordinary dose—followed by small amounts of another drug, called citrovorum factor, that acts as an antidote, preferentially protecting normal cells from total devastation. Later, Dr. Djerassi collaborated with Dr. Norman Jaffe at the Sidney Farber Cancer Center in Boston in the use of high doses of methotrexate followed by the citrovorum factor "rescue" to treat children with advanced osteogenic sarcoma—children in whom the cancer had recurred after surgical removal of the original tumor. In 1972, Dr. Jaffe and Dr. Emil Frei III decided to use this treatment right after surgery instead of waiting for the later appearance of obvious metastases, because in the vast majority of patients the cancer had apparently already spread by the time of surgery, although these metastases were not visible to the surgeon.

The first seventeen children so treated were all alive twenty-one months later and only one had detectable spread of the cancer. Senator Edward Kennedy's teen-age son Edward, Jr., was treated this way after his right leg was amputated above the knee in November 1973 to treat a related cancer of the cartilage. The boy completed methotrexate therapy in June 1975 with no evidence of recurrent cancer.

Then doctors at Memorial Sloan-Kettering decided to try, not only to destroy metastases with methotrexate and thus save lives, but also to save the limbs of children with osteogenic sarcoma. Instead of using methotrexate after surgery, Dr. Gerald Rosen tried it before surgery to reduce the size of the tumor. In this way, the surgeon was able to avoid amputation in most cases. Instead, only sections of bone were removed and replaced by metal rods.

In Boston, where Drs. Frei and Jaffe are also using this limb-saving approach, a 17-year-old boy who had osteogenic sarcoma in his left arm now has both his arms and a large measure of hope thanks to this progress. After four weeks of therapy with high doses of methotrexate and citrovorum factor rescue, in January 1975 surgeons removed a six and a half inch portion of upper arm bone and adjacent muscle, replacing the bone with a metal rod. Had the doctors used the earlier standard treatment, they would have had to amputate the left arm and remove much of his left shoulder to clear the area of cancer cells. When they finally did operate, the doctors were especially encouraged by the fact that they could find no living cancer cells in the section of bone they removed. Today the boy has full use of his left hand and is capable of lifting a weight of eighteen pounds with that arm. His doctors have been unable to find any trace of cancer elsewhere nor any evidence of local recurrence fifteen months later.

Other drugs, including adriamycin, have also been found effective in warding off recurrences of osteogenic sarcoma. Several centers are now using adriamycin plus methotrexate and citrovorum factor rescue, saving the limb wherever possible. But Dr. Rosen and others caution that the treatment is risky and complicated. They urge that all children with this disease be referred to a pediatric cancer center where the latest techniques can be most effectively applied by a team of experts.

Dr. Frank J. Rauscher, Jr., former director of the National Cancer Institute, recently remarked, "Cancer chemotherapy is in the early flush of adolescence and based on what we now know we think it has a very bright future." The cancers that have thus far proved most responsive to drug treatment are among the less common forms of cancer in this country, responsible for about 8 percent of total cancer deaths. But the understanding and encouragement that have come from this success are stimulating efforts to apply the new principles of chemotherapy to the nation's leading cancer killers. Toward this end the National Cancer Institute spent $65 million in fiscal 1976 in the search for and testing of new anticancer drugs or new ways of using old drugs. Dr. Rauscher has said that it costs more than $25 million to develop just one anticancer drug to the point where it can be used effectively in patients. In 1974, the institute screened more than 51,000 new agents against animal cancers—34,000 synthetic compounds and 17,000 natural products from microorganisms, plants, or animals. That same year, more than 20,000 cancer patients and more than 400 hospitals participated in studies of chemotherapeutic agents.

SUPPORTIVE THERAPY

The success of modern cancer therapy, particularly the use of massive doses of anticancer drugs, often depends on a number of vital supportive measures to counter the life-threatening effects of the treatment or the disease. These behind-the-scenes measures rarely get the credit they deserve in helping to save the patient's life, despite the fact that without them the best therapy in the world is often worthless. However, in 1972, when the Albert and Mary Lasker Foundation gave its annual medical research awards to sixteen pioneers in cancer chemotherapy, one of the prizes honored Dr. Isaac Djerassi for his development and perfection of transfusion techniques to counter the effects of leukemia and chemotherapy on patients' bone marrow where blood cells are formed. Dr. Djerassi developed equipment that can process whole blood from a donor and separate out the white blood cells crucial to fighting infections and the platelets needed for blood clotting, both of which are usually in short supply in patients treated with large doses of anticancer drugs, as a result of both the drug's effects and the cancer itself. The rest of the blood, the red cells and plasma, can then be returned to the donor, whose body would promptly replace the donated white cells and platelets.

Another way of fighting life-threatening infections in the cancer patient whose natural immunity has been compromised by his disease, by anticancer drugs, or by radiation therapy, involves the use of isolation rooms in which air flow is carefully controlled to prevent the patient from being exposed to anyone else's germs. At the National Cancer Institute, these so-called laminar air flow rooms (the air flows in one direction away from the patient) are kept 99.97 percent sterile. The patient is examined, talked to, and treated through a transparent vinyl curtain that is fitted with glove ports. Anyone who must enter the room uses sterilized gowns, gloves, boots, masks, and caps and stands "downwind" from the patient. Everything given to the patient, including all meals and utensils, must first be sterilized.

For some cancer patients, the dose of drugs or amount of radiation—and hence, the effectiveness of therapy—is limited by the fact that the patient is already malnourished as a result of the effects of his progressive disease on his body organs and appetite and can not withstand any further nutrient loss that may result from side effects of treatment. To counter this, cancer researchers at the University of Pennsylvania developed a means of injecting a highly nutritious solution directly into the patients' veins. The solution contains amino acids (the building blocks of protein), fats, and carbohydrates in a "predigested" form. The technique, called hyperalimentation, has succeeded in breaking the "vicious cycle" in which a malnourished cancer patient's only hope for cure or relief is a treatment which produces further malnutrition. Studies at the M.D. Anderson Hospital in Houston have indicated that the patient whose nutritional state is improved by hyperalimentation also experiences an improvement in his body's immune defenses, perhaps enabling him to better fight off his cancer as well as infections.

IMMUNOTHERAPY

Medical scientists now have clear evidence that the immunological defense system—the "army" of cells and antibodies that attack such foreign invaders as bacteria, viruses, and organ transplants—is also a potentially useful weapon against cancer, which in certain important ways is "foreign" to the bodies of the people in which it arises.

Cancer patients usually have poor immunological defenses, and it is thought that this lack of "strength" to reject cancer cells is partly responsible for the cancer growing unchecked. Researchers have also found that cancer cells often have a way of "hiding" from the immune system, donning a biochemical disguise that prevents the system from recognizing their foreignness. Surely, they reasoned, some way could be found to get around these problems and marshal the forces of immunology to favor the survival of the patient, rather than the cancer. In the last decade, slow but steady progress in this direction has been made, although the problem turned out to be far more complex than anyone had imagined at the outset. Thus far, all immunological treatments against cancer are experimental and largely reserved for those patients for whom the other, more conventional methods of treatment have failed, or they are used as an adjunct to conventional therapy.

There are three main approaches to immunotherapy for cancer. One is to try to jolt the immune system into action by injecting a stimulant, such as an extract of bacteria. The revved up immunological defenses would then presumably attack the cancer. This is called nonspecific immunotherapy. It has been the most widely studied, and the most successful, so far. The best researched approach to this has involved injections of an extract of the tuberculosis bacteria, called BCG, used as a vaccine against tuberculosis in many parts of the world. When BCG is injected directly into melanomas, a lethal form of skin cancer, the lesions often shrink or disappear. Sometimes even uninjected lesions disappear in patients who have had other lesions treated with BCG. In fourteen studies of BCG therapy, 58 percent of patients have benefited, some remaining free of cancer for several years and a few achieving apparent cure. Sometimes the immunotherapy is combined with surgery. But for this immunotherapy approach to work, the patients must be "immunocompetent" to begin with; that is, they must be capable of summoning up the forces of their immune system. BCG is also being tested in the treatment of acute leukemias where, when combined with chemotherapy, the BCG treatment seems to prolong the time that patients remain free of disease. BCG is also being tested against some of the more common cancers, such as cancer of the breast, colon, and lung. Therapy with BCG is not without hazards. Patients may experience fever, chills and abscesses, liver problems and jaundice, as well as other difficulties. A few deaths have been reported related to BCG therapy.

A second approach to immunotherapy is called active, or specific, immunization with "vaccines" prepared from the patient's own tumor. In most studies this has involved inactivating the tumor cells in some way, such as with heat or radiation, so that they cannot multiply, and then injecting them back into the patient. Sometimes the tumor cells in the "vaccine" are treated with a substance that is thought to help the immune system recognize their foreignness. Tests of this approach to therapy appear promising but thus far are inconclusive.

The third method, passive immunotherapy, has also not yet demonstrated conclusive effectiveness. Passive immunotherapy may involve such approaches as 1) preparing an antiserum to the patient's tumor cells; 2) injecting white blood cells that have first been "sensitized" to the cancer cells and therefore are likely to attack them in the patient; or 3) administering extracts from sensitized cells, such as a substance called transfer factor, which somehow arouses an immunological attack against the cancer. Transfer factor has been used, with some success, in treating osteogenic sarcoma, the often lethal bone cancer that has also begun to yield to combination chemotherapy.

Dr. Stephen K. Carter, then deputy director of the National Cancer Institute's Division of Cancer Treatment, concluded in November 1975, "There can be no doubt that immunotherapy has tremendous potential . . . as a new treatment modality in cancer." However, he added, right now its "potency" is limited, and much further study is needed before it can be widely useful. Dr. Carter, who is now (1976) director of the Northern California Cancer

Program in Palo Alto, predicted that immunotherapy will play its greatest role as a supplement to other cancer therapies to help wipe out tiny hidden colonies of cancer cells that may escape treatment with surgery, radiation, or chemotherapy.

OTHER APPROACHES TO CANCER TREATMENT

Phil, a roofer by trade, was plagued by a backache that he could not get rid of. He just hadn't felt well for weeks. Finally, he went to a doctor, who ordered a blood test. The diagnosis was acute myelocytic leukemia (AML), which before combination chemotherapy was nearly always rapidly fatal.

Although drug therapy has saved or prolonged the lives of a number of AML victims, for Phil the drugs simply did not work. His leukemic cells, initially knocked out by the drugs, quickly reappeared in his blood and bone marrow. A new round of drugs was no more successful, and Phil faced imminent death. But one chance remained—a 2 percent chance that Phil's life could be saved by a new and still experimental treatment. It involved total destruction of Phil's leukemic bone marrow, followed by a transplant of healthy bone marrow from someone in Phil's family. The success of the treatment—in fact, the only way it could be attempted at all—depended entirely on whether a marrow donor could be found whose tissues biochemically matched Phil's. Luckily his older brother Gary turned out to be an excellent match.

First, Phil was given very high doses of radiation therapy over his entire body to kill off all his bone marrow cells. Ordinarily, such treatment would be rapidly fatal because the person would be unable to manufacture any blood cells—red blood cells to carry oxygen, platelets to help the blood clot, and white blood cells to combat infection. But Phil was placed in a sterile isolation room to prevent infection and given transfusions of red blood cells and platelets. Then a large hypodermic needle was used to extract marrow from his brother's hipbone. The marrow was injected into one of Phil's veins, and it "took"—that is, it established itself in the core of Phil's bones and started manufacturing blood cells. Within two weeks new white cells were found in Phil's blood and they were healthy cells. There was no sign of leukemia anywhere.

But the treatment was not that simple. Although the tissues of the two brothers were well matched, they were not perfectly matched (only identical twins have perfectly matched tissues), and once Gary's bone marrow took over in Phil, it started making cells that attacked Phil's tissues as foreign. This is called "graft versus host" reaction, and it can be and often is life-threatening. But Phil weathered the crisis, aided by treatments to counter the reaction, and no further rejection has occurred. Gary's bone marrow has apparently accepted Phil as its own. Three years later, according to a report in *Today's Health* magazine, there is still no sign that Phil's cancer has returned.

The doctor who treated Phil, Dr. E. Donnall Thomas at the University of Washington in Seattle, was a pioneer in bone marrow transplantation. Thus far he has done forty-six such transplants for Phil's type of leukemia, with slowly increasing success. Thirteen of the patients are still alive. At the outset, bone marrow transplants were restricted to identical twins, but now that doctors are better able to control graft-versus-host reaction, they are trying and in some cases succeeding with transplants between well-matched siblings. But even when the donor and recipient are well-matched and graft-versus-host is overcome, there remains another problem with bone marrow transplants in treating leukemia. About 30 percent of patients develop a recurrence of their disease anyway, possibly because the radiation prior to transplantation failed to kill off every last leukemic cell or perhaps because the same factor that caused the leukemia in the first place caused it a second time in the new marrow. These are some of the difficulties that need to be overcome before bone marrow transplantation can become anything more than the last-ditch effort it now is in the treatment of leukemia.

During the last century some physicians have observed that an occasional cancer patient experienced a temporary reduction or complete disappearance of his cancer following a severe, fever-inducing infection. Often the infection was erysipelas, a skin infection caused by bacteria called streptococci. Some cancer patients were deliberately given erysipelas, and of those who survived the infection, a rare few were cured of their cancers. To avoid the danger of a fatal infection, the late Dr. William B. Coley of Memorial Hospital in New York injected patients with the poisons extracted from dead erysipelas streptococci and another bacterium, a combination that came to be known as "Coley's mixed toxins." In 1893 he reported that some of his patients were completely rid of their cancers. But in part because the therapy often involved severe and possibly fatal side effects, it never became an accepted treatment. It is now thought by some that Dr. Coley may have anticipated immunotherapy of cancer, and that the actual anticancer effect of his mixed toxins may be to give a boost to the immune system, something like what BCG does. But it is also possible that part or all the effect results from the high fevers that usually accompany the therapy.

Recently, cancer researchers here and abroad have taken a new look at the century-old idea that hyperthermia (very high temperature) can kill cancer cells. Some have treated cancers by temporarily diverting the blood flowing to the cancer area and heating the diverted blood to well above normal body temperature before it is returned to the patient's body. The result, when this therapy has been used in treating cancer of the bladder or melanoma of the hands or feet, has been considerable improvement in the patient's survival chances.

Other advanced cancer patients have been subjected to hot oil baths and encasement in hot melted wax, which as it hardens, raises the body temperature to over 107 degrees. A few patients, who initially had only weeks to live, experienced dramatic although temporary relief from the symptoms of their disease.

Still another approach to treating cancer with heat involves the use of radio waves directed at known sites of tumor. When the radio waves are absorbed by tissue, they are converted to heat energy. Because cancerous tissue is not as well supplied as normal tissue by cooling blood vessels, the cancer heats up more than surrounding normal tissue. At Veterans Administration Hospital in Brooklyn, New York, in a preliminary test on twenty-one patients with various types of advanced cancers, the radio wave therapy destroyed the treated cancer or substantially reduced the size of the tumor, although no patient was permanently helped by the procedure.

These experimental treatments are described, not because they are ready—or ever will be ready—for use by large numbers of cancer patients, but to demonstrate the willingness of legitimate cancer researchers to explore seemingly far-fetched ideas in the search for new and more effective cancer treatments. But one essential criterion must be satisfied before such a treatment idea is pursued—there must be some sound biological or medical reason to believe it will work. With all the as yet untested treatments that have suggested an anticancer effect either in occasional patients or in experiments on laboratory animals, it is a cruel hoax to attempt to treat cancer patients with a remedy that has nothing more going for it than someone's say-so that it will work. This problem will be discussed at length in the section on cancer quackery.

SPONTANEOUS REGRESSION

In extremely rare cases—perhaps one in 100,000—a patient's cancer will shrink or disappear for no apparent reason. Either no treatment was given that could account for the change or the treatment received was known not to have been effective. Yet the patient's cancer comes under control, at least temporarily and sometimes permanently. This phenomenon is called "spontaneous regression." It has been closely scrutinized in recent years for possible clues to more effective cancer treatments. If the causes of spontaneous regression of some cancers can be understood, perhaps the forces could purposively be marshaled to treat the overwhelming majority of cancer patients whose disease would progress unrelentingly without treatment.

At a 1974 meeting on the subject sponsored by the Maryland division of the American Cancer Society, cancer researchers said that the 176 cases of spontaneous regression that have been thoroughly studied suggest that a variety of factors may be involved, including a sudden awakening of the immune system, a response to the trauma of surgery, high fever, infection, a change in natural hormone production, blood transfusions, miscellaneous drugs and chemicals that are not known to affect cancer, and a change in psychological state.

Dr. Edward F. Lewison, breast cancer expert at Johns Hopkins Hospital, relates that, according to authoritative church legends, St. Peregrine was suffering from a cancer of his leg and was advised by his surgeons that amputation was necessary. The night before surgery, he prayed to be saved from amputation. In his dreams that night he imagined he was cured. Upon awakening, he found his vision to be true—he was miraculously and spontaneously cured of his cancer. He lived a long fruitful life, dying in 1346 at the age of 80 without further evidence of cancer. He was canonized in 1726 as St. Peregrine and has become the patron saint of cancer.

Dr. Lewison, who during his career in treating breast cancer has encountered twelve cases of spontaneous regression of this disease, tells of one woman who was operated on for extensive breast cancer in 1956 at the age of 35. She was well until 1959 when she developed metastases to her bones. Her condition improved some after treatment with radiation therapy, hormone therapy, and removal of her ovaries. In 1961 she became an alcoholic and stopped her hormone therapy. During the next 10 years, she alternated between bouts of severe alcoholism and use of a special drug called Antabuse to help her quit drinking. Gradually, all evidence of cancer disappeared from her bones despite the lack of further treatment for her cancer.

In 1971 she fell from a third story window and died. An autopsy showed a high level of alcohol in her blood and small nests of cancer cells in her bone marrow—a sign that although she still had cancer, somehow it was being held in check. To this day, no one knows why her cancer regressed and stayed quiescent for a decade. Neither alcohol nor Antabuse are known to have any anticancer effects.

In another intriguing case, a 57-year-old man with cancer of the rectum that could not be completely removed by surgery (only pieces of his tumor could be removed) did well for eighteen months when a large tumor recurred at the site of previous surgery. He refused to be hospitalized and soon thereafter developed a severe psychosis and became completely disoriented. At the same time, his rectal cancer began to regress and in six months the man was completely healthy, with both his cancer and his psychosis gone. Seven years later he was still fine.

In relating this case, Dr. Alfred Ketcham, then at the National Cancer Institute, pointed out that psychological factors may play a role in determining how a patient's body responds to a cancer. He suggested that this interaction between mind and body may help to explain the occasional effectiveness of some unproven but widely touted "cancer cures." If the patient believes strongly enough in the curative value of a purported remedy, the cancer may in very rare circumstances spontaneously regress. The "cure" is then attributed to that remedy, although the agent may have had no direct anticancer effect.

Still, for the vast majority of cancer patients, the most certain path to a cure lies in methods of treatment that have been established as effective through careful, well-controlled studies. Despite occasional seemingly miraculous cures, cancer is not a disease that one can count on to disappear of its own accord. If you are told you have cancer, your best bet is to find as fast as possible the best treatment available for your type of cancer. This is not always an easy job, but as described in a later section, various procedures have been established to help assure that every cancer patient can get the best that medicine currently has to offer toward a cure.

7. Childhood Cancer Treatment

In November 1973, another in a long series of tragedies struck the famous Kennedy family. This time it was young Teddy Kennedy, Jr., the 12-year-old son of Massachusetts Senator Edward M. Kennedy, who had been bothered by a painful swelling in his right leg. Teddy's leg had to be amputated above the knee to treat a cancer called chondrosarcoma which arose in the cartilage below his knee. Although this form of cancer is less lethal than most bone cancers, the boy was given powerful anticancer drugs every three weeks for a year and a half following surgery to kill off any stray cancer cells that might cause a recurrence of his disease.

Today, Ted is a healthy and active teen-ager. He was fitted with an artificial leg right after surgery. He walks aided by a cane and he skis—his family's favorite sport—using special ski poles and a ski that fits onto his artificial leg. The chances that he is completely cured are considered excellent.

Many physicians in practice today were taught that most cancers in children were incurable and that the best they could do was make the child's remaining life as pleasant as possible and help the family adjust to its impending loss. But in the last 10 years, medical researchers have achieved a complete reversal in the formerly hopeless prognosis associated with most childhood cancers.

In fact, at a few centers that specialize in treating cancer in children, more than half the young victims treated since the late 1960s have apparently been cured. And, it is widely believed that among children now being treated for cancer, the cure rate will be even higher. Some childhood cancers which previously were fatal in more than three-fourths of cases now are being apparently cured 80 or 90 percent of the time. According to Dr. Sidney L. Arje, Vice President for Professional Education of the American Cancer Society, today "cures are possible in almost every type of childhood cancer." Even in apparently hopeless cases, "there are too many reports of extremely good responses" for the doctor to give up on any child with cancer, Dr. Arje says. "Unfortunately," he added in a bulletin to educate health professionals, "misconceptions about the role of cancer in childhood mortality and pessimism about its prognosis are still popular and have handicapped early diagnosis and proper management. The problem of childhood cancer is not only larger than supposed, it is also more solvable. Some of the most important new advances in cancer management have been made against those cancers which often attack children."

Dr. Donald Pinkel of Milwaukee Children's Hospital, who has been a leader in developing potentially curative therapy for childhood leukemia, points out that "when a child is saved from cancer, a whole lifetime is preserved, not a few twilight years. Although only 1 percent of cancer occurs in children, the potential number of productive years of life to be saved by eliminating childhood and adolescent cancer deaths is nearly equal to that to be saved by eradicating adult cancer mortality."

Cancer is a relatively rare disease in children, but at the same time it is more common than many people think. In any given year, only one child in 8,000 is likely to get cancer. A pediatrician might practice for ten or twenty years before encountering one case of cancer—if any—among his young patients. As a result, both doctors and parents are often not alert to the signs of cancer in children. Yet cancer kills more children between the ages of one and fifteen than any other disease in the United States. In 1938 cancer ranked tenth among the causes of death in children. But by 1968 with the control of infectious diseases, cancer killed more children in this age group than any other cause except accidents. All told, cancer annually strikes more than 6,500 American youngsters, and more than 3,000 children die each year of cancer.

Childhood cancers are quite different from those that affect adults. They tend to grow more rapidly and they are concentrated in different organ systems. The most common cancers in children involve the blood and lymph systems (leukemia and lymphoma), the brain and central nervous system, the bones and connective tissue, the kidneys, and the eyes. Children rarely get the cancers of the lung, breast, or colon, which are the most common cancers in adults.

In all likelihood, the causes of cancer in children are also quite different from those in adults. A child hasn't lived long enough to have developed cancer because of years of exposure to a cancer-causing agent. Rather, childhood cancers are more likely related to some prenatal influence, such as exposure to radiation or a cancer-causing hormone, to a defect in the immune system, or, perhaps, to exposure to some as-yet-unidentified infectious agent or some totally unrecognized cause.

While the biological differences between adult and childhood cancers thwarted earlier attempts to cure cancers in children using surgery or radiation, the differences have proved an asset to modern treatment with chemotherapy and combination therapy. Now, in fact, the principles developed for effectively treating cancer in children are being adapted and applied to attack the more resistant cancers in adults. But before these principles can be used to treat childhood cancer, the disease must first be diagnosed. Because parents and doctors tend not to "think cancer" when dealing with a child, and because the symptoms of childhood cancers are often vague and mimic other less serious conditions, many children's cancers are not diagnosed until they are rather advanced and less curable than they might otherwise be. Following is a description of the most common forms of cancer in children, their likely symptoms, and a summary of the progress that has been made in treating them.

● *Leukemia,* a cancer arising in the blood-forming tissues, is the most frequent type of cancer in children, with acute lymphocytic leukemia (ALL) accounting for about 45 percent of childhood leukemias. It is most likely to occur in children below the age of six. The symptoms and signs at first are vague—the child may be tired, pale, and listless. Later he may develop rashes and swollen lymph glands in the neck and groin. He may also bruise very easily. Any child with such findings should have a complete blood test, which would reveal abnormal blood cells if the child had leukemia. Leukemia is one cancer where the stage at which the disease is diagnosed does not seem to make much difference in the effectiveness of therapy, so long as the child is not so sick that he cannot withstand the side effects of the vigorous anticancer treatment.

Progress in treating leukemia, once fatal within a few years in 99 percent of cases, has been one of the most remarkable achievements of modern cancer therapy. Today, more than half of children who receive the most up-to-date treatment can look forward to being alive and well five years later, and in all probability, most of these children will be permanently cured. The treatment, as described in the section on chemotherapy, involves a combination of antileukemia drugs plus chemical or radiation therapy to the spinal column, the most common site of recurrence. With modern chemotherapy, more than 95 percent of children will experience at least a temporary disappearance of their leukemia. Since the 1940s when these drugs were introduced, there has been a four- to six-fold increase in the average length of time children survive following a diagnosis of leukemia.

● *Neuroblastoma*, a cancer of the central nervous system, is the next most common type of childhood cancer. Neuroblastoma arises in certain nerve fibers of the body, usually in the abdomen. One of the first warning signs may be a swelling of the abdomen. There is also a simple urine test available to detect this cancer, which occurs most commonly in infants and very young children. If detected early and treated, 80 percent of children with neuroblastoma are alive and well five years later. Unfortunately, more than half of neuroblastomas currently are not diagnosed until after the cancer has spread beyond the site in which it arose.

● *Brain cancers* are difficult to detect early in very young children. One sign may be a strange squint or enlarged head. Other symptoms include severe headache, blurred or double vision, dizziness, difficulty in walking and unexplained nausea and vomiting. Some brain cancers are quite curable if treatment is begun early.

● *Wilms's tumor*, a kidney cancer, is now being cured in 80 percent of patients using a combination of surgery, radiation therapy, and chemotherapy. In fact, the focus of therapy now is to reduce the amount of treatment used (to minimize side effects) without compromising the children's survival chances. Wilms's tumor usually occurs before the age of seven and is first noticed as a swelling or lump in the abdomen.

● *Bone cancers* more commonly affect teen-agers, mostly occurring in the lower leg or forearm. The swelling and pain that may accompany them are often dismissed at first as a minor injury or "growing pain." If such symptoms last more than a week or two, they should be checked out thoroughly by a physician. The recent progress in treating bone cancers (the most common form is called osteogenic sarcoma, which until a few years ago was lethal in 80 percent of patients within two years of diagnosis) was outlined in the section on chemotherapy. Powerful anticancer drugs, when combined with surgery, have thus far kept more than 80 percent of children alive and well for at least two years after their cancers were found, the longest they have been followed at the time of this writing. For Ewing's sarcoma, another bone cancer in children, that formerly was fatal in more than 90 percent of cases, about half of children with seemingly localized cancer can be saved by treatment with combination chemotherapy and radiation. The early results of the latest treatment approaches suggest that an even higher cure rate is now possible.

● *Eye cancer,* or retinoblastoma, usually occurs in children under the age of four. The first symptom may be a widening of the pupil of the eye. Later a pearly glint, commonly called a cat's eye reflex, may be noted. Surgery or radiation therapy, sometimes in combination with drugs, can cure 85 percent of youngsters with this cancer. The vision in the affected eye can often be preserved. This cancer runs in families, so that if one child in a family has developed it, other young children in the family should be watched closely for early signs. In families that carry the disease, children have a 50–50 chance of developing retinoblastoma.

● *Lymphomas*—Hodgkin's disease and lymphosarcoma—are most frequently treated with radiation or a combination of radiation and chemotherapy. The chances of survival have increased dramatically since the early 1960s. In all cases of Hodgkin's disease, there is now an 80 percent chance of being alive and well for at least five years after diagnosis, and nearly all such patients remain well indefinitely. Lymphoma patients develop tumors mostly in their lymph nodes, and these tumors are initially small and difficult to detect.

Regular medical examinations—so-called well-child checkups—and prompt investigation of any symptoms that may develop between regular exams are the keys to effective control of cancer in children. Dr. Arje recommends that infants (between birth and 1 year of age) should be examined every month; children 1 to 4 years old, at least twice a year; and children 5 to 14 years old, at least once a year. Nearly half the children who get cancer are under the age of 5, so regular preschool checkups are extremely important (for the complete well-being of the child and not just to detect cancer). Dr. Arje urges doctors and parents alike to raise their cancer-consciousness when it comes to children. Better, he says, to have the doctor think you are overly concerned about cancer than to miss a diagnosis of early cancer in your child.

Once such a diagnosis is made, the decision on where and how to treat the cancer is critical to your child's chances for recovery and a long and healthy life. To maximize the chance for cure, the first treatment your child receives must be the best available to totally eradicate his disease. The best place to receive such treatment is in a cancer center or major medical center or institution where there are teams that specialize in treating cancer in children. Nowhere has the effectiveness of the team approach to cancer treatment been more effectively demonstrated than in treating childhood cancer. A cancer therapy team consists of a variety of physician specialists, supported by specially trained nurses and assistants, who work together to plan and carry out the treatment strategy that will most effectively destroy the cancer with the least harm to the child. The team must be able to deal rapidly and effectively with complications of therapy as well as unexpected simultaneous illnesses.

A 5-year-old boy being treated with potent drugs to kill his leukemic cells suddenly develops appendicitis, and must undergo emergency surgery at a time when the anticancer drugs are already impairing his body's ability to cope with physical stress. An 11-year-old boy with Ewing's sarcoma is found to have rheumatic fever while undergoing cancer treatment with radiation therapy and chemotherapy. The cancer team must be able to call on and work with other experts within the medical complex to help them in such complicated cases. The team also must work with the child's pediatrician at home, since after the initial therapy much of the follow-up treatment is done on an outpatient basis. But treatment must do more than cure the cancer. It must also preserve as much as possible the integrity of the child's future health, both physical and emotional. The child should be returned to as near normal a life as possible after treatment of the cancer.

At many hospitals parents are intimately involved in caring for their children with cancer, often living in hotels or other facilities on or near the hospital grounds and coming to the hospital each day to assist in feeding, entertaining, and even treating the child. That way, says Dr. Jordan Wilbur of Stanford Children's Hospital in Palto Alto, California, "even when the child dies of his disease, his family has the satisfaction of knowing they contributed to his possible survival in every way they could." And, Dr. Wilbur says, when the child survives—as more than 50 percent of them could—close parental involvement in treatment makes it easier for the child and his family to carry on their life afterward because the emotional scars left by the disease and its treatment are kept to a minimum.

Children's cancer specialists are always looking for ways to improve the treatment, both to cure more patients and diminish damaging side effects. "Cure is not enough." That's how Dr. Giulio J. D'Angio, formerly chairman of the department of radiation therapy at Memorial Sloan-Kettering Cancer Center and now at the University of Pennsylvania, sums up the current approach to treating cancer in children. "The relentless, aggressive attack against childhood cancer has led to a crescendo of success, and medicine can take justifiable pride in the progress made," Dr. D'Angio told a National Conference on Childhood Cancer sponsored by the American Cancer Society in 1974. But, he added, "those concerned with the malignant diseases of childhood are not satisfied with these results." He explained that sometimes the powerful treatments used to cure cancer in children have unfortunate, delayed side effects—problems which develop years after the cancer has been successfully eradicated. Among these problems may be disturbances in growth, damage to body tissues, such as the liver, kidneys, and reproductive organs, and the development of second cancers.

"The child cured of cancer must be followed for life, not so much to detect late recurrence of disease, but to permit early diagnosis of any side effects of treatment," Dr. D'Angio emphasizes. In one study of 414 children who had been successfully treated for cancer, nineteen developed second, unrelated cancers. Under ordinary circumstances, only one person in 414 would be expected to get a second cancer. In all but two cases, the patients had received radiation therapy to treat their original cancer. Thus, says Dr. D'Angio, while the main emphasis in treating childhood cancers is properly on improving survival rates, "there is a parallel effort to refine treatment, reducing it to the minimum necessary to achieve cure." The focus is on finding the least hazardous agents used in the lowest possible dosage to achieve the same high or even higher cure rates than are currently being attained.

Despite difficulties of long-term side effects, the vast majority of children whose cancers are successfully treated apparently go on to lead full and healthy lives—working, marrying, raising families. One study of forty-six such survivors of childhood cancer—seventeen men and twenty-nine women—showed that among them they had parented ninty-two children. The children of the former cancer patients have been free of cancer and other major diseases. They were no more likely than other people's children to suffer from birth defects. In fact, the miscarriage rate among the former cancer patients was much lower than that found in the general population, where about one in five pregnancies is miscarried.

As Dr. D'Angio sums up the progress so far in treating cancer in children: "We are near the end of a long tunnel, looking back to the blackness of no hope and no cure." The goal now is "to insure that the increasing number of successfully treated children of today do not become the chronically ill adults of tomorrow."

8. How to Find the Best Treatment

"The worst thing to do when you're told you have cancer is to give up. Instead, you should take a realistic, positive attitude and get the best care you possibly can. If you have cancer, you should be treated by a physician who knows the best available therapy for your disease." The words are those of Michael Finamore, the young New Jersey man described earlier who was cured of acute leukemia by experimental therapy attempted at a leading center for cancer research and treatment.

His sentiments are shared by many experts in the field. Dr. Audrey Evans, director of pediatric cancer at the Children's Hospital in Philadelphia, says that for cancer in children, "The family should insist on being referred to a specialist for treatment. There is a better chance of cure if you go to a center with a program for children with cancer." Modern cancer therapy is anything but simple and the techniques and strategies are changing rapidly. Even cancer specialists must work very hard to keep up with the latest innovations.

As you have seen, modern cancer therapy can also be quite dangerous, so it is important that it be applied by physicians qualified to give such treatment and in hospitals that have all the necessary expertise and supportive care readily available to deal with side effects. It is also extremely important for every cancer patient to get the optimal treatment the first time around. Once cancer recurs, the chances for eventual cure are greatly diminished.

Officials at the National Cancer Institute say that currently many patients with life-threatening but potentially curable cancers may not be getting the best therapy for their diseases because they do not get to doctors who know how to properly diagnose and treat cancer. The officials estimate that at least 100,000 additional lives might be saved each year if existing information about early diagnosis and prompt and adequate treatment were applied to all cancer patients.

Dr. Vincent DeVita, director of cancer treatment at the National Cancer Institute, suggests that patients get a second, independent medical opinion when told they have cancer, especially when the first doctor's opinion is that "nothing can be done." It is important, though, that a patient not waste a lot of time going from doctor to doctor hoping to find one who will tell him what he wants to hear whether it is true or not—that he doesn't really have cancer or that the radical treatment his doctor recommended is unnecessary. If a patient does not have or know of a doctor to whom he can turn, the patient can ask his local unit of the American Cancer Society for guidance to a qualified physician. In addition, the National Cancer Institute has established an Office of Cancer Communications to help cancer patients and their physicians find the names and addresses of cancer specialists nearest home. Each year this office handles many thousands of inquiries about cancer from the general public, most of them about where to go for treatment. Your physician can also obtain a consultation about the management of your case with a cancer specialist on the staff of the Institute's Clinical Center or at a major hospital, medical school, or facility designated as a comprehensive cancer center.

The best current therapy for your cancer may already be available through the physician who initially cares for you. But in cases where there is a need for advanced or complicated treatment, the Institute can guide you or your physician to the best nearby source of such specialized care.

In some cases, the Institute may tell you of an experimental treatment program it is sponsoring. You need not be afraid to be a "guinea pig" by taking part in an Institute-sponsored experimental program since you will receive, at the least, the best currently accepted treatment for your cancer and, at the most, you may receive an experimental new therapy that may be even more effective.

The best available therapy may not be able to cure every cancer patient, but it can often cause a temporary shrinkage or disappearance of cancer and give patients many precious months, and sometimes years, of good life. One patient who was glad he didn't accept the hopeless attitude of his doctor was Delos Smith, long-time science editor for the United Press International. When told that he had inoperable lung cancer, currently an incurable and rapidly fatal disease, Delos was sent home to die. Instead, he went to Memorial Sloan-Kettering Cancer Center where intensive radiation therapy led to the temporary but complete disappearance of the large tumor in his lung and knocked out a metastasis in his thigh bone. Then daily chemotherapy was used to kill off stray cancer colonies. After recovering from a series of complications, Delos was back at work and writing, among other things, the story of his battle against cancer, an article which served as an inspiration to countless cancer patients and won for Delos a prestigious writing award. At the time his article was printed, in October 1972, he had already lived at least six months longer than had been expected, and he was still "free of obvious disease." In his article Delos called his extended life "useful and enjoyable." It was also a productive life for more than a year before cancer finally claimed it.

To his dying day Delos Smith maintained that in treating cancer today, there was no room for what he called "therapeutic nihilism"—giving up on the patient before all possible beneficial treatments had been tried. He pointed out that the survival statistics in some cases may be highly unfavorable, but "being based on large numbers, statistics forecast for large numbers. They can't forecast for any individual." Like Michael Finamore, Dr. Evans, and many others, Delos Smith urged every cancer patient to get treated at a hospital where the team approach is used to apply the latest and most effective treatments. Even though knowledgeable physicians recognize that cure in every case is presently an unrealizable goal, they also know that if you don't shoot for cure, you're less likely to achieve it. By setting their sights high, they maximize the chances for survival for every cancer patient they treat. National Cancer Institute officials are certain that the death toll from cancer could be substantially reduced if all cancer patients were treated "aggressively" using the full range of available treatment techniques.

There are currently eighteen "comprehensive cancer centers" designated by the National Cancer Institute, and more will be established if warranted within the coming years. The specialists at a comprehensive cancer center are equipped to provide up-to-date treatment for all types of cancer. The centers provide care for patients at the request of the family physician. They make or confirm the diagnosis, plan or administer the therapy, and help local physicians provide follow-up care for their patients after they leave the center.

Dr. Frank J. Rauscher, Jr., former director of the National Cancer Institute and now (1976) Senior Vice President for Research at the American Cancer Society, emphasizes that there is no need for all patients to be "funneled into a cancer center" for treatment. For most cases, he says, community physicians who are experienced in treating cancer can do an excellent job. He views the role of the comprehensive cancer center as that of a "quarterback" to help patients receive the best possible care at the local level. Only when highly sophisticated treatment is needed, such as for a child with leukemia or bone cancer, should the patient be referred to a cancer center for therapy, Dr. Rauscher explains.

Dr. DeVita points out that bigness does not necessarily mean good care. "Personally," he says, "I would prefer to go to a doctor with experience in the cancer I had, however small the group in which he practiced, than to a big center which might not have that expertise." He defines a "center" at which patients can get good cancer treatment as "a group of physicians who are interested, experienced, and capable in caring for cancer at a particular anatomical location."

Many of the comprehensive cancer centers have established telephone "hot lines" to answer doctors' questions about how to deal with specific patients. Some centers receive hundreds of calls every week from local physicians who want expert guidance. About 60 percent of these calls result in patients being admitted to a comprehensive center for treatment. Comprehensive cancer centers also try to involve community physicians and local hospitals in the latest methods of treatment so that wherever possible, the cancer patient can get the best treatment available without having to leave his home town. In addition to the eighteen comprehensive centers, there are dozens of smaller centers, each one specializing in treating particular types of cancer, and 420 institutions which participate in clinical tests of new cancer treatments directed by the National Cancer Institute.

The goal of the national cancer treatment program is to establish enough hospital programs that specialize in cancer treatment in various parts of the country so that the vast majority of the American people will live within 120 miles of such a hospital. To accomplish this, many smaller community treatment facilities are needed. The American Cancer Society, the American College of Surgeons, and the National Cancer Institute have been working together to establish approved cancer programs in hospitals throughout the nation. By 1976 more than 750 hospitals had such approved multidisciplinary programs.

Through a system of regional treatment networks involving 120 community hospitals, the National Cancer Institute is also conducting specialized education programs for community physicians and other health workers to teach them how to apply the latest and most effective treatments for such cancers as childhood leukemia, Hodgkin's disease, lymphoma, breast cancer, and cancers of the head and neck. To help doctors keep up with the latest developments in cancer research, the Institute has established a computerized "Cancerline" which links physicians and scientists at 450 research centers throughout the country with summaries of the results of 50,000 cancer research projects published since 1963. More than 15,000 new abstracts are added each year. This information bank, which is reachable by telephone, also provides the descriptions of about 10,000 on-going research projects, including nearly 1,000 summaries of the experimental treatment programs for cancer patients.

The American Cancer Society has for decades been a leader in educating health professionals about cancer. The society's educational efforts emphasize the cultivation of a hopeful attitude about cancer—a belief in the curability of cancer and in the importance of early detection and prompt and adequate treatment. Several times a year, the Society holds national conferences where the latest facts about cancer prevention, detection, diagnosis, treatment, and rehabilitation are discussed. The Society publishes *Ca—A Cancer Journal for Clinicians* six times a year and distributes 380,000 copies of each issue free to physicians and medical students throughout the country. The Society also supports the publication of "Cancer," a monthly medical journal for physicians and scientists with special interests in cancer. Many professional educational booklets have been prepared by the Society on the prevention, detection, diagnosis, and treatment of cancer. These booklets are distributed without charge to physicians, dentists, nurses, and other health professionals. The Society also makes professional films and audio cassettes on various aspects of cancer.

Since 1948 the Cancer Society has supported a clinical fellowship program to give resident physicians and dentists special training in oncology. The aim of these professional education efforts is to speed the widespread application of existing knowledge so that more cancer patients can be saved.

Another part of the National Cancer Institute's Cancer Control Program involves the establishment of seventeen cancer information centers around the country where the general public and health professionals can, by calling a toll-free number, obtain information about cancer causes, detection, and treatment, assistance in locating community resources, and referrals to cancer experts in their region. Local units of the American Cancer Society can also provide such information. The appendix contains lists of medical facilities where up-to-date treatment or guidance about proper treatment can be obtained.

9. The Courage to Live

Jean Marie was 20 years old and in Florida on vacation from her job at a Minneapolis day-care center, where she worked with pre-school children. Suddenly she realized how extraordinarily tired she was—tired and weak and depressed. She went horseback riding one day and came back covered with bruises. She was black and blue from head to toe. "Surely," she thought, "this isn't normal." As soon as her vacation ended, Jean Marie visited the family doctor. He sent her directly to the hospital for tests, which revealed that she was suffering from acute myelocytic leukemia, a disease which until very recently was almost universally fatal in a matter of months.

The hematologist who examined Jean Marie's blood said that if she had waited much longer to receive medical care, she might not have survived. He also told the young woman's family that even with treatment, the prospects may not be good. An experimental anticancer drug, daunomycin, would give her a 50–50 chance of remission (disappearance) of her cancer, but how long the remission would last no one knew.

The family gathered around and, with the doctor, broke the news to Jean Marie. "Oh, damn!" she blurted out and threw everything in reach onto the floor. Everyone cried, then Jean's younger brother said, "We're all with you, even the dogs," and Jean Marie decided she was going to fight for all she was worth.

To prevent an infection her body might be unable to fight off, she was placed in isolation in a sterile laminar air flow room where nothing reached her that wasn't first sterilized. She received a huge bundle of mail each day, some of which melted in the sterilizer, but Jean Marie insisted on seeing every good wish. Once she was in isolation, the round of painful injections, transfusions, and seemingly endless tests of blood and bone marrow began. Despite the precautions, Jean Marie developed an infection, with raging fevers and convulsions. She had to be placed in cooling blankets to control her body temperature. She couldn't keep food down. "If I ate one string bean, I thought I was doing well," she recalls. Her

128

long blond hair all fell out, and she became so weak she couldn't lift the receiver of the sterile phone by her bedside. "We had a special speaker installed so we could talk to her," her father says. "We kept the family members on rotation twenty-four hours a day so she was never without someone to talk to." Jean Marie needed 125 transfusions before she left the hospital a month later with her disease in partial remission.

"Even then, I was already feeling better. On my last day in the hospital I ordered a steak—and ate it—and I was able to sit up and walk around a little," Jean Marie says proudly. The doctors said there would be less dangerous germs at home than in the hospital, but they ordered her to remain confined to her bedroom, which had been scrubbed clean. An electronic air purifier completely changed the air in her room every three minutes. All visitors had to wear masks, no one outside the immediate family could see her, and everything she was given was first sterilized. Gradually, Jean Marie was allowed out—first to the rest of the house and finally outdoors.

While she was confined to her home, a hospital nurse visited regularly to test Jean Marie's blood. "Gradually, there were fewer and fewer leukemic cells, and one day, I was looking at a carton of 2 percent milk and I said—'That's what I am, 2 percent.' Only 2 percent of my white blood cells were leukemic cells." Eventually even that 2 percent disappeared, and about a month after leaving the hospital Jean Marie was in what doctors call complete remission—there was no sign of leukemia either in her blood or in her bone marrow, which had previously spewed forth millions of leukemic cells each day. At this time, she was placed on maintenance chemotherapy, a drug called mercaptopurine which she is still taking for two-week periods with two weeks' rest in between. The pills make her feel tired and nauseous and it is hard at times for her to study for the university courses she is now taking. But monthly blood tests and periodic marrow tests have shown no sign two years later that her leukemia has returned. Meanwhile, she is enjoying life as much as she can. An outdoor person, she swims a lot in summer and has taken up badminton. She travels around Minnesota, visiting some of its more than 10,000 lakes. And she maintains an active social life, with a steady stream of boyfriends.

"Some people treat me differently when they first find out I've had leukemia, but they soon learn how to handle it. I've discovered that when people ask me how I am, they really want to know. When I first got out of the hospital, I had horrible nightmares, and the bad dreams still come back every now and then. Sometimes I'm nervous, sometimes scared. I realize how easy it is to die and that makes me impatient. I don't want to have to wait to do anything."

But Jean Marie says she has also learned a lot about cancer and how to beat it. Her message to other cancer patients: "Really hang in there. You have to have a positive attitude. When I was in the hospital I didn't think about dying. I thought, this is something I have to get over. I had a lot of people who hung in there with me, too."

She also warns against quack remedies. "Everybody came at me from all angles. They offered what they thought was good advice— Laetrile, faith healing, asparagus, vitamins—here, take three worms. My dad even bought a juicer and whipped up some brew." (The juicer was also used to prepare nutritious shakes to rebuild Jean Marie's strength.) Her advice to other patients is to get the best therapy possible from qualified physicians who are experienced in treating cancer. She even has an ace in the hole if the antileukemic drugs don't keep her disease in check. Her sister has the same tissue type as she, and if all else fails, doctors will attempt to transplant to her some of her sister's healthy bone marrow.

Just as he reached his fiftieth birthday, John K. started to get thick through the middle—which is not particularly unusual for a man his age, although he had been slim all his life. His family teased him about his "beer belly," as they called it, until one day it seemed as if he could hear the "beer" sloshing around inside him when he moved. John's wife pointed out that he really hadn't been his usual energetic self for several months following a bout with flu from which he never quite recovered. He went to see his doctor who put John in the hospital for a series of tests and X-rays. He drained some of the fluid that had collected in John's "beer belly" and found that it contained albumin, a protein that had leaked out from his liver and the lining of the abdominal cavity.

Exploratory surgery followed. Two gallons of the protein-rich fluid were drained from his abdomen and behind it the surgeon found a massive cancer. The surgeon sewed John back up and said there was nothing *he* could do because this was not a disease that could be managed surgically. John had lymphosarcoma, a cancer affecting the lymph tissue. Swollen lymph nodes then appeared over parts of his body like bunches of grapes. He became grey and thin, his weight dropping to only 126 pounds. Without treatment, his life expectancy could be measured in several months. John was very depressed. "He didn't want to see anyone or have anyone see him," Mrs. K. recalls. "He wouldn't even open his mail. He was really down, but we just kept coming to see him. We didn't ask his permission."

Neither John's family nor his doctor was ready to give up. The doctor told him, "You have lymphosarcoma. Until recently it was considered incurable. We are going to do everything we can to stop it." New treatments, the doctor explained, using radiation and combination chemotherapy have increased the proportion of patients in which the disease can be controlled. "The treatment will be hard on you, but it's your only chance," he said.

John first received ten radiation treatments to shrink the abdominal tumor. Then the doctors let him rest. He was a very sick man. The fluid returned to his abdominal cavity and another two gallons were drained off. In eight or nine days, the fluid had to be drained again; ten days later, a third draining was done, then in two weeks, a fourth. But each time there was less fluid than the time before and it built up more slowly. John began to feel—and to look—better.

Even so, Mrs. K. says, "After he got home from the hospital, I had an awful time getting him out of the house. He didn't want people to see him, so we would wait until dark and I would go for a walk with him."

Then the chemotherapy began—injections of vincristine followed by twenty-two pills a day of prednisone and cytoxan, for five days. John had to drink at least two and a half quarts of liquid a day to keep toxic substances from the destroyed cancer cells draining out of his system and to dilute the drugs as they passed through his kidneys. He lost his hair and got tingling sensations in his fingers and toes. Three weeks later he began a second round of chemotherapy; then a month later, a third.

Bit by bit the lymph nodes swollen with cancer cells began to go down. For a year John had chemotherapy every month, then every second month, and after a year and a half of treatment, all the lumps had disappeared. Three years after John first became ill, the doctor did a complete workup and could find no evidence of cancer. He told John, "To me, you're a perfectly healthy specimen," and stopped the chemotherapy. Now, six months later, John feels well and is working harder than ever.

The year John got sick, he lost his job, not because of his cancer but because his job was eliminated. Nonetheless, as a cancer patient and a middle-aged man, it was not easy to get another job. He was out of work for over a year and that compounded his depression. "He did a lot of crying; he didn't think he would make it. It was a very hard year," Mrs. K. says. But finally he was able to find work, although he no longer had seniority and had to start at the bottom of the ladder with the new company.

"When something like this happens you get a different perspective on life," says Mrs. K. "We've always been a close family. But now we're even closer. And we appreciate everything more—everything that's done, everything we have. Not a day goes by when John doesn't say 'Thank God I see another day' in the morning and 'Thank God I've had another day' before he goes to bed.

"The doctor had told us, 'You need a lot of prayer, a lot of faith.' Now John tells people, 'You have to believe you are going to get there. You have to believe it's going to work.'

"You also have to have the family in there with you. The kids—everyone—was great. They just kept coming and being there when they were needed. The strength of the family was very important."

10. A Treatment Controversy: Breast Cancer

In the 1880s, Dr. William Halsted, a Baltimore surgeon, developed an operation that in the decades since has remained the standard treatment for breast cancer—the Halsted radical mastectomy. It involves removal of the entire breast, the underlying muscles of the chest wall, and the lymph nodes in the armpit.

Among the approximately 50 percent of breast cancer patients whose disease is still confined to the region of the breast at the time it is discovered, the Halsted radical is a curative operation in the vast majority of cases. For the remaining patients in whom cancer has already spread beyond the breast and armpit, the surgery cannot cure, but it can often prolong the patient's life for months or years. Nonetheless, in recent years, the Halsted radical has been the subject of intense debate within the medical profession and among women who may get breast cancer. Many articles have appeared in medical and lay publications advocating less radical operations as equally effective in curing women with breast cancer and less damaging to the patients' physical appearance and emotional state.

In a society where breasts are idolized as the epitome of femininity and sexual attractiveness, these claims have drawn the interest of many thousands of women who face the prospect of losing a breast to cancer surgery. Indeed, women have come into their doctors' offices waving articles from this or that magazine or newspaper, demanding the less radical type of surgery or radiation therapy. Some women in need of urgent surgical attention for cancer "shop around" from doctor to doctor until they find one willing to administer the kind of treatment the articles recommend. What most of these women fail to realize is that the claims that simple surgery or radiation therapy is as effective in curing breast cancer as the more radical operation are based on incomplete evidence.

One day perhaps less extensive treatment for breast cancer will be firmly established as equally effective as radical surgery, but right now the evidence is far from unequivocal, and what evidence there is strongly suggests that in the long run, radical surgery may save significantly more lives. The question, then, for women facing possible breast cancer surgery boils down to this: Is preserving both your breasts more important than maximizing your chances of living a full and healthy life? For women who have thought this question through carefully, discussing it with family members or close friends as well as with their doctors, the overwhelming majority opt for the very best chance to live, a radical or modified radical mastectomy, over the alternative—keeping both breasts but possibly diminishing chances for survival. In making this choice, it is helpful to understand the nature of the various approaches to breast cancer treatment. Following is a description of the surgical procedures:

- Extended Radical or Supra-radical Mastectomy—removal of the entire breast, the underlying chest muscles, the lymph nodes in the armpit, and internal mammary chain of lymph nodes which lie beneath the breastbone inside the chest.
- Halsted Radical Mastectomy—removal as a single unit of the entire breast, chest muscles, and lymph nodes in the armpit.
- Modified Radical Mastectomy—removal of the entire breast and many of the lymph nodes in the armpit but only partial or no removal of the chest muscles.
- Simple or Total Mastectomy—removal of the entire breast but leaving the chest muscles and lymph nodes intact.

All of the above procedures involve complete removal of the breast. Depending on the nature of the patient's cancer, particularly with regard to how early in the natural progression of the disease the cancer is discovered and treated, each of these procedures has a place in generally accepted medical practice.

Other operations have been advocated by some cancer specialists in which the breast is not removed. The techniques are known by a variety of names, including lumpectomy, tylectomy, local excision, and partial mastectomy. All involve removal of the malignant tumor with a varying amount of surrounding tissue but without removing the entire breast. As an alternative to any kind of breast surgery, other than biopsy, a few specialists advocate radiation therapy as the sole treatment for breast cancer. Radiation therapy sometimes must be used when the cancer is so large that it cannot be encompassed surgically or the patient is so ill that surgery is unsafe. In other cases, radiation is used as the primary treatment (usually combined with surgical removal of the lump) when the woman simply refuses to undergo a mastectomy. The use of radiation therapy as a primary treatment for early breast cancer has been suggested by a few small studies on selected patients over the last two decades and is common treatment in Europe, but it has yet to be definitely proved as effective as mastectomy in the long run.

What are the factors that influence the decision as to which treatment to use? How is a woman to know what to do? Maybe she thinks her surgeon doesn't really understand what a breast can mean to a woman. In truth, what guides the surgeon is not a callous attitude but a desire to cure as many of his patients as possible. Therefore, in most cases, he will choose either a simple, modified radical, or radical mastectomy as the most effective treatment for the patient, the exact choice depending on the individual case. To understand why, it is helpful to know something about the nature of breast cancer and how it grows and spreads.

Breast cancers arise inside the milk ducts of the breast. In the earliest stage, it is called an in situ (noninfiltrating) cancer because it has not yet invaded the wall of the milk duct. At this stage, breast cancer is virtually 100 percent curable by removal of the breast—simple (total) mastectomy.

It is best to remove the entire breast even for very early cancer because of another characteristic of breast cancer—its tendency to arise in more than one location of the same breast at the same time. Thus, on a mammogram (breast X-ray) the doctor may see only one suspicious spot, but after removing the breast the pathologist who does a detailed microscopic examination is highly likely to find several other in situ cancers, and possibly small, more advanced cancers.

In treating in situ breast cancer, some surgeons perform what is called a subcutaneous mastectomy. They remove the underlying breast tissue, leaving a bag of skin of the breast and the nipple. Then they replace the removed tissue with a silicone implant. However, lesser surgery that removes only one focus of in situ cancer is not as likely to cure as a total mastectomy. In one study in which only partial mastectomy was done to treat in situ cancer, 30 percent of the women later developed invasive cancer in the same breast. When the invasive cancer appeared, there was no longer the assurance of a nearly 100 percent chance of cure.

A few doctors say that an in situ breast cancer, once diagnosed by biopsy, can be followed periodically by physical examination and mammogram, with mastectomy done only if a lump appears which proves to be invasive cancer. Most breast cancer surgeons say, however, that this is like living on a powder keg, and once the in situ cancer, which is curable by mastectomy, begins to invade the wall of the milk duct, a cure can no longer be guaranteed. When the cancer has invaded the wall of the milk duct, it is called invasive cancer. At this point, there is the possibility that cancer cells could enter the lymph system or blood vessels and travel to other parts of the body.

The earlier in its life an invasive breast cancer is treated, the less likely it will already have spread beyond the breast. Also, the initial area of spread is usually to the lymph nodes near the breast, especially those in the armpit. Cancer cells may stay in these nodes for a long time before any break loose and travel to other parts of the body. The only way the surgeon can know for sure whether there are any cancer cells in the lymph nodes is to remove them and have them studied microscopically by a pathologist. In 30 to 40 percent of cases where the surgeon thinks (on the basis of feeling the armpit) that there is no cancer in the nodes, the pathologist finds cancer under the microscope. This does not mean that the surgeon is a poor diagnostician; it simply means there is no way to know for certain unless the nodes are removed and examined microscopically.

Presently, 90 percent of breast cancers are diagnosed after they have become invasive and thus may have already spread to the nodes. This is the reason surgeons prefer to do a radical or modified radical mastectomy for most cases of breast cancer. Otherwise, if they did not remove the lymph nodes, they would unwittingly be leaving behind cancer cells in one-half or more of their patients, including in 30 to 40 percent of those patients who were thought on the basis of a physical examination to have no cancer in their nodes. These cancer cells in the nodes could then break away and establish cancer colonies—metastases—elsewhere in the body. At that point, chances for cure are very low. When a patient is found to have cancer in the lymph nodes—and sometimes even when the nodes are free of cancer, postoperative radiation therapy may be given in selected cases to kill any cancer cells that might remain in the area after surgery. However, radiation treatments after breast cancer surgery do not prolong survival and are no longer advised as routine therapy for all—or even most—patients.

In the last few years, preliminary results of several studies have indicated that for patients with breast cancer who have cancer in the nodes, postoperative chemotherapy can significantly reduce the risk of recurrence of their cancer during the first two years after surgery. (See "Chemotherapy" in Chapter 6.) It is not yet known whether women so treated will have an increased life expectancy, but the early study findings strongly suggest that their chances of survival will be improved by the drugs. Unlike radiation, which can only affect the region of the breast, chemotherapy is a systemic treatment potentially able to knock out hidden colonies of cancer in remote parts of the body. In any event, the precise kind of surgery and follow-up treatment for breast cancer must be individualized, depending on such factors as the type, size, location, and extent of tumor, all of which influence the probability that cancer has already spread to the nodes or beyond. The age and general condition of the patient may also influence the surgeon's decision about the extent of surgery.

With this understanding of how breast cancer develops and can threaten life, let's look at some statistics comparing the results of radical mastectomy with other types of surgery or radiation therapy. The studies of different kinds of treatment have pointed to one essential fact—for breast cancer an adequate comparison must involve 10 years of follow-up after treatment. After five years, no firm conclusions can be drawn.

In one such study, patients who were thought to have no cancer in their lymph nodes (so-called clinical stage I) were treated either with radical mastectomy, simple mastectomy, or radiation therapy without surgery. After five years, survival in all three groups was the same.

But after ten years, the survival figures were as follows: 70 percent in the radical mastectomy group; 39 percent in the simple mastectomy group, and 30 percent in the radiation group. The researchers showed that when early breast cancer was treated by radical mastectomy, 15 percent of the patients were cured (who would otherwise have died) because their lymph nodes were removed at the time of surgery. Since each year tens of thousands of women are diagnosed as having seemingly early breast cancer, the potential saving in lives as a result of radical surgery is enormous.

Mastectomy may seem to be a primitive way to treat breast cancer. But right now, medicine does not have a better way of proven equal effectiveness. A few carefully formulated studies are presently underway to determine whether less than radical surgery or mastectomy can work just as well in certain groups of patients. But it will be many years before the result of these studies are fully known. In the meantime most surgeons recommend that removal of the entire breast—most often by radical or modified radical mastectomy—is the acceptable surgical treatment for operable breast cancer. In fact, it seems likely that long before the con-troversy over the extent of breast cancer surgery is resolved, the argument will become moot for two reasons: as early detection programs become more and more widely used, the disease will be detected at earlier stages that require less drastic surgery to achieve cure; and, as the value of postoperative chemotherapy becomes better established, it may be possible to achieve the same or better cure rates with lesser surgery plus postoperative drugs.

Some women, when told they should have a biopsy to check out a suspicious lesion in their breast, have objected to the fact that doctors ask them to sign a consent form agreeing in advance to have their breast removed should the biopsy show the presence of cancer. Since four out of five biopsied lesions turn out not to be cancer, these women ask why five women should have to suffer preparing themselves for the possible loss of a breast when only one will actually have her breast removed. Why not have the bi-opsy first, examine the findings, prepare only these women who have a positive finding of cancer for a mastectomy, and do the surgery a few days later?

Surgeons point out that the main advantage of doing the biopsy and mastectomy as one procedure is that the woman has only one hospitalization, and is put under anesthesia, with its attendant hazards, only once. They add that if the pathologist has any doubt at all about whether cancer is present in the biopsy specimen, a mastectomy will not be done at that time. Instead, the woman is allowed to wake up and await the final report of the pathologist.

For women who insist on knowing the results of the biopsy before consenting to a mastectomy, surgeons have found that the chance for cure is not reduced if the operation is done as a two-step procedure—first the biopsy, and then a separate operation for the mastectomy should it be necessary. However, most women prefer to have the matter all taken care of at once rather than face two trips to the operating room.

The most important thing, if you find a lump or are told you need a breast biopsy, is not to delay in getting proper medical treatment—either because you fear what a biopsy might show and the treatment that might ensue or because you are shopping around for a doctor who will give you exactly what you order in the way of therapy. Delay increases the possibility that your can-cer, if indeed it is a cancer, will spread beyond the breast, thus greatly reducing your chance of cure.

11. Quacks Can't Cure Cancer

Linda Epping was an 8-year-old California girl with a muscle cancer called rhabdomyosarcoma affecting her left eye, a disease that doctors at the University of California Medical Center in Los Angeles were fairly certain they could cure by surgically removing the eye and surrounding tissue. However, in the hospital waiting room one day before the surgery, a woman told Linda's parents of a chiropractor who had supposedly cured her son of brain cancer without operating.

Mr. and Mrs. Epping, who were dreading the surgery to begin with, decided to leave the hospital and take Linda to this "miracle healer." The chiropractor, Marvin Phillips, was not licensed to treat cancer but he told Linda's parents he could cure their daughter by "chemical balancing of the body." He treated Linda with vitamins, huge quantities of pills he never identified, enemas, iodine solutions, daily skeletal "adjustments" in his office, and special exercises. Despite the unorthodox remedies, which cost the Eppings $739, Linda's cancer continued to grow, pushing her eye out of its socket, until finally her parents realized the worthlessness of the "therapy." But then it was too late. Precious time had been wasted, and Linda died of her cancer soon after the Eppings brought her back to the University of California Medical Center. The doctors there said her death was a needless tragedy that could have been averted had her parents stuck with conventional, potentially curative therapy.

The chiropractor who cost Linda her life was brought to trial, convicted of second degree murder and sentenced to jail. But this was an unusual result. The law rarely catches up with cancer quacks. Most go on, year after year, preying on the fears and hopes of cancer patients and occasionally working "miraculous cures" in persons who only think they have cancer but were undoubtedly perfectly healthy to begin with.

Americans throw away between two and three billion dollars a year on worthless potions, devices, and ceremonies that are pur-

ported to be able to rid them of their cancers, according to estimates of the U.S. Food and Drug Administration. Many of these
people are dying and desperate and feel they could not die in
peace unless they knew they had "tried everything," even the
seemingly unreasonable and unlikely. But many others, like Linda
Epping, initially had an excellent chance to be cured of their
cancers, but in choosing to throw away their money on cancer
quacks, they also threw away their lives.

Why do people go to cancer quacks? Largely out of ignorance
and fear, like Linda's parents. Being told you or someone you love
has cancer is like being hit by a truck. The news is stunning and
often leads to irrational thinking and behavior. For many, it is the
most frightening diagnosis they could think of, because to them it
spells a prolonged, painful experience ending in certain death.

As you have already read, a diagnosis of cancer is far from an
automatic death sentence—one in three cancer patients is now
being saved and one in two could be saved with currently available methods of early diagnosis and treatment. And in many more
cases, useful life can be prolonged. But when a person is filled with
fear, it is hard for him to think clearly and consider facts ration-
ally. To the mind beclouded by fear, the cancer specialist who says
he thinks there is a good chance for cure surely must be lying.
Didn't Mrs. X, who lived on the next block, die of the very same
kind of cancer four years ago? He forgets that every patient is
different and that Mrs. X did not even go to a doctor until her
cancer was so far advanced that she could hardly function. He also
forgets that rapid progress is being made in the treatment of several kinds of cancers, and in four years cancer researchers could
have greatly changed the odds of survival. A person thinking such
thoughts is a sitting duck for a cancer quack who promises a sure
cure, especially if that "cure" can be achieved with a far less traumatic treatment than the cancer specialist would have used.

Many patients dread the surgery, radiation therapy, and
drugs that are the hallmarks of modern, effective cancer treatment.
They fear the disfigurement of surgery and the toxic effects of
radiation and drugs. Thus, someone who promises a cure through
a special diet or "harmless" injection or merely the laying on of
hands seems very attractive in the face of the alternatives offered by
legitimate medicine. The pitfall, of course, is that while legitimate
medicine can offer a real chance for cure, the quack offers nothing
more than a false hope. It *can* hurt to use a "harmless" or nontoxic
unproven remedy because in treating cancer, time is of the essence. If the patient wastes time with an unproven—albeit "harmless"—remedy which has no effect on his cancer, when he finally

gets to a legitimate therapist his cancer may be beyond the possibility of cure.

Some people fear the expense of legitimate cancer treatment and are attracted by the seeming low cost of therapy offered by cancer quacks. (Surely, some think, if this healer isn't charging much, he could hardly be a crook.) Unfortunately, while it costs an average of about $2,000 to treat a curable case of cancer, it can cost $20,000 or more to care for an incurable cancer patient, and many people who start out with the quack's cheap "cure" end up having to spend far more to die than they would have had to spend to live in the hands of a competent cancer therapist.

Some persons are generally distrustful of doctors and will try any and every purported remedy they can get their hands on, so long as it doesn't come from a man (or woman) in a white coat. But while for nonfatal diseases, the patient is not likely to be particularly harmed by following a "special diet" described in a magazine or book before he visits a doctor, for a cancer patient dallying around for weeks or months with some unproven remedy could make the difference between life and death.

Still another—and probably quite common—reason cancer patients go to quacks is that they believe or know their own competent doctors have given up hope for their recovery. Such a patient —or his family—is likely to clutch at any straw that rekindles hope for survival, the quack's main—but false—selling pitch. It would be far more constructive for the patient and his family if someone on the medical staff helped them to accept and adjust to the inevitable instead of relinquishing them to the false promises of the cancer quack. Others advise doctors that, while it is wise as well as honest to be realistic about a patient's survival chances, it is also important never to strip that patient of his last vestiges of hope. Many doctors have heard their terminal patients say something like, "I know I'm dying, Doctor, but I'm still praying for a miracle that will make me well."

Dr. Emil J. Freireich, a cancer chemotherapist at M.D. Anderson Hospital and Tumor Institute in Houston, urges physicians to take a lesson from the quack in the art of positive thinking. As he told a cancer conference in 1975, "The physicians have to replace what quacks do in some areas. They must be positive and believe that the treatment they give will work. Physicians have to make patients feel better by letting them know that they are getting the very best care available. They must avoid hopelessness. No one wants to be told that nothing will help him. That just sends him off to the quack across the street."

How can you recognize a cancer quack? This is not always easy for the layman. Quacks usually present a professional facade, appearing in medical garb and using pseudo-scientific terms to impress prospective patients. They tend to be warm, friendly, enthusiastic, and concerned, assuring the patient that he can be cured by the treatment offered.

Some quacks sport an "M.D." after their names and are quite professional in appearance and manner. Others use the title "doctor" to create an aura of medical mystique. They may hold advanced degrees in other fields, such as physics or biochemistry. Some hold multiple unusual—but not medical—degrees, such as N.D. (for Doctor of Naturopathy), Ph.N. (Philosopher of Naturopathy), DABB-A (Diplomate of the American Board of Bio-Analysts), or Ms.D. (Doctor of Metaphysics), and others. Still others are simply businessmen.

There are usually certain hallmarks that characterize the cancer quack's trade. They include the following:

● A monolithic, or "one type," attitude toward the treatment of cancer—whatever kind of cancer you may have, the treatment is pretty much the same. In fact, different types of cancer will respond differently to the same therapy. There is no form of therapy that is universally effective against all cancers.
● Quacks tend to be isolated from established scientific or medical facilities and colleagues. Because their treatment approaches have never been shown effective to the satisfaction of knowledgeable experts in cancer therapy, quacks tend to avoid—and to be shunned by—competent medical specialists.
● Quacks tend to use unorthodox methods of making their "discoveries" known. Instead of publishing in reputable scientific journals or presenting their findings to meetings of their medical peers, they take the "publicity" route. They get their theories published in popular magazines and newspapers and present reports to groups of laymen, who are in no position to critically and scientifically evaluate their statements.
● They usually claim they are being persecuted by organized medicine or science. They may charge that the American Medical Association, the American Cancer Society, the Food and Drug Administration, the National Cancer Institute—indeed, the entire medical "establishment"—are out to get them. They say such things as, "I can't get my papers published in scientific journals because those in the cancer establishment don't really want to see it cured. That would cost them their jobs." In fact, they can't get their papers published (or presented at a reputable professional meeting) because the reports are simply scienti-

1

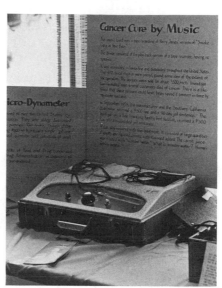

2

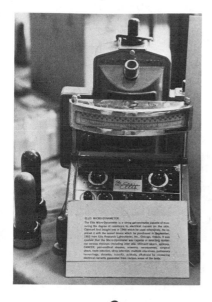

3

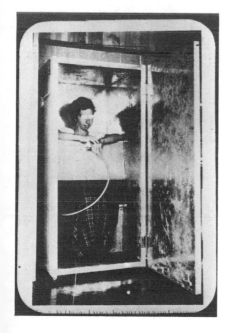

Quack cancer devices come in many different forms, but they all share the characteristic of doing nothing to treat the patient's cancer and of robbing the patient of valuable time during which effective treatments may be applied. Among the devices for which false curative claims have been made are 1) the "Ellis Micro-Dynameter," which has been seized by the California Department of Health, 2) the "Cancer Cure by Music" which gained its promoter a $500 fine and a 90-day jail sentence, and 3) the "Orgone Energy Accelerator," a zinc-lined pine box in which the patient sits to absorb "orgone energy."

fically worthless. If anything, they tend to be anecdotal accounts of a patient here and a patient there who felt better or whose tumor seemed to have temporarily shrunk following the purported cure. Rarely is there any objective evidence of effectiveness. And rarely does the quack give credit to any legitimate cancer therapy the patient may be getting simultaneously.

● The quack's methods are often couched in secrecy. Either the treatment itself or the way it is prepared is kept a trade secret. Components are not named, or at least not properly named with a designation that would be meaningful to any other scientist who is an expert in the field. The quack is also usually reluctant to let legitimate scientists try his method in an attempt to establish its effectiveness. He may claim, "Others wouldn't do it right, and then they'd say it didn't work. I'd rather keep it to myself until I'm sure it will get a fair trial." But when would that magic moment come? For a quack, probably never.

● The medical records they keep—if they keep any—are usually totally inadequate. Often, the patient's "cancer" has not been confirmed by biopsy or other direct means. The quack often uses a phony diagnostic test (there is no one blood or urine test or machine that can tell for certain whether a person has cancer), and as a result, many of the miracle "cures" he claims were never cancers in the first place. Yet the patient, convinced he had had cancer and is now cured, becomes a living testimonial for the "truth" of the quack's claim.

● The quack relies on testimonials from patients and endorsements from prominent persons—actors, legislators, writers—who, out of ignorance or friendship, are only too ready to attach their prestige to the quack's claims. None of these supporters has the training or experience to evaluate the effectiveness of a cancer therapy or the validity of a scientific experiment. Sometimes quacks are able to convince gullible, nouveau riche foundations to espouse and publish their misinformation, or the quack forms his own phony foundation with a high-sounding name.

● Quacks often challenge established theories and attack prominent scientists as making false claims or wanting only to promote themselves, not cure cancer. Quacks are quick to liken themselves to such historic figures as Columbus, Galileo, and Copernicus, who were initially persecuted for their ideas but eventually proven right.

The ingredients of quackery are as wide-ranging as one's imagination. They include raw foods (for example, the "grape cure"), special diets (Max Gerson's hourly drinks of vegetable and calves' liver juices followed by coffee enemas), natural products (cobwebs saturated with arsenic powder as a poultice to "draw out" the cancer, or extracts of apricot pits), corrosive agents, bizarre devices (such as "Orgone Energy Device" which is said to "harness cosmic energy from the universe"), and a host of "vaccines," cell therapies, and anticancer serums.

Indeed, unproven cancer remedies must be as old as the disease itself. Old-time physicians had nothing but unproven remedies, so there was nothing to be lost by using them. In 1748 Virginia's House of Burgesses, with George Washington and James Madison present, passed a resolution to appoint a committee to test Mary Johnson's "receipt of curing cancer," which consisted of garden sorrel, celandine, persimmon bark, and spring water. The report of the committee, giving the testimony of many witnesses that this concoction had cured them of cancer, was read to the House of Burgesses, and Mrs. Johnson was subsequently voted a reward of one hundred pounds. A rather complete list of modern-day versions of Mary Johnson's "receipt" is contained in the American Cancer Society's book, "Unproven Methods of Cancer Management." The book or reprints from it may be obtained from your local unit or division of the American Cancer Society (see Appendix).

Most but not all unproven methods of cancer management involve purported cures. In addition to cures, there are some unproven gadgets and tests, such as the Kanfer Neuromuscular or Handwriting Test, that are supposed to detect hidden cancers or establish a diagnosis of cancer. Other unproven agents, including the infamous Laetrile, prepared from the extracts of apricot pits, are not claimed to cure cancer (at least by their "scientific" proponents) but merely to reduce cancerous growths and alleviate the sickness and pain associated with advanced cancer.

Laetrile is one of a handful of unproven cancer remedies to have captured the imagination of large numbers of people in recent years. Others include Krebiozen, which in the 1950s and 1960s was promoted by a prestigious Illinois scientist, Dr. Andrew Ivy. There was also the Rand cancer vaccine, developed by a wealthy Cleveland businessman in the mid 1960s.

The Federal Government, claiming that Krebiozen was nothing more than the simple chemical creatine dissolved in mineral oil and had no effect against cancer, brought Dr. Ivy, Stevan Durovic, the developer of Krebiozen, and two of their associates to trial. The Government lost the jury trial, but no one ever proved that Krebiozen had any anticancer value. The publicity that surrounded the case probably brought countless more patients to Dr. Ivy's door, since he was forbidden by law to ship the "medicine" out of his home state.

The Rand cancer vaccine created a lesser flurry. National notoriety followed a page one story in the *Cleveland Plain Dealer* in August 1966, written by the financial editor who had been attracted by the rapid climb in the stock of the Rand Development Corporation (a wholly different organization from the Rand Corporation). "A cure for cancer, long hoped for, may be imminent," the uncritical story began. Subsequent versions appeared in papers throughout the country. Cleveland's Academy of Medicine protested, "Such premature publicity on totally inadequate medical evidence is simply the cruelest torture for cancer patients and their loved ones. True medical discoveries require long checking and rechecking."

But the Rand vaccine was too hot to be squelched by one sane voice. The flames were further fed by a two-part series in *Pageant* Magazine. "At Last! Scientists Report Anti-Cancer Vaccine. Claim 12 Dying Patients Saved in First Experiments! 75 doctors in 35 Ohio hospitals now attacking all kinds of cancers in hundreds of cases," the magazine proclaimed on its cover. Patients flocked to Cleveland for this miracle cure. It was shipped illegally to New York and Miami. Finally, the Government obtained an injunction against its manufacture, claiming that Rand had violated federal regulations governing the testing of new medicinal substances in man. Rand apparently never could—or never tried to—satisfy government testing requirements (which serve to establish whether a substance is both safe and effective for use in man), and eventually, the Rand cancer vaccine went the way of all fake cancer cures—it died.

But there is one unproven cancer remedy that simply refuses to die, no matter how many studies show it doesn't work, no matter how strictly laws are enforced, no matter what legitimate cancer specialists say. That substance is Laetrile, also known as amygdalin, Vitamin B-17, Cyto H-3, KH-3, and Aprikern. In May 1976, a Federal grand jury in San Diego indicted nineteen persons, including eight Americans, for smuggling Laetrile across the Mexican border to supply thousands of cancer patients with the illegal drug. Laetrile has going for it one of the most persuasive and persistent lobbying groups—the relatives of former cancer patients. The odd thing is that in nearly all cases, these former patients were not "cured" by Laetrile at all. The vast majority of them died of their disease, and those who did not die were undoubtedly saved as a result of other, legitimate cancer therapies they received at the same time. But even though the Laetrile did not cure, the surviving friends and relatives continue to swear that it works. "If only we'd tried it sooner, I'm sure that Laetrile would have cured him (or her)," is the all-too-familiar lament.

Yet there is no evidence that Laetrile can cure cancer whether used early or late in the disease. There is not even evidence that it can prolong the lives of cancer patients. Even its leading medical proponents do not claim that it cures, merely that it can reduce the size of cancerous tumors, alleviate pain, and restore some vitality to the dying patient. "She was carried into the clinic on a stretcher and she walked out with a cane." "My husband, who had to be given morphine twice a day to relieve his pain, was able to stop all pain killers for the first time in weeks." "My wife's appetite returned and she even talked about going back to work." Such experiences can be very convincing to someone who is dying: "If I am feeling so much better, Laetrile must be curing my cancer. If only I'd tried it sooner, I could have been completely cured." The patient then dies, convinced—along with his friends and relatives—that the Laetrile *was* working, only it was started too late.

And so the myth persists. Thousands of American cancer patients journey to Mexico every year searching for its miracles. Others obtain it illegally in the United States from doctors, pharmacists, health food stores. Some experience a brief respite from the miseries of their cancer, followed by rapid death. But there are no cures, at least not from Laetrile.

Laetrile's proponents charge that this "miraculous" natural substance, which is supposed to kill cancer cells by releasing cyanide inside them, has never been given a fair trial in the United States. But Laetrile's opponents reply that there is no basis—either biological in laboratory animals or medical in patients—on which to justify vast expenditures of valuable time and money for a well-organized, controlled test in cancer patients. In such a test, some patients would be given Laetrile and others a dummy substance, or placebo, that they think is Laetrile; still a third and fourth group might receive drugs known to be biologically active against cancer. Then the results in the various groups would be compared.

This sounds fairly straightforward—and indeed, it is the way tests are actually conducted on nearly all new anticancer treatments. But Laetrile lacks one essential prerequisite: it has never been clearly shown in a reproducible way to be active against cancer in any test system—whether the cancer cells are growing in a laboratory dish, a mouse, rat, hamster, or guinea pig. Every known drug that attacks cancer in human beings has been shown to also attack cancer in at least one—and usually several—of the test systems in which Laetrile has been tried and found wanting. In the face of such failures, officials at the National Cancer Institute, which supports most of the country's cancer research and nearly all testing of new anticancer drugs, felt that diverting time and money to test Laetrile was unjustified when they have hundreds of other chemicals which do attack cancers in animals waiting to be tested in cancer patients. However, in 1977, more than half a dozen states legalized the use of Laetrile in an attempt to bypass Federal restrictions, and with growing thousands of patients using the substance, legally or otherwise, the Cancer Institute decided to consider doing a carefully controlled clinical trial. The trial, if and when it is done, will examine Laetrile's purported harmlessness and ability to alleviate pain, as well as any effect it might have against human cancers.

The Laetrile lobby is likely to persist, whether or not Laetrile is ever given a "fair trial" and no matter how such a "trial" might turn out. Proponents of Laetrile write books about its miraculous effects and saturate newspapers and magazines with press releases about its wonders. Some are not averse to telephoning the relatives of cancer patients and calling them "murderers" unless they try Laetrile. This kind of preying on people's fears and desperation is contemptible beyond words.

Certain organized groups, some of them with prestigious-sounding names, have traditionally supported unproven methods of cancer treatment and detection (and some also have made unsupported claims about substances purported to cause cancer). The American Cancer Society lists among these organizations the following:

● The International Association of Cancer Victims and Friends, Inc. Founded in 1963 by Cecile Hoffman, who claimed her life had been saved by Laetrile (she died six years later of metastatic breast cancer), this organization now has thousands of members with chapters throughout the nation. The association holds meetings to promote unproven methods of cancer management and freedom of choice in therapy for cancer patients.
● The Cancer Control Society. Formed in 1973 as a dissident faction of the previously mentioned association, this group favors legislative and court action against governmental restrictions on unproven remedies.
● The Committee for Freedom of Choice in Cancer Therapy, Inc. This group emphasizes constitutional rights and freedoms, and its members direct cancer patients to unproven remedies available outside the country.
● The National Health Federation (best known, perhaps, for its

opposition to fluoridation of drinking water, which it says causes cancer). Claiming more than 10,000 members, this group lobbies strenuously in Congress for and against health-related legislation. Its theme is promotion of personal choice, including the freedom to choose unproven cancer remedies.

● The Independent Citizens Research Foundation for the Study of Degenerative Diseases, Inc. This organization considers cancer a "symptom" of disturbed body chemistry and raises funds to support the work of "free, independent scientists, groups and clinics in their research on cancer." It has distributed promotional information on such unproven methods as Krebiozen and the Max Gerson diet.

These and other organizations are frequently behind the publication of books and magazines that promote unproven methods of cancer management. Among the magazines that oppose the so-called "medical monopoly" and often promote such means of cancer treatment are the *Herald of Health, The National Health Federation Bulletin, Prevention, The Cancer News Journal, The Cancer Control Journal,* and *The March of Truth on Cancer.*

Among the many books that have been written about alleged cancer cures—some of them well-enough written to give the reader the impression that the reports are factual—are *Has Doctor Max Gerson a True Cancer Cure?, Laetrile: Control for Cancer, The Incredible Story of Krebiozen: A Matter of Life and Death, Vitamin B-17: Forbidden Weapon Against Cancer,* and *World Without Cancer.*

What can be done to control cancer quackery? First and foremost is for you, if you are a cancer patient or friend or relative of a cancer patient, to resist being lured by false or unsubstantiated promises and hearsay. While your doctor may not always know all the answers, he is virtually guaranteed to know a good deal more than any promoter of an unproven cancer remedy. If you have any doubts about the legitimacy of a cancer therapy you are considering or have been given, check it out with your doctor or with the American Cancer Society, which maintains an up-to-date list of unproven methods of cancer management. The American Cancer Society, as well as the American Medical Association, the United States Food and Drug Administration, the National Cancer Institute, and researchers at leading cancer research centers across the nation are active in investigating, regulating or reporting on such unproven methods.

The Food and Drug Administration regulates the testing of all anticancer drugs. Before such drugs can be tested on human beings, they must be shown to be safe and effective against animal cancers. Only then can clinical trials (tests on patients) be started. At first, only about ten patients can receive the therapy until such procedures as proper dosage and methods of administration are established. Then tests can be expanded to perhaps a hundred patients to measure the agent's effectiveness as a therapy or preventive. Finally, extensive tests are done on thousands of patients at many different centers to more clearly assess the agent's safety, effectiveness and most desirable dosage and treatment schedule. Only if an agent proceeds logically through these steps and passes the final test can it be approved for marketing and general use in cancer patients. Most of the organized tests of possible anticancer agents are supported and coordinated by the Federal Government's National Cancer Institute, in Bethesda, Maryland, a part of the National Institutes of Health. The United States Postal Service investigates worthless cancer tests and treatments that are promoted through the mails. These investigations have resulted in the conviction of quacks who use the mails to defraud the public. The United States Customs Service conducts antismuggling activities to keep unproven cancer remedies from entering the country.

But the Federal government, including the Food and Drug Administration, can only regulate items that cross state lines. It has no control over an unproven method used entirely within the borders of one state, even though patients may come from all over the United States, and even from foreign countries, to obtain it in that state. To stem this source of cancer quackery, state laws must be enacted.

In 1966 the American Cancer Society formulated a State Model Cancer Act which was instrumental in the enactment of anti-quackery laws now enforced in nine states. Presently, purveyors of unproven remedies in California are subject to a possible felony conviction. The use of unproven methods is also a criminal offense in Colorado, Illinois, Kentucky, Maryland, Nevada, North Dakota, Ohio, and Pennsylvania.

The Society and the American Medical Association also provide information to the public and the medical profession on cancer quackery and cultism. In 1969 the Society produced a television film, "Journey into Darkness," to alert the public to the problem of quackery. But once again, the most effective weapon against cancer quackery is you, an informed public. Once people understand that cancer can be detected and treated with proven methods —with the highest chances for cure when the cancer is diagnosed early and treated promptly and appropriately—they will be loathe to waste precious time and money on worthless "remedies."

Part III
LIVING AFTER CANCER

12. Rehabilitating the Cancer Patient

The American Heart Association was holding a seminar and the day for us medical writers had begun at the crack of dawn and proceeded at a hectic clip through mid-afternoon. After filing our respective stories for the next day's newspapers, several of us gathered at poolside to catch the last rays of fading sunlight. The air was chilly and the breeze was up, but Herb Black, medical writer for the Boston *Globe*, and I decided to restore our souls with a swim around the kidney-shaped pool. Refreshed by the brisk swim, we sat back in lounge chairs for a chat.

Twenty minutes had passed before I noticed a slight bulge mid-abdomen on one side of Herb's bathing trunks. Then I remembered that six years earlier in 1968 Herb had had surgery for rectal cancer. His surgery was life-saving, but as in most such cases, it left him with a colostomy—a new opening called a "stoma" in his abdomen through which his body wastes are discharged. The bulge I'd noticed was a colostomy bag, used by some colostomy patients all the time and by others on occasion, to collect the wastes. I thought as I talked to Herb that he seemed hardly conscious of his condition—he worked, played, traveled, and socialized just like the rest of us. I wondered to myself whether I could be so successful at living after cancer.

At a National Conference on Human Values and Cancer held in 1972 by the American Cancer Society, a film prepared by the Cox Broadcasting Corporation of Atlanta pointed out that the cancer patient worries a great deal about the quality of his survival. "Will I be able to go back to normal living? Do the things I did before? Or am I going to have to hide at home? Afraid to face my neighbors? Knowing my friends will think I'm some kind of freak?" The narrator gave some examples: "One woman, recovering from a mastectomy was so ashamed about her disfigurement, she said she felt like half-man, half-woman. Another who seemed to take it in stride was worried about her attractiveness to her husband . . .

153

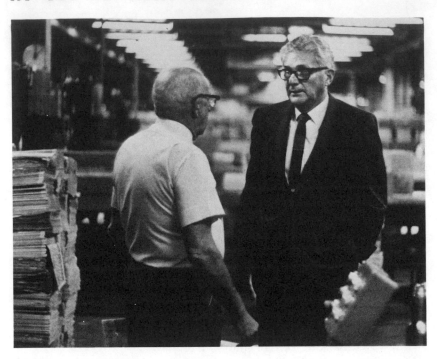

Herbert Black (right), medical writer for the *Boston Globe*, had surgery which cured his rectal cancer in 1968. He quickly returned to his active life despite a colostomy.

whether she could keep his love. To still another, nothing would ever be the same. How can I wear low-necked dresses? Play golf and tennis? The fact that she was still alive was overshadowed by the kind of life she envisioned."

Many a colostomy patient, the narrator continued, "sees nothing but problems in his future. Can he ever really be sure about that odor? Be active enough to hold down his job again? Or even get that job back? And what's to keep people from finding out that he's different? Problems also abound for many a laryngectomee (a person whose voice box was removed). Speak again? Without sounding like a mechanical man? And, as one laryngectomee put it, "What about that stoma, that damned hole in my neck? How do I hide that so I at least look normal?"

When told that surgery will give them an excellent chance for survival, many cancer patients think, "Survival for what? To live as a partial person? Without an arm, or leg, or gut, or breast, or voice box? What kind of life is that?" But Herb Black and hundreds of thousands of other cancer survivors have clearly proved that life after cancer need not be a mere shadow of one's former existence. It can be just as rich, fulfilling, and rewarding—and some former cancer patients say even more so—as life before cancer. True, there may be some added inconveniences, but most people find them a small price to pay for a second chance at living.

This is certainly not meant to belittle the trauma, both physical and emotional, of cancer surgery. For all but the rarest of patients, it is hardly like having a tooth pulled or a hernia repaired. Shock, depression, and anxiety are common and to be expected following a cancer operation. Adjustments in living, thinking, and feeling are nearly always necessary, and for some people these adjustments represent an enormous challenge to what had heretofore been the very essence of their existence. But the adjustments—even the most profound adjustments—can be made successfully, and many patients say that afterward you can be that much more of a person for having met the challenge. Making a healthy adjustment to living after cancer depends on many factors, including the nature of your job, the support you get from family and friends, your general approach to life and the quality of rehabilitation services offered by your hospital or available in your community. But probably the most important determinant is your attitude.

Herb Black recalls how he reacted to the description of the proposed treatment for his rectal cancer, "I told the surgeon I would prefer a colostomy and a chance to continue writing on medicine for *The Globe* to the alternative—starting my career all over again as a police reporter for the *Pearly Gates Gazette!*"

Four years later, he told the American Cancer Society's Conference on Human Values and Cancer, "It seems to me now that that simple reaction helped to sustain me through surgery, hospitalization, the trial of learning to control a stoma and my return to work. It is the only attitude toward a colostomy that makes sense to me. For me a stoma was a life-saving device and not a 'scarlet letter.' It was a chance to continue doing what I wanted to do." He added, "There has been no social stigma as far as I am concerned. There has been no withdrawing from other people—no loss of mobility."

Adjusting to life after cancer is a process that ideally should begin before your cancer is even treated. Doctors have found that much of patients' fear and anxiety about cancer surgery and profound emotional reactions after surgery result from a lack of understanding of the procedure and how they will be able to adapt to their disability. Herb, whose surgeon helped him to prepare mentally for a major rearrangement of his organs, urges doctors to explain to their patients the extent of surgery prior to the operation so that they can come to terms with themselves before the event. "I know I would have been resentful, angry and uncooperative if I had not been brought through to realization by degrees," he said. "Instead, I was grateful that I had been told that the quality of life need not be destroyed. I was ready to cope with the colostomy after surgery."

But the heart of rehabilitation comes after surgery—and the sooner it is started, the better. No matter how good the patient's attitude may be beforehand, he still needs a great deal of encouragement and support afterward—assurance that he is still loved and wanted, that he will be able to cope, that life after cancer will not be a living death. One source of encouragement for Herb came in the form of a young, attractive nurse who was herself an ostomate (the word used to describe people for whom new body openings have been created).

The nurse explained to him what it was like to live with a stoma. She taught him how to manage one, and she displayed through the personal experience of her life how well a person can get along despite this handicap. In a word, Herb said, she was "priceless." He was also aided by his wife, who had herself been a nurse at one time. She was comforting and patient and not put off by his initial awkwardness in caring for his stoma.

As more and more cancer patients survive their disease, rehabilitation after cancer becomes an increasingly more important part of cancer treatment. Traditionally, rehabilitation efforts were focused only on those patients whose condition had stabilized and were expected to live for a long time afterward. In recent years, however, doctors have come to realize that all cancer patients must be "rehabilitated" to the greatest extent possible, starting from the moment the patient enters the hospital. As part of the new emphasis on rehabilitation, the National Cancer Act of 1971 requires that rehabilitation efforts be a part of every cancer control program that receives funds under the act.

Patients who have a long life expectancy should receive appropriate training in how to compensate for their disability and should have any structural defects repaired or replaced to restore them to a full life. Patients who face slowly progressive disease and disability also need physical and psychological support so that they can live as fully and happily as possible during the years they have left. And patients with advanced cancer, whose life expectancy may be measured in months, should be helped to live as comfortably and independently as possible for as long as they can.

Dr. J. Herbert Dietz, consultant to the rehabilitation program at Memorial Hospital for Cancer and Allied Diseases in New York, urges early rehabilitation therapy to help eliminate "periods of hopelessness, frustration and despair." He says, for example, for cancers of the bone and connective tissue, where amputation is necessary, training before surgery in the use of crutches or a walker has been found to speed rehabilitation afterward. Such patients are now likely to be fitted with an artificial limb either at the time of surgery or soon afterward, before they leave the hospital.

The breast cancer patient is best started on exercises shortly after her mastectomy to preserve the proper function of her arm and shoulder. She also is greatly boosted by the use of a temporary prosthesis—or "falsie"—to replace her lost breast (a more accurately molded permanent breast prosthesis is fitted after the wound has healed completely).

In patients who are to lose all or part of a lung, preoperative training in breathing control and coughing techniques are very helpful, followed by a moderate exercise program that begins on the first day after surgery, Dr. Dietz reports. For some patients with cancers of the face or mouth, reconstruction with a temporary or permanent prosthesis can now be done at the time of the cancer surgery so that the patient's defect is less obvious and psychologically damaging. Modern plastics can be molded and stained into highly realistic facial parts that closely resemble the shape, size, and color of people's natural cheeks, noses, and jaws. These parts are applied with adhesive to fill in the gaps left by surgery to give the patient a visage with which he can better face the world and himself. They can be removed for cleaning, but essentially they serve as permanent prostheses that last for several years before they must be replaced.

To illustrate the range of possibilities in rehabilitating cancer patients, Dr. Dietz describes a 49-year-old man who had bladder cancer that had spread throughout his pelvis, necessitating amputation at the waist. The man was fitted with a prosthesis consisting of hips and legs and was taught how to stand and walk. He later took driver training and obtained a driver's license after passing a road test. Four and a half years after his surgery he was well and active, functioning quite independently.

Jim Doty, who in 1970 underwent surgery and radiation treatment for cancer of the testicle, tells what it means to face cancer at the age of 33. "What went through my mind when I was told? First, I wanted to know whether I was going to live or die. Then, if I was going to live, I wanted to know how much I was going to lose. In my case, I was lucky. It was just the lymph nodes and the testicle." Jim was assured he could lead a normal life after his cancer treatment. But to most of us, Jim's life after cancer was hardly "normal." Not only did he continue as an insurance broker and the father of three small children, but he went into training as a marathon swimmer. And four years after his surgery, Jim took the big plunge into the English Channel and attempted to swim across it. Although he didn't make it to the other side, he did succeed in becoming a fully rehabilitated, cured cancer patient. Jim, who also served as president of the Boston unit of the American Cancer Society, says that now he wants "to help others who've been hit by cancer. I want them to know that they don't have to curl up and die."

Another cancer patient who refused to let cancer interfere with her life and career is Marguerite Piazza, singing star of stage, television, and the Metropolitan Opera. In mid-career Miss Piazza, a beautiful woman and recently widowed mother of six, developed a spot on her cheek that wouldn't go away. It turned out to be a melanoma, a skin cancer that can be rapidly fatal. Her surgeon put it to her bluntly, "I will have to mutilate you. Either you can be very beautiful in a coffin, or you can have an excellent chance to live a long life, with not so much beauty." For Miss Piazza, there was no decision. "My children needed me alive," she says. The operation took five hours. She lost her right cheek and the lymph

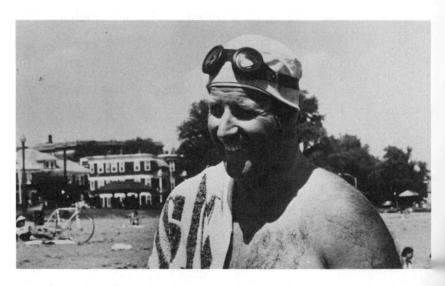

Jim Doty of Dedham, Mass., attempted to swim the English Channel in 1974, four years after having surgery and radiation treatment for cancer of the testicle.

nodes in her neck. She decided afterward that she was not going to hide. Four months after her operation, she sang the National Anthem at the Inaugural Gala for former President Nixon. Then she did a benefit performance, which went off swimmingly, convincing her that she was "winning the fight with cancer." In the months following the benefit, she underwent five plastic surgery procedures to rebuild her face and neck, and a year after her cancer surgery she opened at the St. Regis Hotel, a sensation to ear and eye.

Another who made a comeback after conquering melanoma was defensive line-backer Jack Pardee, who in 1972—seven years after undergoing an 11-hour operation involving his right biceps and the adjacent lymph nodes in his arm and chest—led the Washington Redskins all the way to the Super Bowl. In his spare time, he devotes his efforts to educating others to have regular checkups for cancer.

MASTECTOMY AND REACH TO RECOVERY

Nearly every week for the past year I have played tennis with Ellen M.; Ellen is the 38-year-old mother of Katie and Denise, wife of Jim, singing star and instrumentalist for a neighborhood theatre group, and part-time student working toward a graduate degree in sociology. A tall, blond, pretty woman whose blue eyes crinkle when she smiles—which is often—Ellen is quite a sight on the tennis court. Her knit tennis dresses reveal a slender, well-proportioned figure that not infrequently distracts the men on adjacent courts. She also plays a pretty good game of tennis, with an especially strong serve and forearm. She is a veritable tiger at the net.

It is hard to realize that only a year before we began our regular tennis games, Ellen had had a mastectomy. Ellen and an estimated 72,000 other American women were diagnosed as having breast cancer that year and most had a mastectomy. Now every year another 90,000 go through a similar experience. Approximately half of them will live five or more years after their surgery, with most permanently cured of their disease. The price these women have to pay for their second chance at life is the loss of a highly visible part of their bodies, a part that has been endowed in our culture with emotional trappings and a significance that goes far beyond its main biological function.

Few will deny that we live in a bosom-oriented society, where a woman's sex appeal is often measured by the size and shape of a two-part organ that was really intended by nature for nurturing the young. How sexy can a woman be when one of those parts is lost? Will her man still want her? Will she be able to stand herself? It is hardly unexpected that many women who have undergone a mastectomy at first feel defective, incomplete, even mutilated. Added to the loss of a breast is the fact that for most women at this time, mastectomy means radical mastectomy—the loss, not just of the breast, but of the nearby lymph nodes and the chest muscles underlying the breast, with the result that one side of the chest is somewhat flatter than the other and the arm on that side has a tendency to swell because the lymph nodes that drain excess fluid from the arm have been removed.

In 1952 a spunky, tireless lady named Terese Lasser found herself faced with just these problems. Mrs. Lasser had always lived in a whirlwind. Mother of two, amanuensis for her husband's first edition of *Your Income Tax*, Mrs. Lasser loved to go dancing, give parties, swim, and play golf. During her college days (after her marriage to J. K. Lasser), she squeezed in volunteer work in several hospitals and later drove an ambulance for the American Red Cross. Mrs. Lasser simply did not have time to be sick. But when she awoke from the anesthesia and was told that her right breast had been removed, she says, "I wanted to shrivel up and die." The questions ran unbidden through her mind, "How could I face life, a scarred woman? How could I go on, forever unfit for work or play? How could I look in a mirror again, knowing what I must see there and hating it—sensing the revulsion in others and enduring the pity behind their curious stares? How could such a life be worth living? And—most tormenting thought of all—what about my husband? He was devoted to me—I was as confident of his love as any woman ever is confident. But after this, what? Suppose, in spite of his love and his devotion, he should be repelled by me? Was it possible for a man to desire a woman who wasn't whole? Suppose all my husband could feel for me now, all he would ever be able to feel, was pity—so that never again would he need me, or reach for me as a man reaches for a woman? If that were to be so, better not to be alive at all . . ."

And there she was, as countless thousands of women have been before and since, in "a valley of despair, desolate, solitary, swept by anguish, darkened by confusion." She "ached to talk to another woman who had had the same experience and come through it, and so could counsel, and reassure and understand! But no such woman was available."[1]

---

[1] *Reach to Recovery*, Terese Lasser and William Kendall Clarke, Simon and Schuster, 1972, pages 20–22.

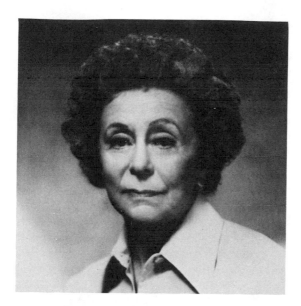

Terese Lasser founded the Reach to Recovery program to help rehabilitate mastectomy patients after her own mastectomy in 1952. She remains national consultant and coordinator for the program, which is now sponsored by the American Cancer Society.

Out of Mrs. Lasser's experience, a program was born to help spare other women with mastectomies the same doubts, fears, and anxieties, and to see to it that they need not be alone and in despair. This program, which Mrs. Lasser called Reach to Recovery, was born modestly in 1953 and grew steadily until 1969 when it merged with the American Cancer Society and mushroomed into an international network of carefully selected and trained volunteers. Today, at the request of the surgeon, more than 6,500 women—all of them former mastectomy patients themselves—visit women recovering from mastectomy at some 2,500 hospitals across the nation. In 1975 alone more than 50,000 mastectomy patients were assisted by such volunteers. These volunteers are, first, living, flesh-and-blood proof of how well a mastectomy patient can look and how good the quality of her life can be. Second, they are the bearers of crucial information, not only for the patient but also for the patient's husband and children, to help dispel fears and misconceptions about mastectomy and smooth the patient's transition back to a full, normal life. Third, the Reach to Recovery volunteer is the source of a temporary breast form (to be worn under the patient's old bra) and a list of where to purchase a permanent prosthesis and special clothing (such as bathing suits) for mastectomy patients. Last—but certainly not least—she gives the patient a kit which includes a rubber ball and a plastic rope and instructions on how to exercise her arm and shoulder so that no mobility is lost and the chances of swelling are reduced. The Reach to Recovery manual found inside the kit is realistic and practical yet hopeful and inspiring. In addition to exercises and dressing tips, it gives helpful hints on such topics as sex after mastectomy, rebuilding your self-image, appreciating your femininity, and dealing with children's questions. No mastectomy patient—even if her surgery was years ago—should be without this manual. A copy can be obtained from the Reach to Recovery program of your local unit of the American Cancer Society. Reach to Recovery publications have been transcribed in Braille by the Jewish Guild for the Blind. They can be borrowed postage-free from the Guild at 15 West 65 Street, New York, New York 10023, as well as from local units of the Cancer Society.

In short, the Reach to Recovery program emphasizes the importance of adopting a constructive approach to life and shows the mastectomy patient how to go about it: how to return to her previous lifestyle as career woman, homemaker, mother; how to resume stylish dressing; how to gain full motion and control of the operated arm and shoulder; and how to talk about her surgery with friends, neighbors, and family.

Marvella Bayh, wife of Senator Birch Bayh of Indiana, tells what a visit from a Reach to Recovery volunteer meant to her. In 1971 when she underwent a modified radical mastectomy (the chest muscles were not removed), Mrs. Bayh, a former Oklahoma beauty queen, was 38, her son Evan was 15, and her husband was campaigning for the 1972 Presidential nomination. Her first thought after surgery was "Will I survive?" Only later did she think about losing a part of her body. She cried to her husband, "I'm only 38 years old, and I'm going to go through the rest of my life with only one breast." To which Senator Bayh replied, "I'm five years older than you are, and I've gone through my life without any."

"He let me know that he married *me* and loved *me*—the me that no bodily amputation can change," she recalled three years later. He also dropped out of the Presidential race and gave her the support and attention she needed during her recovery.

Further vital support came from the Reach to Recovery volunteer who visited Mrs. Bayh in the hospital. As she described it two years later in *Medical Tribune,* a newspaper for physicians, "About five or six days after the operation, my hair had lost its set, and I was feeling quite dowdy when an attractive, well-dressed lady entered my room and identified herself as a representative of Reach to Recovery. As my visitor began discussing the postoperative exercises which would be most important to my recovery, I noticed that she had a lovely figure and that she was wearing a form-fitting blouse. I thought, 'How can she understand the problem which I face?'

"To my amazement my visitor mentioned that she and all other Reach to Recovery volunteers had undergone a mastectomy. My reaction to her visit changed immediately. All of a sudden there was someone who could answer all my questions, from her own firsthand experience. I realized that what I had been told about regaining my vitality and resuming a normal lifestyle was absolutely true. In many respects the visit from the Reach to Recovery volunteer was the turning point in my recuperation. Here was someone who not only cared but who fully understood what I was experiencing and was ready and anxious to help me through the period of adjustment."

Unfortunately, however, not every mastectomy patient has the opportunity to benefit from such a visit. A Reach to Recovery volunteer will only go to see a patient at the request of the patient's doctor. Some doctors still do not know about Reach to Recovery or misunderstand its goals and methods, mistakenly thinking the volunteer will discuss medical questions, which she won't, or somehow interfere with the doctor-patient relationship. If you or someone you know is in the hospital following a mastectomy and the doctor has not contacted Reach to Recovery, the patient or the patient's family would do well to ask the doctor about it.

Dr. Arthur I. Holleb, the medical consultant for this book, and a former breast cancer surgeon at Memorial Sloan-Kettering Cancer Center before he joined the American Cancer Society staff as Senior Vice-President for Medical Affairs, recalls that before Reach to Recovery he thought he had been "doing a pretty good job of providing the 'pat on the back,' the reassuring 'Don't worry, my dear; everything will be like it was before.' Little did I know!" In the introduction to *Reach to Recovery*, the book Mrs. Lasser wrote in 1972 with William Kendall Clarke, Dr. Holleb said that it has long been the custom of doctors "to discourage patients from discussing their operations with other patients," thinking that this approach was in the patients' best interests. "Most of us who specialized in breast surgery apparently did not recognize that so much more assistance could be given to the woman who had lost a breast."

As Mrs. Bayh has pointed out, "Reach to Recovery is not a substitute for high-quality medical care, nor can it replace the treasured support of loved ones during the period of crisis. By limiting its volunteers to those who themselves had a mastectomy, by being candid, by offering literature which has guidance not only for patients but for their husbands and children, by offering hope where there is despair, Reach to Recovery can play a truly significant role in the recovery of women who undergo breast surgery. I know, I've been there."

Mrs. Bayh says that following her surgery, she returned to a full and happy life, serving, among other things, as Co-chairperson of the National American Cancer Society Crusade in 1974. But, she adds, her brush with cancer left an indelible mark on her life, "When I'm out for a walk I don't rush so fast; I take time to stop and watch the squirrels play. I see the beauty of the clouds and the colors of the sunset more clearly. I believe I've been able to put into proper perspective material achievements that used to seem so important."

Mrs. Bayh's experience is not unique. Dr. Thomas J. Craig and his colleagues at the Johns Hopkins Hospital in Baltimore questioned 134 women who had undergone mastectomies (most of them at least five years earlier) and 260 other women, matched for age and race, who had not had breast cancer. The researchers found that the vast majority of both groups (84 percent of mastectomy patients and 89 percent of the others) rated themselves as "happy" and that approximately equal proportions participated in recreational activities—sports and social functions. Only 4 percent of the mastectomy patients reported any physical disability related to their surgery. In fact, a slightly higher percentage of the mastectomy patients were employed. Other similar studies have shown that more than 80 percent of mastectomy patients resume their preoperative responsibilities within two years of surgery.

A Connecticut woman who had a radical mastectomy five years ago has continued her strenuous life as an underwater photographer. Julia Child, the famous expert in French cookery, became a household word through a public television series that began years after her mastectomy. She says, "We have such a breast fetish in this country that women are led to believe that they're absolutely useless without them. Sexuality is really a matter of attitude, not equipment."

Merla Zellerbach, a columnist for the San Francisco Chronicle, considered her two mastectomies this way, "I can't help feeling angry when I hear people speak of a mastectomy as a tragedy or disaster. A mastectomy is not horrible, shameful, or the end of a woman's sex appeal. It's a second chance at life." Part of Ms. Zellerbach's attitude stems from the reassurances from her husband, Fred Goerner, that the surgery had changed nothing between them. To the husbands of mastectomees, Mr. Goerner says, "Remember only to say, 'I love you. Get well. We've got a life to live.' "

The husband of another mastectomee, David Sawyer, met and married Patricia after her breast was removed. "It's been eleven years since the operation. We lead a most active life—Pat plays tennis, swims, wears all the clothes she likes." Mr. Sawyer works as a husband-volunteer in a Reach to Recovery program, which tries to get men to express their feelings about the operation. He points out that the husband of a mastectomy patient also has fears. A husband may, for example, be afraid to initiate sexual activity after his wife's surgery lest she feel he is pushing her. The wife, however, may interpret his lack of initiative as a sign of disgust and rejection. Mr. Sawyer says these feelings must be discussed openly. Sex need not change after breast surgery, at least, not for the worse. In fact, he reports, "For some couples, sex is better after surgery because of the new understanding that has developed."

Mrs. Lasser tells of one woman whose life was completely turned around by her mastectomy—turned in a much more positive direction. The woman, who was unmarried and in her midthirties, had been more or less a recluse—grossly overweight and shy and antisocial. Just before her operation, she came across an article which Mrs. Lasser had written two years earlier, just two years after her own breast operation. "It gave me hope that I could come through it like you did," she recalled. "I knew then exactly what I had to do to help myself—change my attitude, believe in myself, have faith in other people, live life instead of hiding from it." Five weeks after surgery, a much thinner and happier woman was out square-dancing. She hardly sat out a dance all evening.

The physical rehabilitation of the mastectomy patient is just as crucial to her recovery as her attitude. The exercises developed and described by Mrs. Lasser are mainly "reaching" exercises—hence, the title of the program, Reach to Recovery. The exercises include hair brushing, paper crumpling, wall reaching, rubber-ball squeezing and tossing, and rope pulling and jumping.

Other groups besides Reach to Recovery provide postmastectomy exercise programs. Good rehabilitation programs are conducted at most cancer hospitals—the National Cancer Act requires that rehabilitation be part of every federally supported cancer control program. In addition, in New York, the Young Men's and Young Women's Hebrew Association (YM-YWHA) holds weekly

evening classes, teaching exercises in and out of the water to increase strength in the arm and shoulder, prevent or reduce swelling, and improve general muscle tone.

In California, Diana Welch, a dancing teacher at the University
of Santa Clara, conducts a free ballet class for mastectomy patients.
The program has been endorsed by the American Cancer Society,
as well as by doctors and physical therapists. It not only helps the
woman regain and maintain mobility, but since ballet has long
been associated with feminine grace and beauty, it also helps restore the feeling of lost femininity that often accompanies mastectomy. According to a report by United Press International, the
course evolved because one of Miss Welch's regular ballet students
was trying to lift the spirits of her mother, who had had a mastectomy some months earlier. The mother was depressed and had
severe stiffening of the left shoulder that prevented her from raising her arm above her head. At the daughter's suggestion, her
mother attended one of Miss Welch's classes. The mother reports,
"I left the studio after that first day feeling better than I had since
the operation. I went back the next week and then the next. After
three weeks of ballet, my doctors agreed that I had improved
tremendously. It wasn't only what it did for the arm, but also what
it did for the spirit."

In addition to physical and emotional rehabilitation after mastectomy, an increasing number of women are seeking cosmetic
rehabilitation—plastic surgery to construct a new breast. Although
breast reconstruction after mastectomy rarely produces a "cosmetic
triumph," as one surgeon put it, the effects on the woman's psyche
and spirits are often astounding. A variety of techniques are now
available for breast reconstruction. Most use a silicone implant
under the skin, one uses transplanted tissue from the abdomen.
Some are completed in one operation, others require several; some
reconstruct a nipple, others simply create a "breast mound."
Whatever the technique, breast reconstruction is not suitable for
all patients. If you have already had a mastectomy, you may check
with your surgeon as to its possibility and advisability for you. If
you face the possibility of mastectomy, it is best to discuss breast
reconstruction if you think you might be interested in it before
biopsy and surgery because it could affect the technique the surgeon uses in removing your breast. It is also important to check
with the carrier of your medical insurance policy, since most
companies currently do not cover breast reconstruction (a policy
which breast surgeons generally regard as insensitive and inane),
and the surgery and hospitalization involved can cost the patient
several thousand dollars.

OSTOMIES

When cancer strikes the colon, rectum, bladder, or larynx, the surgery that offers the best chance for cure may involve removal of the organ and the creation of a new body opening, called a stoma. Patients with such stomas are commonly referred to as "ostomates." In most cases when the cancer is diagnosed early and can be treated effectively by less radical surgery or by some other form of therapy, such as radiation, a stoma is not necessary. But should a stoma turn out to be the result of cancer surgery for you or someone you know, it is not necessarily—as Herb Black's case so clearly showed—a portent of doom. Nor is it a sentence to a lifetime of incapacitation or withdrawal from society.

Abdominal Ostomies

More than one million persons have abdominal ostomies—openings in their abdomens for their intestines or bladder. Most but not all ostomies are a result of cancer treatment (some, for example, are created for children with birth defects). More than 100,000 persons become ostomates each year.

There are hardly enough physicians, nurses, and therapists trained in rehabilitation to provide adequate aid for all ostomates, so here again, volunteer organizations try to fill in the gap. The American Cancer Society as part of its Ostomy Rehabilitation Program, works with the United Ostomy Association, Inc., at 1111 Wilshire Boulevard, Los Angeles, California 90017. The association, with 20,000 members, consists of more than 270 local chapters around the nation, all staffed by volunteers who themselves are ostomates. The American Cancer Society also has Colostomy Volunteer Visitor Programs of its own. At the doctor's request, the volunteer visits the new ostomate in the hospital. He teaches him how to care for his stoma and gives dietary and other useful advice. The visitor concentrates on the future: When does the patient plan to return to work? What are his favorite hobbies? Will he visit the local ostomy group where he can meet with others who have had similar experiences and perhaps become a trained volunteer himself? The patient is given several pamphlets that will help him to care for his stoma after leaving the hospital and erase some of his doubts about his future. As with the Reach to Recovery volunteer for mastectomy patients, the visiting ostomate provides a vivid example of the quality of life possible with a stoma.

There are doctors, nurses, business executives, stenographers, professional athletes, ballet dancers, lawyers, truck drivers, telephone operators, firemen, policemen, mailmen, deep-sea divers, test pilots, waitresses, public officials, actors, and housewives, among others, who have had ostomies. With few exceptions ostomates can do all the things they did before surgery. One possible exception is heavy lifting and heavy contact sports, although there are plenty of ostomates who do one or both of these. If you have a stoma, you can also wear almost everything you wore before, including tight clothing and bathing suits (except for bikinis). You can get married, and in many cases be sexually active and have babies. You can shower, bathe, swim, camp out, climb mountains, travel and play sports.

Persons with stomas for the bladder (urostomies) or small intestine (ileostomies) have to wear appliances to receive body wastes. When properly fitted, they are completely odor-free. Persons with colostomies (stomas for the large intestine) often manage well without an appliance, using only a small patch to cover the stoma. They are able to control odor through proper diet (avoiding especially gassy foods) or deodorants used externally or taken by mouth. Most colostomy patients can be trained to control their eliminations through well-timed enemas (called "irrigations") that clean out the intestinal tract. Some people irrigate once a day, some every other day, and still others every third day. But many, with practice and patience, can master bowel control and colostomy regularity that frees them from worry about accidents and odors. In special circumstances, such as while traveling or when the digestive tract is upset by illness or nervous tension, a colostomy bag can be worn as additional insurance. It is important that the new ostomate give himself time to adjust to his stoma and learn how to care for it properly. As with mastectomy, the support, encouragement, and understanding of family members can be crucial to a good adjustment for the ostomate.

Laryngectomies

Another type of stoma presenting an entirely different kind of rehabilitation problem, can result from surgery for cancer of the larynx, or voice box. Approximately one-third of patients with laryngeal cancer must undergo surgery that involves removal of the larynx. There are 30,000 "laryngectomees" in the United States, with more than 4,000 new ones each year.

The great trauma of this surgery is not so much the stoma as the fact that the natural voice is lost and a whole new way of speaking —called esophageal speech—must be learned. Following a laryngectomy, people naturally worry about whether they will ever again be able to speak intelligibly, use a telephone, keep their jobs, and maintain their dignity. But as many laryngectomees have dramatically demonstrated, the possibilities are enormous— if the person is well-motivated. Anne G. Lanpher, who now works as a volunteer for the American Cancer Society division in Washington, D.C., said she learned esophageal speech well enough to return to her job as a high school French teacher six months after her laryngectomy. The discipline required by the teaching and periodic checkups with a speech therapist helped to further improve her voice as time went on. Another laryngectomee so perfected esophageal speech that she was able to become a long-distance telephone operator. A general practitioner and surgeon in Cleveland learned esophageal speech in six weeks and returned to his busy practice. Not only does he deal effectively with two or more dozen patients a day, but he also teaches laryngectomee rehabilitation to nurses and instructs surgical residents at his hospital, where he served as president of the medical staff.

The larynx is located at the upper end of the trachea, or windpipe. When the larynx is removed, there is no longer any connection between the mouth and the lungs. Instead, to get air into and

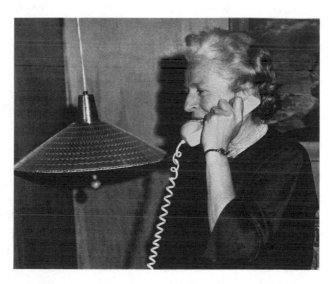

Anne G. Lanpher of Alexandria, Virginia, learned esophageal speech after her larynx was removed for cancer in 1960. Six months after surgery she returned to her job as a French teacher; later she taught speech to other laryngectomy patients.

out of the lungs the surgeon places the opening of the trachea in the lower front part of the neck. The mouth remains connected to the esophagus and the rest of the digestive tract, so the laryngectomee is able to eat and drink normally. The patient can breathe, cough, and "sneeze" through the opening, or stoma, but he can't expel air from his lungs into his mouth for speaking. Normally, speech is produced by forcing air from the lungs through the larynx, where the vocal cords vibrate to produce sound which is then molded in the mouth into recognizable words.

Because air inhaled through the stoma goes directly to the lungs, the laryngectomee is advised to avoid jobs or activities that involve extreme heat or cold or gases, fumes, or dusts. He is also unable to swim, since there is nothing to stop the water from flowing through the stoma into his lungs. The laryngectomee loses much of his sense of taste and smell (although it returns to some extent as time passes), he is unable to sing or laugh out loud, and because he has no way of temporarily locking in his breath, he may be unable to lift heavy loads or to strain hard.

But he can learn to speak again. The technique of esophageal speech involves taking air into the esophagus by locking the tongue to the roof of the mouth. When the air is forced back up, it causes the walls of the esophagus and the pharynx (throat) to vibrate. This, in turn, causes the column of air in the passages to vibrate, creating a low-pitched sound. It is this sound that is molded—just as the sound from vocal cords would be—by the patient's tongue, lips, teeth, and palate into recognizable words and sounds. A person's esophageal voice tends to be huskier and deeper and more of a monotone than the normal voice had been. When Anne Lanpher uttered her first words in esophageal speech to her older son, he clapped her on the shoulder and said, "Hi, Tallulah." Some laryngectomees can learn recognizable esophageal speech in a few weeks; for others, mastery takes months or a year. At least two-thirds of laryngetomees are able to master esophageal speech. The technique can be learned even by patients who have been speechless for years. For patients who are simply unable or unwilling to learn this new way of speaking, there are a number of artificial devices available to create a voice for them, including an electronic larynx and a mechanical prosthesis that fits into the stoma and uses inhaled air to create a voice. There are also electronic amplifiers for persons whose esophageal speech is not loud enough.

Pete B., a 40-year-old football coach for an Indiana high school, used both esophageal speech and a prosthesis so that he could continue with his job after surgery for laryngeal cancer in May

1973. Pete used his prosthesis to give him a more authoritative voice while coaching, and three months after his operation, he was back coaching his team through an all-win fall season. Pete also learned esophageal speech, which he uses at home and on other occasions less demanding than coaching.

As with the mastectomee and the ostomate, there is for the laryngectomee a nationwide network of volunteers to ease them through their adjustment to life after laryngeal cancer. These volunteers all have had laryngectomies themselves and are representatives of such groups as Lost Chord, Anamilo, or New Voice Clubs, sponsored by the American Cancer Society. These clubs—there are more than 200 of them—are affiliated with the International Association of Laryngectomees (I.A.L.), which maintains a registry of esophageal speech instructors and holds seminars for prospective teachers. I.A.L. has an executive office at The American Cancer Society headquarters at 777 Third Avenue, New York, New York 10017.

Larynegectomy groups help to teach new laryngectomy patients how to talk, how to shower, how to dress and how to resume their previous lifestyles as quickly as possible. The volunteers are living proof that successful rehabilitation is possible after a laryngectomy. At the request of a physician, an I.A.L. volunteer will visit a new laryngectomee in the hospital, bringing a kit that contains a pad and pencil, a magic slate, bibs to cover the stoma, and an assortment of informative and inspiring brochures and reprints. The visitor may also show a film, "To Speak Again," produced by the District of Columbia Division of the American Cancer Society. During the hospital visit, new laryngectomees and their spouses are urged to participate in the local I.A.L. club, which can be a continuing source of practical and psychological help.

A further service provided by the American Cancer Society for laryngectomy patients is free instruction in esophageal speech. In most cases, these courses are taught by a professional speech pathologist, who may also work with local club members who have mastered the technique. Sometimes club members alone provide the instruction. In most urban areas, esophageal speech instruction is also available through speech clinics at universities and hospitals, as well as from speech therapists in private practice. Speech lessons cannot start until the surgeon decides that the wound has healed adequately, which may take several weeks. In the meantime, to avoid developing bad habits—such as whispering—the new laryngectomee is urged to do all his communicating in writing or by using an artificial larynx temporarily. Once lessons start, the new voice will sound rough and gutteral—this improves with time and

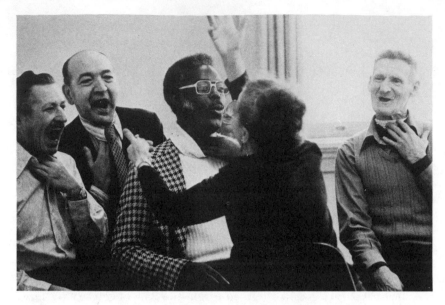

A therapist at the National Hospital for Speech Disorders in New York helps laryngectomy patients learn a new way of speaking. Such programs are offered free to cancer patients throughout the country.

practice—but you can be sure that no matter how rough the sound, it will be music to the ears of the family after the patient has been silent for a month or more. The visit from the I.A.L. volunteer is often a critical factor in motivating the new laryngectomee to learn esophageal speech. As one patient said to his visitor, "I want to learn to talk as well as you do so that I can help someone else as much as this visit has helped me."

Nor does the laryngectomee have to be concerned about putting people off with his "unsightly" stoma. Ties, high-necked clothing, scarves, jewelry and tiny bibs can be used to cover the stoma lightly as long as they allow air to pass through readily.

Socially, most laryngectomees seem to do quite well after surgery. In an American Cancer Society survey, two out of three laryngectomees questioned said they now have as many or more friends as they had before surgery. Two out of three who had not retired also returned to their jobs.

13. Back to Work: Job Discrimination

Having a job he or she can return to is often crucial to the successful rehabilitation of the cancer patient. Anne Lanpher, the Washington, D.C., woman who underwent a laryngectomy, credits her school principal's insistence that she return to work as a main reason for her persistence in learning excellent esophageal speech. As she stated in *The Climate of Hope*, by Walter Ross, the two crucial factors in recovery after cancer are "the security you get from your family, the feeling of being loved; and job security, the feeling of being useful." She said she felt constantly "buoyed up" by the support she got from her students and principal. As one symbol of acceptance, she was surprised at her first Christmas back to work by a present constructed by the principal, her students, and an electronics teacher—an amplification system for her classroom so that she would not have to strain to make herself heard.

But some cancer patients are unable to return to their old jobs after treatment, either because of their disability or because they had to leave their jobs when they became ill. Other patients seek new jobs because they move to a new location or they wish to get ahead in their fields. Many such persons soon discover that the working world can be a cold and hostile place to someone who had been a cancer patient. The scenario is often like this—the person is interviewed, his references are checked, he is told he is qualified, and he is promised the job. He may even start working. But then comes the employment medical exam and suddenly the job evaporates. Sometimes the prospective employer is straightforward. He may tell the applicant that the company has a "five-year survival" rule—no hiring of cancer patients until five disease-free years have elapsed since treatment—or that the company's insurance rates would be raised by the hiring of a former cancer patient. More often, nothing specific is said—the person is simply never called back and he never knows whether it was because someone better qualified was hired in his stead or because he had

had cancer. Even the patient who does return to his old job some-times faces subtle discrimination, finding himself passed over at promotion time, or being denied the assignments that would most likely lead to his advancement.

Job discrimination is an especially painful form of bias after cancer because it can severely impair the rehabilitation of an otherwise successfully treated patient. In addition to the psycholog-ical handicap of trying to regain a sense of self after cancer and being unable to find a job, the former cancer patient is often burdened by debts incurred as a result of treatment or wages lost during his illness. Dr. Robert J. McKenna, a California cancer surgeon who heads the American Cancer Society's committee that is now studying employment problems of cancer patients, says the consequences of such discrimination are that "industry loses a qual-ified employee, the government loses tax dollars, and another family is forced to go on welfare." Dr. McKenna estimates that the job bias against cancer patients costs the nation's economy $500 million a year.

Some former patients finally resort to lying about their medical history if they have no apparent scars that cannot be otherwise accounted for, and others are discouraged from seeking proper treatment for their cancers. Dr. McKenna tells of one woman who was between jobs when she was found to have breast cancer. She refused to have her breast removed because she was afraid she would be unable to get a job afterward. A 22-year-old college graduate was twice turned down for teaching jobs because he had had leukemia. Desperate for work, he decided to lie about his medical history and easily got the next job he applied for. In five years on the job, he missed only two days of work. Finally his illness returned and he was forced to tell his employer, who said that he "could not have found a better teacher" but admitted that if he had known about the illness to begin with, "I would not have hired him."

Because most employable cancer patients are very anxious to work, they often go to great lengths to maintain their normal work schedules. One engineer was careful to schedule his chemo-therapy treatments for Friday afternoons so that he would not miss work. He was sick from the side effects of the drugs all week-end, but always well enough to go to work by Monday. Another patient, a woman executive, went to work every day during the six weeks of radiation therapy she needed following a mastectomy. She said her husband treated it all so matter-of-factly, dropping her off at her office every day, that she never even realized that many people don't even try to work while coping with the side effects of radiation treatments.

Contrary to the belief that cancer patients are disabled permanently or for long periods, surgeons report that up to 85 percent could return to work as soon as they have recovered from surgery. In a study of Bell System employees, cancer developed at a rate of 167 cases per 100,000 employees. Of the total cancer patients, 81 percent returned to work after cancer treatment, missing on the average eighty days of work. Fifteen percent of the patients died. Only four percent went on disability or claimed their pensions. Company officials concluded that while disability from cancer can be prolonged, it is far less common a problem compared to other diseases. They added that they especially welcomed the return to work of a valued older employee who has recovered from cancer. The Bell System, in fact, has begun employing persons directly from college campuses without requiring a preemployment medical exam, on the assumption that if the individual is well enough to complete his college work, he is well enough to be employed. This policy, company officials report, has not adversely affected their insurance ratings or stability of the worker population.

In 1957 the Metropolitan Life Insurance Company knowingly hired its first employee with a history of treated cancer. Subsequently, seventy-three other such employees—out of 150 applicants with a cancer history—were hired and their subsequent employment records were studied. The company found that worker turnover, absenteeism, and deaths during employment were no more frequent among the cancer patients than among other employees of the same age. Job performance was also acceptable. The cancer patients cost the company no more than other employees. Forty-three of the seventy-four former cancer patients had been treated for their diseases less than five years before they were hired. Only one patient had to go on disability because her cancer recurred. Two others developed a second cancer, but were able to return to work following surgery. The company concluded, "The selective hiring of persons who have been treated for cancer, in positions for which they are physically qualified, is a sound industrial practice." In selecting employees, Metropolitan Life relied on the most recent studies of survival rates achieved by various types of cancer patients undergoing specific types of treatment. Thus, on a statistical basis, if the patient's chance of survival was considered good, his history of cancer did not disqualify him for the job.

Nonselective policies, which in effect prevent the hiring of any former cancer patient until it is fairly certain he is permanently cured, discriminate unfairly against patients who have a good prognosis and are able and willing to work right after cancer treatment. Joyce Arkhurst, who had recently been treated for a very tiny, highly curable breast cancer, was denied a job at the United Nations because the international agency has a "five-year" rule. Those who interviewed Mrs. Arkhurst told her she was highly qualified for the job but that she was not given medical clearance. Dr. McKenna, who wrote to the United Nations asking them to reconsider their arbitrary rule, said, "The five-year policy of many companies is absurd. What is a person supposed to do for those five years—watch television and go hungry?" For Mrs. Arkhurst, the nonselective policy was particularly trying—she was seeking only a two-year position to begin with, and the chances of her suffering a recurrence of her cancer during those two years were practically nil. But still she did not get the job.

In another arbitrary application of a "five-year rule," a 22-year-old woman who had been successfully treated for a rare cancer of the reproductive tract a year and a half earlier was denied a job as a VISTA volunteer in Nashville. Following her cancer treatment, she had completed college and worked for five months. Struck by the irony that the Government was willing to let her go on welfare but not to be a productive volunteer with VISTA, the young woman said, "I thought the major battle of my life—fighting cancer—was behind me. Now it looks as if it has only just begun."

In the face of such rules, the former cancer patient who wants to work is often relegated to only part-time or substitute status with no job security. Those who are able to often are forced to go into business for themselves to avoid preemployment physicals. Dr. John F. Potter, who heads the Department of Oncology at Georgetown University Medical Center, believes that it even makes good economic sense to employ a cancer patient who has less than a normal life expectancy. It costs society a lot less to give the cancer patient a job than to support him until he dies, Dr. Potter points out. Certainly, he adds, for the effectively treated cancer patient, the low death rate simply does not justify the kind of job discrimination that exists.

Job discrimination against cancer patients has many and varied roots. According to Dr. McKenna, they include a fear that the employee who has had cancer will have endless periods of sick leave and then die before the employer can get much work out of him, a fear that his disease is contagious and will spread to other employees, and a concern about increased costs of insurance, workmen's compensation claims, pensions and other fringe benefits paid for by the company. As the Metropolitan Life study showed, for the most part these concerns are baseless. There is no evidence that a former cancer patient is more costly to a company than other employees, and there is certainly no evidence that cancer is contagious. Yet this fear of "catching cancer" prevails. Dr. William M. Markel, Vice-President for Service and Rehabilitation at the American Cancer Society, says he has even heard of other employees being afraid to use the same telephone that a former patient has used.

What is the solution to this problem? One important factor is public education to dispel misinformation and irrational fears about cancer. The American Cancer Society spends a major portion of its annual budget of nearly $100 million toward this end. And by the efforts of such groups as the Society's committee headed by Dr. McKenna, employers should become better informed about the liability—or lack of it—involved in hiring cancer patients. The Society will focus on educating company personnel departments and medical directors and will encourage doctors to "go to bat" for their patients, Dr. McKenna said.

In the meantime from the patient's standpoint, Dr. McKenna advises, "Don't quit your job if you get cancer. If you have to look for a new job after cancer treatment, consider taking a part-time position if no permanent job is offered." One woman worked for a large international organization on a six-months basis, with her temporary position renewed every six months until five years from the date of her cancer surgery, when she became a permanent employee.

Another solution—one that is being used with increasing success—is to legally appeal a job rejection based on health status. The Federal Government and nearly half the states now have laws granting equal job opportunities to Americans with medical disabilities, including a history of cancer. The only requirement for employment is that the person is able to perform the job in question at the time he applies for it. No judgment is allowed at the time of employment about the person's future suitability for the job or whether his present health status will prevail for any length of time. You do not need a lawyer to fight for a job under these laws. The responsible commission in each state will act as your representative if you file a complaint that you have been denied a job unfairly because you had been treated for cancer.

To find out about the law in your state, check with the human rights commission or fair employment practices commission or its equivalent in the state where you live. If you are a cancer patient and there is a law in your state barring job discrimination against the handicapped, it should cover you. Most of these laws are quite new, and as a result many employers do not know about them. Sometimes, just informing your prospective employer about the existence of such a law will get you the job you seek.

Former cancer patients also often have difficulty getting medical and life insurance. If insurance is granted, the person is placed in a "high risk" group and forced to pay higher premiums for the same coverage. If you have a job which has a group insurance policy, it will cover you at normal premium levels, because the group rate absorbs the high-risk along with the low-risk insurees. The best bet for good insurance coverage is to be certain you have a good policy from the start, before you or someone in your immediate family gets cancer.

14. The Cost in Dollars

Mrs. W. was 32 years old and had been treated for cancer for four years. She received a kidney transplant which failed. She then spent nine months at a prestigious medical clinic, followed by six months at a medical school hospital, where she finally died. Her husband then faced a $25,000 debt incurred as a result of his wife's prolonged illness.

For Mrs. V. of Queens, New York, the more than $7,500 in hospital and physician costs involved in the amputation of her leg for the treatment of cancer were almost the least of her financial worries. These costs were partly covered by medical insurance, and the doctor has told the V's not to worry about the bill—to pay whenever they can. But as Mrs. V. explained to a reporter for the New York *Daily News*, now she needs an artificial limb, which can cost several thousand dollars. And the 35-year-old woman is also going to need a car with special controls so that she can continue to function adequately as a homemaker and mother of five children.

It is not unusual for a family's life savings to be wiped out by the costs of caring for a patient with cancer. When these were savings earmarked for retirement or to underwrite the children's education, the financial devastation is especially tragic. Kitty Hanson tells in the *Daily News* of one retired couple not yet eligible for Medicare who had been living on an income of $3,100 a year when cancer struck the husband. The medical bills mounted to $35,000. They spent their savings, sold their home, and cashed in their life insurance policies to pay. After paying $26,500 of their bills, they were penniless and finally qualified for Medicaid, which paid the remainder.

Cancer pays little attention to a person's pocketbook when it strikes. It does not discriminate between rich and poor, and it hits especially hard at the middle class. The poor may qualify for Medicaid, and Medicare helps to offset the medical costs of persons over age 65. But younger, middle-income persons must rely on their own resources. For them a good medical insurance pol-

179

icy may be their only safeguard against financial disaster caused by a prolonged, costly illness. Dr. Sidney Cutler of the biometry branch of the National Cancer Institute has analyzed the hospital costs for typical cancer patients. Based on 3,151 patients whose cancers were diagnosed in 1969 and who were followed for two years thereafter, Dr. Cutler found that in the first twenty-four months of his disease the average cancer patient spends twenty-six days in the hospital at a total hospital cost of $2,289. One in eight patients is hospitalized for fifty days or more, and for 15 percent of patients the hospital costs come to $4,000 or more in the first two years of illness. When doctor's fees and the costs of out-patient care, nursing and homemaker services, and the like are added to this, the cost of cancer is virtually doubled, Dr. Cutler estimated. And in the five years since these data were collected, inflation has increased this total cost by more than one-third.

Considering only hospitalization costs, Dr. Cutler found that for the total group of patients who were 65 years of age or older, Medicare paid 83 percent of the bill. For patients under 65, 40 percent was paid for by Blue Cross, 32 percent by other insurance plans, 11 percent by the patients themselves, 11 percent by Medicaid and welfare, and 6 percent by other sources. Elderly persons who are covered by Medicare under the present law cannot afford to assume that this federal program will pay all the costs that cancer might entail. Medicare benefits can run out rapidly, and if the senior citizen is not medically indigent and thus eligible for Medicaid thereafter, he should purchase a supplemental insurance policy in order to be adequately protected in the event of prolonged illness.

Eligibility for Medicaid varies from state to state. Each state sets its maximum income level (depending on family size) for eligibilty, plus the amount of savings that can be retained to cover burial costs. Some states allow the Medicaid recipient to own his home, regardless of its worth, and to have a small savings account in addition to the burial fund. In most states, the Medicaid recipient is allowed to own a car and equipment needed to earn a living. However, even Medicaid coverage may not be unlimited; as states run short of funds, they are putting limits on the length of hospital coverage.

Most people today are covered by one or another form of private medical insurance, either by a group policy obtained through an employer or union or by an individually purchased policy, or both. It is very important to know precisely how well you are covered by your insurance in order to avoid financial disaster in the event of a lengthy, costly bout with cancer or some other extended illness. Dr. William M. Markel, Vice-President for Service and Rehabilitation at the American Cancer Society, advises that you check with your insurance agent or company to be sure you understand the benefits and how long they would last. If your policy is through your job or union, a personnel officer should be able to go over its terms with you. Also, you should carefully read the policy yourself to be certain you understand its terms and limitations.

According to experts at the American Cancer Society and the National Cancer Institute, the characteristics of an insurance policy you should examine include the following:

● The number of days of hospitalization covered. A policy should cover at least thirty days in the hospital.
● Out-patient coverage, for such things as chemotherapy and radiation therapy, which are generally given on an outpatient basis. Currently coverage in this area is spotty.
● Home health benefits, such as visiting nurses and homemakers. The majority of Blue Cross plans offer some payment for these services.
● Deductibles—the percentage of the costs the individual has to pay. Generally, policies that have a lot of deductibles have better long-term coverage. Most people are able to pay for the first $500 or $1,000 of costs, so a policy with no deductible for the first $500 of illness is not so important. It is far better to have a policy that requires you to pay some percent at the outset but that continues to cover you for catastrophic illnesses.
● Coinsurance—the hospitalization period after which the individual must pick up a share of the costs.

Some 35,000 cancer patients participate each year in studies of new treatment methods sponsored by the National Cancer Institute of the Federal Government. To pay for this treatment, the Institute-sponsored programs obtain whatever reimbursement they can from private and governmental insurance. But whatever is not picked up by insurers is paid for by the Institute itself out of tax monies paid by American citizens. In 1975 the Institute paid an average of $1,000 for each patient in its study programs. Thus, study participants can have all their hospital, doctor, drug and other treatment-related costs totally paid for.

Don't wait until cancer strikes to determine how well you will be able to pay for treatment. Then it may be too late, for if you find your coverage to be inadequate, you will have great difficulty getting additional insurance after a diagnosis of cancer. Find out now how well covered you are and consider purchasing a new or additional policy if you find your present coverage is not what it should be.

15. Helping the Patient Cope with Cancer

It is the rare individual who greets a diagnosis of cancer with equanimity. More likely the reaction is one of shock, anger, and intense fear: fear of the unknown, pain, disfigurement, helplessness, and dependency; fear of losing one's lifestyle, self-image, and self-respect; and, most important, fear of death. All too often, the cancer patient is left alone with his crushing fears. Just when he most needs support, he finds himself deserted. He is surrounded by a wall of silence. Neither family nor friends will mention the word cancer, and his doctor seems too busy and remote to discuss such matters. Everyone seems determined to distract him from his "morbid" thoughts. No one seems willing to stop long enough to help him talk through his fears and find ways to overcome them.

Cancer patients often find themselves socially and emotionally isolated. As one patient reported, "I felt very secure while I was in the hospital. But once I came home, I found that my friends and relatives sort of deserted me. They felt ill at ease and didn't come around." Just when he most needs psychological support—a feeling of intactness, belonging, being the same person he was before —the cancer patient often faces withdrawal and isolation.

Cancer has a greater emotional impact than any other disease that afflicts man, and fighting cancer is as much an emotional battle as it is a war with surgical tools, potent drugs and ionizing radiation. If the emotional battle is lost, a clinical victory can be an empty one. Dr. Morton Bard, psychologist at The City University of New York, notes that many of the lives saved by advances in medical science and technology are doomed to psychological invalidism. As he has described some of cancer's emotional victims:

● Ten years after successful cancer surgery, a previously dynamic corporation president is unnecessarily confined to a wheelchair with a nurse in round-the-clock attendance.

● A colostomy patient has spent the six years since her operation as, she says, "a prisoner in my bathroom," compulsively irrigating her colostomy for twelve hours every other day.
● A 35-year-old mother of three remains a virtual recluse five years after a mastectomy successfully halted her breast cancer.
● A successful businessman sold his business at a loss, became a nonfunctioning invalid and settled down to await death. He was free of cancer and still waiting eleven years later.

Throughout human history, Dr. Bard says, cancer has carried with it "a burden of frightening, superstitious, moral and even demonic implications . . . Cancer is commonly perceived as an always fatal and particularly loathsome disease, not 'clean' and uncomplicated like, for example, the frequently more fatal heart disease." When such distorted impressions are superimposed on the real burdens and threats of cancer, it is little wonder that the cancer patient finds himself weighted down by the extreme emotional stress of his illness. There are many ways of coping with this stress. Some people with strong inner resources handle it well on their own. Others need the help of family, friends, and professionals. The important thing to realize is that the psychic and social stresses of cancer must be dealt with—they cannot be brushed aside as unimportant any more than one would ignore the physical treatment of the disease. "Without successful emotional rehabilitation, neither successful treatment of the tumor nor successful physical rehabilitation has great meaning," Dr. Jordan R. Wilbur, pediatric oncologist at Stanford Medical Center, said. "The goal must be to return the cancer patient to a normal lifestyle as much as possible."

A person's reactions to cancer are likely to vary according to his age, the type of cancer and its prognosis, and the kind of treatment necessary to halt the disease. For an adolescent, whose normal concerns focus on establishing a stable self-image and a sense of belonging, a diagnosis of cancer—which rocks that image and sets him apart as different from others—carries more than its usual psychological burden. For a young woman, a diagnosis of breast cancer and the consequent need to remove the breast may represent a psychic threat more severe than death itself. Can anyone love a mutilated woman? Can I love myself? Often, a new definition of self becomes necessary, and many women report that the physical destruction involved in mastectomy caused them to dig deep within themselves and come up with a much more enduring and lovable self-concept than physical beauty. The parents of young children may worry about the youngsters' reaction to parental illness and to the aftereffects of treatment, in addition to such concerns as who will care for the family and whether the patient will live long enough to raise his children to independence. Older people may be concerned about becoming dependent on others and disrupting the lives of their grown children.

Reactions to a diagnosis of cancer also depend on the kind of coping patterns people have used throughout their lives. Some people are "confronters"—they meet challenges head-on and strive mightily to continue with life as usual despite new obstacles. Others are "deniers"—they push the thought of cancer promptly out of their minds, sometimes to the point of further endangering their health by avoiding the proper treatment for cancer. Typical of the "confronters" is one self-assured 72-year-old widow. Three months after her husband died of cancer of the esophagus, she noticed a little blood in her stool. She went to a doctor immediately and a cancer of the colon was diagnosed. She talked about her worries and concerns and cried for a few days after surgery, but she maintained confidence that she would soon resume her usual lifestyle, which included swimming and flying a plane. And she did.

Confronters have built into their psyches the essential ingredient for the emotional rehabilitation of cancer patients. That ingredient is hope. Hope is an inner resource, something that stems from how a person regards himself and his influence on the world around him. Hope does not grow out of deceptions and little white lies and evasions about the patient's diagnosis and prospects. Indeed, there have been patients who were told that nothing could be done and they had only a short time to live, who nevertheless clung to that last shred of hope and occasionally proved the doctors wrong in their estimate. For example, one eight-year-old boy who had had surgery for thyroid cancer later developed metastases in his lungs and was virtually given up for dead by both his parents and physicians. However, the boy recovered and ten years later, he was racing for the University of California track team. Neither does having hope mean that the patient is unrealistic about his disease and its likely outcome. Just the bare possibility of one chance in a thousand may help some patients endure psychologically the trials of therapy and the increasing disability associated with their disease.

Cancer patients face still another assault to their usual ways of coping with illness. With most kinds of illness, the disease makes you feel sick and the treatment makes you feel better. With cancer in many cases, the patient feels quite well when his illness is diagnosed. It is the treatment that may make him feel sick. "How can

I be getting better when I feel so much worse?" the patient wonders. It is especially trying to maintain a positive outlook under such circumstances.

Yet it is practically axiomatic in medicine that a positive outlook, a "will to live," can significantly improve a patient's chances for recovery. Studies at Johns Hopkins University suggest that a cancer patient's attitudes toward his illness and its treatment can influence the course of his disease. Does the patient think that "cancer equals death and I'm going to die soon" or does he believe "I have a serious illness, but I'm going to lick it; I will fight as hard as I can." The attitudes of patients who had just been diagnosed but not yet treated for cancer were rated by psychologists and psychiatrists who knew nothing about their illnesses. Those patients with the most positive attitudes consistently responded better to subsequent treatment. In accordance with their outlook, people with the identical illness and identical prognosis responded very differently to the same treatment, and the incidence of remissions and cures was much higher in the group with a positive attitude. The so-called "will to live" is more than a figment of the imagination; it can be a vital factor in the success or failure of therapy.

A patient's hope can be kept alive regardless of the outlook. Even after hope for a cure seems dim, there can still be hope that the patient's needs will be met as his disability increases—that he will not be abandoned, that his family will be taken care of, that his pain will be relieved, that he can die with dignity. The future can be kept alive, even if only limited to tomorrow or the next week. And the positive things remaining in the patient's life can be focused on—the activities that can still be enjoyed, the alternatives still available, the symptoms that can be treated.

Annette knew she was dying, but with the help of devoted friends she saw to it that she enjoyed to the greatest extent possible every minute she had left. During her first days in the hospital, she arranged for the continuing care of her elderly, widowed mother after her death. Then she told a nurse, "Now I am ready to go any time." In her remaining days she talked with visitors about the simple things of life, such as the beautiful wild flowers that grew outside her hospital window. One day, a cousin who visited her brought a pocket camera and took her picture against some flowers friends had sent. Delighted with the snapshot, Annette ordered copies made and sent to a few special friends. She read her Bible and poetry and took an interest in the welfare of the nurses who attended her, as well as that of other patients in her hospital wing. Annette died as beautifully as she had lived, quietly in her sleep and with dignity. Her cousin, who had spoken with her only days before, marveled at her attitude, which he described as that of a person who was "simply going on a visit."

Inevitably, in discussing the cancer patient's outlook, the issue arises of how much to tell the patient about his disease. First and foremost looms the pressing question: to tell or not to tell the patient he has cancer. It is ironic how much time is spent debating this question and warning family and friends not to disclose the awful truth when, in fact, surveys have shown that more than 80 percent of patients already know their diagnosis without being told, and 87 percent of people say they would want to know if they were found to have cancer. So the real question becomes, not *whether* to tell, but *what* and *how* to tell. A diagnosis of cancer must be accompanied by reassurance that all that can be done toward conquering the disease will, in fact, be done, that there are treatments available and that there is always hope even in advanced cases. Patients respond well to a feeling of empathy on the part of their doctors—acknowledgment that cancer is a tough break, a tough disease to lick, but with reassurance that it can be licked and that an acceptable life can follow cancer treatment. The doctor should not deceive the patient by giving him uncritical, unrealistic hope, but he should treat the patient as a person with a future, however limited that future might be. Time and again, doctors have remarked that the informed cancer patient is more cooperative and better able to tolerate the effects of treatment. It is not unusual for patients, particularly children, to balk at taking drugs that make them feel sick when they do not know that the reason for the drugs is to combat a potentially fatal illness.

Fourteen-year-old Paula was told she had "anemia" (she really had leukemia). She would be sick, hostile, and withdrawn every time she had to go to the clinic for chemotherapy. Why, she asked angrily, did she have to come for shots all the time when she felt perfectly well? Her parents finally told her the real reason for the treatment and suddenly Paula's symptoms and anger disappeared. She became cheerful and cooperative and willing to talk about herself and her disease. Another teenager with Hodgkin's disease initially refused chemotherapy because it would make her gain weight and lose her hair. When she was told the implications of her refusal and given a choice, she made the decision regarding her own life and body and agreed to accept the temporary change in her looks to gain a chance for survival.

Doctors have found that it is also important, in informing the cancer patient about his illness, to tell no more than the patient really wants to know and to disclose the facts in small doses over a long period of time, giving the patient time to adjust to each step in the disclosure process. Dr. LaSalle D. Leffall, Jr., Professor and Chairman of the Department of Surgery at Howard University College of Medicine in Washington, D.C., says that it is also important that the family be informed about the patient's condition. If the information is imparted to the family in the presence of the patient, then pretenses can be dropped and the conspiracy of silence broken. Dr. Leffall adds that there are some patients who should *not* be told they have cancer. These include very young children (although many doctors think even young children should be told), patients with severe psychiatric disorders, and very infrequent cases where the family members insist that the patient simply could not tolerate being told he has cancer.

But while most doctors now favor informing the patient about his *diagnosis*, most caution against giving any kind of definite *prognosis* to either the patient or the family. Predicting the patient's life expectancy—except in terminal illness when death is but a few days off—is a risky and often inaccurate business. Even patients who were given little hope to live out the week have sometimes rallied and lived for months or years longer.

Irving was a 70-year-old businessman who had neither time nor patience for illness when he needed two major operations to treat a cancer which the doctors thought they could not cure but could control and extend Irving's life. Radioactive needles were implanted in the tumor to help destroy it, but the doctors did not expect him to live very long. A month passed, then two. After five months, Irving decided to move back into his own house. Then when the United States entered World War II, he advertised himself as a 71-year-old retiree looking for a war job. He worked his way up in a tool shop, starting as an assistant and ending as chief buyer. As the eighth decade of his life wore on, he reduced his working time to three days a week so that he could spend more time with his grandchildren. He died at 81 of a heart attack.

When giving a prognosis for cancer, about all that can be said with accuracy are impersonal statistics, something like—"given 100 patients with your disease, half can expect to die within so many months or years. But you are not a statistic; you are an individual patient, and there is no telling where on the spectrum of probabilities you will fall."

Learning to live with cancer is an art, not a science. Each person must find his own way in his own style. What is important to realize is that a way can be found, regardless of the circumstances and prospects. A way can be found to live with cancer even if you know you cannot be cured.

"You don't have to go home to die," says Orville Kelly, a man who should know. Mr. Kelly of Burlington, Iowa, is the 45-year-old father of four young children and a victim since since 1973 of lymphocytic lymphosarcoma. This is a cancer affecting the lymph glands for which there is currently no established cure, although recent drug therapies have held out the promise that some patients may survive this disease. Mr. Kelly received regular chemotherapy, but until recently the treatments have only succeeded in holding his cancer at bay. For the last half year, however, his body has been rid of all apparent signs of cancer.

About four months after he learned he had cancer, Mr. Kelly was driving home from the hospital on a golden autumn evening when he suddenly realized that his fear of death was robbing him of the pleasure of his last days. Since the diagnosis, he had become withdrawn and his wife and children were very nervous.

"Actually, I had given up," Mr. Kelly recalled in the spring of 1976, nearly three years after his cancer was diagnosed. "The covers of my bed were turned back and I was only too willing to go to bed to await the inevitable. I even considered suicide as an easy way out.

"Things had become pretty bad at our home. My wife was sleeping in another room, and I discovered later that she didn't want me to hear her crying at night. I spoke little about my problems because I didn't want to worry my family. There was little communication. They were trying to protect me and I was trying to protect them and nothing was working. The children (then ages 3 through 12) knew something was wrong, but they did not know what," Mr. Kelly told a Reuters reporter. "Driving home that day, I knew I was going to tell them I had cancer and then we were going to have a picnic in the back garden. Now the whole matter of having cancer is in the open and the family can cope with it better. The children are doing better in school now that they know."

Mr. Kelly also started making plans for the future, no matter how short or long it might be. He started making notes for a book on living with cancer. In August of 1975 that book, *Make Today Count*, was published. It is based largely on his experiences through the Make Today Count organization he formed early in 1974 to help other people in a similar predicament. By 1976 there were fifty-four Make Today Count chapters throughout the country helping patients and their families learn to live with cancer and face death with equanimity. Make Today Count, Box 303,

Burlington, Iowa, 52601, is a sharing process, a mutual talking through of problems and grief and arriving at an acceptance that makes it possible to enjoy the time left.

In the spring of 1975 Mr. Kelly got a call—not unlike many others he has received—from the distraught parents of a young boy who, they had just been told, would die of cancer within five years. "There are many children who will die tonight," Mr. Kelly told the father, according to an Associated Press report. "They will die from accidents or illness. Their parents would give anything to have just one of the years your son has left. The question is—are you going to waste those five years with your son, or are you going to make them count?"

Are you going to go home to die, or are you going to continue living as normal a life as possible—enjoying the woods, the flowers, the seashore, the activities you like, the people around you, life?

Mr. Kelly has made hundreds of public appearances all over the nation to help people learn to live with cancer. He answers phone calls from distressed patients and their families day and night. He is always available to help people deal with their grief and learn to Make Today Count.

One woman who has learned well the value of Mr. Kelly's lesson is Linda Hardy. Mrs. Hardy was only 29 when she developed breast cancer. She was the sole support of her three young children, whose father had deserted the family several years earlier. Mrs. Hardy survived three major operations for cancer, and realizing she would eventually die of her disease, she searched for a family who would care for her children after her death. Once her appeal reached television and national newspapers, she was flooded with offers of help, many from people who offered their homes to the children in the event of Linda's death. As Mrs. Hardy told a reporter for the New York *Daily News*, "Now I can wake up with a smile every morning and think—even if this is my last day on earth, I don't have to be afraid of anything any more." But Mrs. Hardy did not waste the years since her illness was first discovered wallowing in self-pity and fear. "At first, I couldn' accept death," she said. "I felt sorry for myself for a while. But right now, I feel so happy inside that it's hard to believe it's going to happen. I'm going to live till I die, and I'm going to be happy." During the years of her illness, Mrs. Hardy worked at part-time jobs, remained active in her church, and made a loving home for her children. "We've been a happy family," she reports. She was still alive and happy in the spring of 1976, four years after her cancer was diagnosed.

Eleven-year-old Amy Timmons also knew how to make today

count. As Amy herself wrote in the fourth year of her illness, "I have acute lymphoblastic leukemia. But *please* don't feel sorry for me. I live a perfectly wonderful life. I go to parties, play games, swing on swings, and for the most part, I am able to do whatever I want. . . . Even though you have leukemia and can still have fun, it's not all fun and games. There are some disadvantages and pain along with having fun. But aren't there disadvantages and pain in every life? You must think of people with leukemia as people with feelings, and you must treat them as people with feelings, not as pitied objects." Amy hardly had time for pity. In addition to her fun and games and pain and disadvantages, she was an honor student, president of her class, and active in the Girl Scouts. She died one month after writing the essay from which the above excerpts were taken. According to her mother, Mrs. Anita A. Timmons, Amy left a legacy of "wonderful memories through pictures of family activities, through her needlework and handicraft gifts to each of us; and we have also kept her diaries, letters, prose, and poetry through which we can know of her struggle with, her curiosity of, and her love for life and living. . . . Amy's eleven and a half years were filled with a lifetime of experiences."

16. The Physical Pain

Cancer is commonly thought of as a painful disease. The word cancer triggers in most people deep-seated fears about death and pain and these fears often intensify the agony associated with a diagnosis of cancer and cause others to avoid cancer patients. In fact, however, only a small proportion of cancer patients experience pain as a serious or chronic problem. Dr. Raymond Houde, who runs the pain clinic at Memorial Hospital for Cancer in New York, points out that except for bone cancers, the vast majority of cancers cause no pain in their early stages. Thus, in patients whose cancers are treated early and cured, the most serious pain they experience is likely to be the temporary result of surgery or other treatment for the disease, and this pain is usually readily controlled by one of many pain-relieving medications.

Pain is more likely to be a problem in patients with advanced cancer. But even there, many patients experience little or no pain. British researchers who operate a hospital for the terminally ill state that as many as half their patients with advanced incurable cancer have no pain or only negligible discomfort. About 10 percent have mild pain that requires some medication and 40 percent experience severe pain, necessitating more potent pain-relieving measures, the researchers report. The pain of advanced cancer can nearly always be well-controlled by such modern methods of pain-relief as powerful drugs, electrical stimulation and interference with the nerves that conduct pain sensations, as well as by what is called "palliative" cancer therapy—the use of such treatments as surgery, radiation therapy and chemotherapy to reduce the size of the tumor that is causing the pain.

The causes of pain in advanced cancer include the following:

● Metastases to the bone. A number of cancers, including cancer of the breast, lung, kidney, and thyroid, commonly spread to the bone in their advanced stages. Pain in the bone is often the first sign that the cancer has metastasized. Sometimes bones that have been weakened by cancer fracture easily, causing more intense pain.

- Growth of the tumor into nerves, blood or lymph vessels, or mechanical pressure of the tumor on such vessels.
- Obstruction of an organ, such as the bowel, by a tumor, or growth of the tumor into relatively inelastic connective tissue.
- Inflammatory reactions to the presence of cancer or death of cancer tissue in a pain-sensitive area of the body.

There are also physical conditions secondary to the cancer—as well as psychic factors—that contribute to the pain associated with this disease. Jeanne Q. Benoliel and Dorothy M. Crowley, both cancer nurses at the University of Washington in Seattle, note that the malnutrition caused by advanced cancer is particularly stressful. Loss of appetite, nausea and vomiting, diarrhea, loss of fluids, and imbalance of body salts—conditions which often accompany advanced cancer—cause patients to become weak and debilitated, physically immobile and increasingly depressed, worried and fearful. These responses often intensify the patient's pain and discomfort. As one leading cancer therapist put it, "Seeing oneself waste away—that's the most painful part of cancer."

"Physical pain is only one cause of suffering in advanced cancer," Dr. Houde explains. "Sometimes threats to the ego as a result of the disease may take predominance over pain or make the pain worse. Weakness, nausea and vomiting, incontinence, fear of invalidism and death can all intensify the patient's feelings of pain."

Other emotional responses stimulated by cancer commonly compound the problem. As nurses Benoliel and Crowley point out, "Guilt frequently accompanies pain, and a surprising number of patients with cancer are plagued with feelings of guilt. As they search for some meaning in the catastrophe which has befallen them, unresolved feelings of ill will toward others, remorse for events of the past, or even feelings that they might have been negligent in seeking medical advice or in caring for their bodies aroused feelings of guilt." Such feelings, the nurses add, "may make it more difficult for the patient to participate effectively in the management of pain, since he sees both the disease and the pain as punishment for a transgression."

Still another emotional factor influencing the experience of pain in cancer patients is anxiety, which can intensify the experience of pain and affect the behavior of persons in contact with the patient in negative ways, often causing them to avoid the patient as much as possible. Seeing another person in pain—especially a person who is dear to you—is extremely anxiety-provoking, and people naturally try to avoid anxiety-provoking situations. Ironically, much of a cancer patient's anxiety involves the fear of being abandoned by friends, relatives, doctors, and nurses as the disease progresses. As one patient told a group of student nurses who asked him to tell them about his pain, "What kind of pain are you interested in? Are you interested in the pain that is racking me right now and from which I will never recover? Are you asking about the pain of my life when I lost my daughter? Are you talking about the pain of my loneliness because I have no one who cares?"

Cancer patients who are in pain may also be anxious about the pain itself. How long will it last? What is causing it? Will it get worse? Will I be able to stand it if it gets worse? In light of such common feelings and fears, it is especially important to assure the cancer patient that he will not have to suffer undue pain, that methods are available to relieve most pain, no matter how severe, and that these methods will be used when and if he needs them. The importance of such assurances of relief to easing the patient's discomfort has been clearly demonstrated time and time again in studies of placebos—"dummy" medications that the patient believes will work but which in fact have no inherent pain-relieving properties. A recent study at the Mayo Clinic in Rochester, Minnesota, showed that fully 39 percent of 112 cancer patients who were given a placebo (milk sugar) "pain killer" experienced significant relief of their pain, simply because they expected the pills to bring relief and because the attention they received from doctors and nurses diminished their anxiety and thus also relieved their pain. There is little doubt, Dr. Houde of Memorial Hospital points out, that the pain of cancer can be greatly relieved "by paying more attention to the patient's emotional needs."

Drugs are the most commonly used direct means of relieving the pain of advanced cancer. When nonnarcotic drugs no longer work adequately, doctors can use codeine and morphine and various combinations of pain-killing and sedative drugs to relieve both pain and anxiety without "knocking the patient out" so that his mind is foggy. Nurses Benoliel and Crowley state that if a patient is "snowed under" with medication, he is cut off from effective social interaction, and this is counterproductive. But neither, they add, is it desirable to wait until the patient's pain returns to the point where he becomes uncomfortable and anxious before he gets the next dose of pain-killer. More and more, doctors who care for patients with advanced cancer are coming to realize that this is no time to worry about whether a patient may become addicted to the drug being used to relieve his pain. It is far more important for the patient to know that he need not worry about being overcome by his pain and that he will not have to beg for pain relief.

In the relatively rare circumstances where drugs no longer work to bring adequate pain relief, other techniques can be used that work directly on the nerves that transmit sensations of pain. For example, if the responsible nerve can be defined, a local anesthetic or nerve-killing agent may be injected directly into the nerve or the nerve may be severed surgically. Radiation or electrical current transmitted through a needle to the central nerve fibers in the spine that carry pain impulses to the brain can also be used to relieve intractable cancer pain. In another use of electricity, electrical stimulation of the skin in the area of the pain creates a vibratory sensation that overcomes pain. This is a technique that the patient controls himself, and can be used safely as often as needed.

Patients dying of cancer often linger for many months, becoming progressively debilitated and increasingly invalided. This lingering adds to the psychic, if not the physical, pain of advanced cancer. But as will be seen in a later section, the way the patient and his family deal with anticipation of death can make an enormous difference in how well it is withstood.

17. Helping the Family Cope with Cancer

Cancer eventually strikes two out of three American families. These families basically have to go through the same process of adjustment to cancer that the patient himself faces. As with the patient, family members are likely to experience shock and anger at the diagnosis, sorrow over "what might have been," and hope for a cure or at least a prolonged remission. One study showed that following the diagnosis of cancer in a child, most parents experience temporary "symptoms and feelings of physical distress, depression, inability to function, anger, hostility, and self-blame."

How well the family copes with cancer depends on many factors, including the initial strength of the family unit, how the members function together, how much love there is and, of course, the circumstances and age of the patient, the kind of cancer and treatment involved, and the prospects for recovery. A diagnosis of cancer in a husband creates problems for the 70-year-old woman with married children which are vastly different from those problems of a 35-year-old mother of three youngsters. Sometimes cancer disrupts typical family roles, such as who earns the income and who cares for the household, necessitating a host of psychological and physical adjustments.

As we have seen in Chapter 12, the family has a vital role to play in easing the adjustment of the patient who has had a mastectomy, colostomy, laryngectomy, or other radical surgery that changes body image or normal functions. If the husband responds to his wife's mastectomy with the remark that he "can't sleep with a woman like that," it's almost guaranteed that the wife will have difficulty accepting her fate.

The effects on families who do not cope well with cancer can range from chronic psychic pain to a nearly paralytic irrational fear. One woman whose husband has had chronic lymphatic leukemia for four years says she is "completely unable to forget" her problem and she lives in constant dread that her four children, whom she has shielded from knowledge of their father's condition, will someday find out and suffer as much as she. She reports, "I have gone to college for two years and then tried to work, but the problem is constantly with me. How does one learn to cope? I will never accept this situation, but I must learn to live with it."

In another family, where both the parents died of cancer, the three grown sons live in dread of having inherited the disease. One brother had to have surgery for treatment of an infection, but for two months he refused to go to the hospital, convinced that he really had a hopeless cancer. The youngest son said that he is afraid to go into a hospital to have his tonsils out or have stitches. He said that since the death of his parents, he has been extremely nervous and a doctor had to prescribe tranquilizers to help him relax.

But cancer seems to have its greatest impact on families when the victim is a child. In such cases, family members often become the secondary victims of cancer. The parents' reaction to the stress of the situation may threaten the stability of their marriage and impair their ability to relate to their other children. Dr. C. M. Binger and his colleagues in San Francisco studied 23 families in which a child had died of leukemia. In approximately half of the families one or more previously well siblings developed such problems as severe bedwetting, headaches, poor school performance, depression, severe separation anxieties, and abdominal pains. In eleven families, at least one member reacted so strongly to the crisis that psychiatric help was needed. None of these people had needed psychiatric care before.

In another study of forty families where a child had leukemia, only one in ten families emerged from the experience essentially intact. Thirty-six families were so disturbed that they no longer functioned effectively as a social unit. In twenty-eight families serious marital difficulties developed, with nine of the marriages ending in divorce soon after the child's death. In eighteen families one of the parents developed a serious drinking problem, and in fifteen families, at least one member required psychiatric treatment whereas none had been needed before the child's illness. Of the ninety-seven surviving children, forty-three experienced one or more adjustment problems, in many cases in school as well as at home. In addition, following the death of the child, thirty-five of the forty families experienced morbid grief reactions, including such abnormal responses as enshrining the room of the dead child, making daily visits to the cemetery, or completely prohibiting mention of the child's name. This study, supported by the American Cancer Society, was conducted by Dr. David M. Kaplan, director of the division of clinical social work at Stanford Medical School. He pointed out that the leukemic child is often better able to handle the situation than his parents are, with the ironic result that "the child with the disease ends up protecting his family."

Mrs. Karen Briscoe calls childhood leukemia a "family disease" because the "tension, fears, fantasies and emotional strain caused by the illness affect every member of the family." Mrs. Briscoe should know. The youngest of her five children succumbed to leukemia in 1971, and besides living through the experience in her own family, Mrs. Briscoe, working through the Kansas Division of the American Cancer Society, has helped countless other families through their own crises with childhood cancer. She points out that "in the past, when a child with leukemia had only a few months to live, families were able to rally and stick together in an all-out effort to make the last days of the dying child happy. But now, due to new and constantly improving chemotherapy, children with leukemia are living two to five years and some longer." The same can be said for children with other kinds of cancers. Of all children with cancer today who receive up-to-date therapy, more than half can expect to live five years or longer.

This extended survival (and sometimes cure) can be a mixed blessing if the family is unable to cope with the resulting stresses and strains. As Mrs. Briscoe has outlined the problems that typically arise:

● Once treatment has begun, communication between family members, and especially between parents, breaks down. "The family that wept and ached and rallied together at the initial diagnosis becomes silent and withdrawn. The illness is rarely mentioned. Deep feelings and fears are seldom discussed."

● The mother usually concentrates almost completely on caring for the sick child. Fathers often feel neglected, causing resentment mixed with guilt. Often, the father leaves the child's care entirely to the mother and he spends longer and longer hours away from home. The mother, in turn, may resent this and feel that the father lacks love and concern for her and the child. In the whirl of this vicious circle, tensions mount and little irritations become big ones.

● Other children in the family may resent the fact that the sick child is always the center of attention. Even if the leukemic child does not get extra gifts or privileges, his parents are likely to respond to him in special ways. Every fever, nosebleed, and bad temper is interpreted as a possible sign that the cancer has returned. At the same time that the well child resents his sick sibling, he also feels guilty because he knows the child is sick. Unable to handle these conflicting feelings, the well child may develop behavioral problems which simply increase the tension in the home.

● Sometimes parents feel guilty, believing that their child got sick because they are being punished for past sins or that they in some way caused the leukemia through neglect or heredity.

Mrs. Briscoe has found that most of the family problems created by childhood leukemia can be alleviated by open and honest communication between family members and between the family and physician. She also found it extremely helpful to talk to and be with the parents of other leukemic children. "It is a wonderful, strangely maddening and magnificently relieving feeling to find that the overpowering problems you thought so uniquely your own are, in fact, shared by most of the others in your situation," she reports.

A number of medical centers that specialize in the treatment of childhood cancer now hold, as part of the treatment program, regular individual and group sessions with parents to help them to understand and anticipate their problems and work through appropriate solutions. In addition, a national volunteer organization called The Candlelighters, composed of parents and friends of children with cancer or who died of cancer, serves a similar function. The organization, which was originally established as a lobbying group, has headquarters at 123 C Street S.E., Washington, D.C. 20003. There are forty-six chapters in thirty states, plus some in Canada and one in England. Several of the chapters are service-oriented, helping parents with such practical problems as driving, baby-sitting, and gathering blood donors, but in all cases the opportunity to share the emotional as well as the physical burdens of childhood cancer is there.

In the course of his research, Dr. Kaplan discovered that a family's difficulties in coping with childhood cancer can be spotted in the first weeks after the illness is diagnosed. The early signs of trouble identified by Dr. Kaplan include the following:

● The parents are united in denying the seriousness of the situation, refusing to acknowledge the fact that their child has a potentially fatal illness.

● The parents' reactions are markedly discrepant. The mother, for example, may cry a lot but the father says, "Don't cry. I don't want to see you crying."

● The parents persist in using euphemisms—like "anemia" or "tumor"—instead of the real name for their child's disease. These parents also may try to shield the child from knowing the seriousness of his illness, sometimes establishing a round-the-clock hospital vigil to be sure no one tells the child his diagnosis.

● Appropriate expressions of sadness, such as crying, are inhibited. Instead, the parents steel themselves to remain in control, not to break down and express their grief.

● One or both parents gets absorbed in a whirlwind of activities, keeping so busy that there's no time to sit down and face the bad news.

● The parents start shopping around for doctors, faith healers, quacks—anyone who will promise a cure.

Dr. Kaplan has also found that if one parent is unable to deal realistically with the problem, it makes it very difficult for other members of the family to do so. He said that families who prepare for the worst are able to make the best of the time that remains. Such families have little difficulty in accepting good news if it should come along. But the reverse is not true—the unprepared family or patient cannot handle later difficulties well.

Dr. Kaplan warns against taking on major new responsibilities or making great changes in life—such as changing jobs or place of residence—when the family is trying to deal with childhood cancer. Such changes merely create new problems and stresses and leave the family with even less energy to deal with the major problem, the sick child. He especially warns against quickly becoming pregnant upon learning that your child has cancer. He tells of one woman who gave birth to a daughter on the same day that her leukemic child entered the hospital for the last time. For months after the child's death, the mother was still unable to care for her new baby. In fact, she was indifferent to and angered by the baby's needs. Dr. Kaplan concluded that families should not make decisions that can be avoided or postponed while under the intense stress of serious illness. His advice to such families is, "Don't just do something, stand there."

Dr. Kaplan was able to identify characteristics of parents who did cope successfully with the crisis of childhood cancer. In addition to avoiding unnecessary additional stresses, such as a new baby, they include the following:

● A realistic concept of their child's illness as something very serious that could ultimately lead to loss of the child.

- The ability to discuss the illness accurately and realistically with other members of the family, friends, and the child himself. These are parents who could say to their child something like, "You are very seriously ill and we are very worried about you. You will have to be under medical care for a long time."
- Free expression of the sad and frightening feelings that serious illness naturally provokes.
- The ability to anticipate the eventual loss of their child and experience the normal grief reactions beforehand.

Parents usually try to protect the child with cancer from knowing what is really wrong with him and that his disease may be fatal. But Dr. Binger and others have found that by the age of four or five most children know they are seriously ill and often anticipate their own death. But when the parents maintain a "conspiracy of silence," the child finds himself alone and afraid with no one to talk to about his feelings and fears. As Dr. Binger reported, "The children who were perhaps the loneliest of all were those who were aware of their diagnosis but at the same time recognized that their parents did not wish them to know. As a result, there was little or no meaningful communication. No one was left to whom the child could openly express his feelings of sadness, fear and anxiety." On the other hand, those parents who talked openly with their children about their illness said that they experienced "a more meaningful relation with their child than they had ever experienced before," Dr. Binger said.

Even the young siblings of the sick child are often aware of the seriousness of the illness but cannot talk to anyone about their anxieties because the family tries to "protect" them from what is going on. The result of this lack of open communication can be traumatic. Dr. Kaplan tells of one child whose identical twin brother died of leukemia before he was three. Years later, the surviving twin said that he ought to go out and "get run over" so he could "be in heaven with Jeffrey." After Jeffrey died, his twin started grinding his teeth, walking and talking in his sleep and sometimes crying out and yelling.

The parents in Dr. Binger's study emphasized the importance of treating the child with cancer "normally" during his illness, with the family living day by day, enjoying the child but not giving special privileges or being overprotective. Such an approach proved its own reward for the Donald H. Dilmore family of Dallas, Texas. The day before Helen, the youngest of their four children, was to be five, Mr. Dilmore said the doctor advised him to give his daughter the best birthday party he could "because she may not live for another year. She has cancer and it is in a location where we cannot operate," although other treatments could be used. Well, happily little Helen did not die—radiation therapy and chemotherapy controlled her cancer and she has now graduated from high school. In the intervening years, her family learned some valuable lessons. They learned, for one thing, to enjoy each day and get the most from it. Helen's chemotherapist had told them, "The more normal you keep things, the less you baby her and watch over her, the better it will be, not only for her but for all of the family." So Helen learned to ride a bike and swim. She took flute lessons, and when these caused headaches and dizziness, she switched on her own to a percussion instrument.

Her father reports, "This attitude has made it much easier for the other kids. No one babies Helen. She is treated equally. Her clothes get borrowed by her sisters, she has her share of responsibilities, and no one is ever reminded that 'Helen has been sick.' She gets no special treatment and no pampering."

After the first time Helen was hospitalized, Mr. Dilmore said that he and his wife realized that the other children were concerned. "We found Don, Jr., looking up 'malignancy' in the *World Book*. Pretty heavy reading for a 10-year-old. They had questions and concerns; they knew something was wrong. We talked about it and didn't try to hide anything, nor did we dwell on it. We told them Helen was very sick and that she might die, but the best thing we could do was to pray for her and not be overly attentive." Mr. Dilmore believes that the positive attitude maintained by Helen and the family helped her to recover. The family still tries to encourage this attitude, he says, "by not reminding her that she has been sick and by letting her live a normal life. The end result has been a family brought closer together, with more understanding and a deeper loyalty to each other. Everyone has made some sacrifice. My wife has spent countless hours in the hospital, trips to the radiologist and other doctors. The other kids have had to give up some things and we have all made some financial sacrifices, but we have had a happy family life—I believe a normal family life—and a better philosophy of how to get more out of life."

18. When the Patient Is Dying

We all knew my mother was dying, or so I thought. We had watched for months as the cancer consumed more and more of her vital energy, causing exhaustion, inability to eat, weight loss, and pain. Yet we all observed an unwritten agreement—the word cancer, let alone death or dying, was never mentioned in my mother's presence. Indeed, it was rarely discussed among ourselves. Three times during the last months of her debilitating illness, she attempted to end her life. We responded by hiding all the knives, scissors and razor blades and locking the medicine chest. But we never once discussed what was on all our minds. We never once gave my mother the opportunity to talk about her fears and the difficulty this once-stalwart woman had in accepting her increasing disabilities and deterioration and what they presaged. And we denied her her last wish—to die with the same dignity with which she had lived for nearly half a century.

We didn't realize how wrong we had been until after her death. My 13-year-old brother went into a state of shock, for, it turned out, he had fully believed the pretense we had all observed and he had expected that she would eventually get well. And I, so firmly wedded to the stoical role that I had adopted to help carry myself and my family through the long, exhausting, painful months of terminal illness, was unable to properly mourn the loss of my mother until more than a year after her death.

Playwright Robert Anderson, whose first wife, Phyllis, died in her thirties after a five-year struggle against breast cancer, says, "For four years, we fought the inevitability of her dying. It would have been easier, far, far less lonely, if she had known. I would want to know. The complicated ruses, deceptions, explanations were incredible. The heartbreak of watching her thinking she was improving, while I knew that any improvement was only temporary. I remember her saying as we woke up one morning, 'I've decided that I am not going to make a slow improvement. I am just going to wake up one morning completely well.' I feel I deprived my wife of the opportunity to share her dying with someone. I played God for four years, trying to arrange her life in a way I thought she would want to lead it in her last years, but actually might not have led it if she had known they were last years . . . had definitely known."

But recriminations and regret were not the only consequences of Mr. Anderson's deception. Two years after his wife's death, he found himself still unable to cope with his loss, "unable to move in any significant way," and he sought psychiatric treatment to help him out of his paralyzed state.

"What man shall live and not see death?" is the question posed in the 89th Psalm. But although death is a normal part of living —and not necessarily the worst thing that can happen to a person —most of us are ill-prepared to deal with it. Today, more than two-thirds of deaths occur in a hospital or some other institutional setting, in alien territory remote from the rest of living. Most children grow to middle age never having seen anyone die. When suddenly faced with their own mortality or the impending death of someone they love, they are at a loss as to how to handle it.

This failure to school people in the art of dying as a part of life has at last been recognized. Starting in the late 1960s, a growing league of professionals has opened up discussion of death and dying, the 20th century's last taboo. The goal of these professionals is to make death less dehumanizing, less psychologically painful, more dignified. This is especially important now that swift deaths from acute illnesses are a relative rarity, and many people die over a period of months or years from chronic diseases like cancer. As we have already seen, protracted illnesses that are ultimately fatal can create stresses on a family that leave deep, permanent scars. But by understanding the emotional dynamics that normally accompany the process of dying, many of these stresses can be alleviated and death can be a far less devastating event for both the person who dies and the people who love him.

Lyn Helton was a poet and the mother of a two-year-old child when bone cancer claimed her life. During the final stages of her illness, she wrote in her diary: "Dying is beautiful. Even at the ripe old age of twenty. It is not easy most of the time, but there is real beauty to be found in knowing that your end is going to catch up with you faster than you expected and that you have to get all your loving and laughter and crying done as soon as you can. I am not afraid to die, not afraid of death, because I have known love." Lyn, whose story was told in the *Reader's Digest* in June 1972, had reached what thanatologists (experts in the psychological

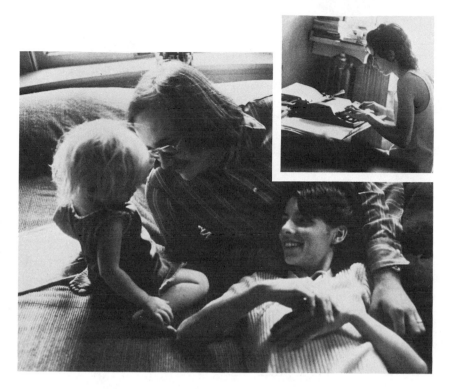

(Jacque) Lyn Helton, who died of bone cancer at the age of 20, spent much of her last months writing and recording her thoughts about life, her illness and her love for her husband, Tom, and daughter, Jennifer, 20 months old. Among them: "I am not afraid to die, not afraid of death, because I have known love."

aspects of death) call the stage of acceptance. She had made her peace, said her goodbyes and was ready to die. Dr. Elisabeth Kübler-Ross, an Illinois psychiatrist, has identified five distinct psychological stages that dying persons typically pass through as their death approaches. The families of dying persons pass through similar stages, and one of the goals of professionals who counsel the dying is to help synchronize these stages for both patient and family.

The first stage is denial: "No, not me." The patient cannot accept the fact that he has a fatal illness. Sometimes patients are unable to pass out of this stage and, as a result, die with much unfinished business. Other times, it is the family that cannot accept the fatal prognosis and may effectively block the efforts of the dying person to come to terms with his mortality.

In most people, however, Dr. Ross had found, denial quickly gives way to anger and rage—the "Why me?" stage. Patients in this stage would do well to be able to scream out their rage. But without a means of expressing anger, the patient may become hard to handle, overly critical, nasty and uncooperative. This reaction is often misinterpreted as ingratitude for what people are trying to do for the patient. And people tend to respond to this seeming ingratitude by making visits shorter and less frequent, the nurse by jabbing in the needle just a little harder. The result is to make the patient feel even more deprived, isolated and rejected.

Following anger, there often comes a period of bargaining: "Yes, me, but . . . if you promise me one more year, God, I promise I'll be a good Christian." Dr. Ross tells of one terminally ill woman who was in intense pain nearly all the time. The woman asked for only one day without pain so that she could leave the hospital and attend her older son's wedding. Through self-hypnosis, her wish was granted. On returning to the hospital she said, "Don't forget, now, I have another son."

The fourth stage is usually depression, a time of mourning over things already lost and of grieving over impending losses. This is when the patient psychologically separates himself from his loved ones. "The worst thing you can do at this stage is call in a psychiatrist," Dr. Ross says. "That implies that the patient is not behaving properly, that he should shape up—'Come on, cheer up. It's not so bad.' Not so bad for whom? A widow is encouraged to grieve, and she has suffered the loss of only one person. A dying person is losing everyone he ever loved—he's a thousand times more sad, and he should be allowed to cry, to mourn the losses he anticipates."

Finally, the dying person may enter the last stage: acceptance. "My time is very close now and it's all right." Dr. Ross says that "this is not a happy stage, but neither is it unhappy. It's almost devoid of feelings, but it's not resignation. It's really a victory." During the stage of acceptance, the person is not likely to talk much anymore. The best thing to do is sit with him quietly and hold his hand, Dr. Ross found.

Not all dying persons go through this orderly progression. Sometimes they skip stages or return to a previous stage. And some do not want to die in a state of acceptance; they want to go out fighting, and they should be allowed to do so, Dr. Ross says. "If you listen to the patient, he will tell you how he wants to die."

She illustrated the progression to the stage of acceptance in the drawings of an eight-year-old boy with an inoperable brain tumor. At first the boy was afraid of death and viewed it as a destructive force. He drew a picture of a large tank with a very small boy holding up a stop sign in front of it. Later, as he came to accept his impending death, he drew a bird with a touch of yellow on one wing. He described it as "a bird of peace flying up to the sky with a little bit of sunshine on my wing."

In general, Dr. Ross has discovered, children are often far ahead of their families in dealing with their impending death, with the family "limping along behind the child and rarely reaching acceptance before the child dies." She emphasizes the importance of dealing honestly with a dying child, and tells of seven-year-old Susie who was dying of leukemia and tired of being lied to about the fate of friends who "disappeared" from her hospital ward. One day Susie tried a frontal attack. She asked everyone she saw, "What's going to happen to me when I die?" The doctor answered, "I hear my page." The nurse said, "You're a bad girl; don't talk like that. Just take your medicine and you'll get well." But the minister replied with a question of his own; "What do you think is going to happen?" Susie answered, "One of these days I will fall asleep and when I wake up I will be with Jesus and my little sister." The minister said, "That must be very beautiful," and at last Susie was satisfied.

In another case, Fred, a 16-year-old boy, was dying of leukemia. His doctor wanted to discuss his illness with him, but Fred's parents forbade it and circumvented the boy's questions. Finally Fred asked the same questions of each of his doctors and nurses, then confronted them all with the discrepancies in their replies. He told his parents that he no longer believed them, that he knew he was going to die and how he wanted his favorite belongings disposed of.

Dr. C. M. Binger, who with his colleagues studied the emotional impact of childhood leukemia, remarked about the "pathetic loneliness of a fatally ill child who has no one with whom he may talk over his serious concerns because his parents are frequently trying to shield him from the diagnosis. Whereas dying adults can express some of their feelings to their spouses, to mature and respected friends, to the clergy or to doctors, the dying child may have to deal alone with his fears, concerns and apprehensions and also cope with his own inner scheme of fantasies and 'white lies' developed by his parents so that meaningful communication between the child and adults is prevented."

"Hope," Dr. Binger noted, "rests not only on life or death." At the beginning of terminal illness, Dr. Ross says, hope is associated with cure, treatment and prolongation of life. But toward the end, hope means different things— like, "I hope my children are going to make it." "I hope God will accept me in His garden." "I hope I will not be deserted."

Actually, for most dying persons, *the fear of abandonment is greater than the fear of death itself.* Too often, once medicine has nothing more to offer the patient in terms of effective treatment, the doctors stop coming around very often. Nurses and visitors feel uncomfortable and keep their visits short and perfunctory, carefully evading all leading questions. The patient feels desperately, frighteningly alone.

Dr. Charles Garfield, a California psychologist who organized the Shanti Project—groups of professional and lay volunteeers who provide companionship and emotional and spiritual support to dying persons and their families—points out that "a patient will often maintain a smiling, happy face even though he is dying because he knows that doctors and nurses respond well to that and won't bother with him unless he does. Instead of the support system helping the patient, the patient is protecting the support system." Dr. Garfield found that patients frequently complain that "they can't talk to their families—that they feel the family has deserted them." Shanti Project volunteers (Shanti means peace in Sanskrit) act as advocates of the dying patient and his family, helping them to establish channels of communication, deal with their feelings, unfinished business, the real and imagined insults of a lifetime, the unsaid "I love you's."

When families are able to reach the stage of acceptance before the patient dies, the period of mourning is usually brief and healthy. But too often the survivors fail to work through their feelings and suffer prolonged and painful grief responses. During the month after her husband died of cancer, Mrs. G. had spent her nights going over and over in her mind the hours of his suffering, wishing she had done this or that for him, wearying herself with sleeplessness and burying herself alive under a tomb of anxiety. Finally, after yet another sleepless night, at five o'clock in the morning she spoke to God. "Lord," she said, "I did all I knew to do for him while he was here, but I can't stand any more of this! What is it you want me to do now?" The Lord answered her, "Why won't you release him to me . . . let me take care of him from now on?"

Mrs. G. then fell sound asleep. She was at peace at last. A similar peace can be, and often is, achieved by persons without religious faith; a peace negotiated on the grounds that all that could be done was done and that, in any case, it's over now and life must go on for the living.

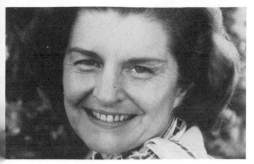

Betty Ford, wife of President Gerald Ford, had a mastectomy for breast cancer in September 1974.

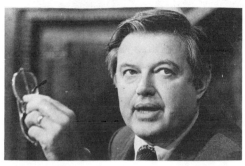

Frank Church, United States Senator from Idaho, cured of testicular cancer in 1948.

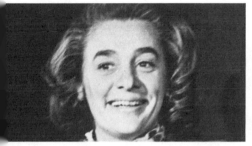

Margaretta (Happy) Rockefeller, wife of Vice President Nelson Rockefeller, had two mastectomies for breast cancer in 1974.

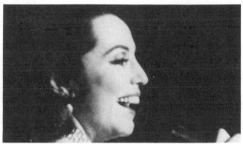

Marguerite Piazza, nightclub entertainer and former Metropolitan Opera singer, cured of melanoma, a serious skin cancer involving the face, in 1969.

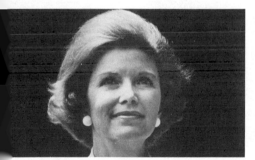

Marvella Bayh, wife of Senator Birch Bayh of Indiana, had a mastectomy for breast cancer in 1971.

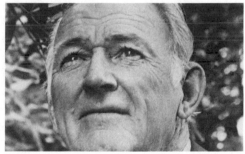

William Gargan, actor, cured of cancer of the larynx in 1960.

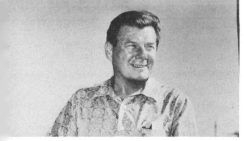

Arthur Godfrey, television and radio personality, cured of lung cancer in 1959.

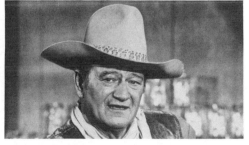

John Wayne, film star, cured of lung cancer in 1964.

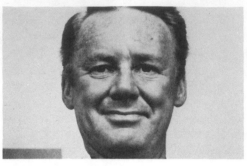

Van Johnson, actor, cured of melanoma in 1963.

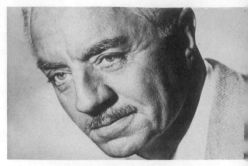

William Powell, film star, cured of recta. cancer in 1938.

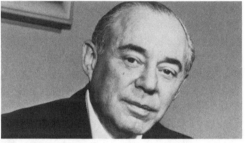

Richard Rodgers, composer, cured of cancer of the jaw in 1958.

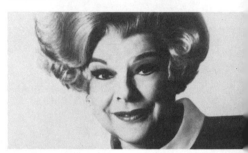

Virginia Graham, television and radio personality, cured of cancer of the uteru in 1951.

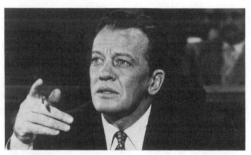

William Talman, television actor, died of lung cancer in 1968. During his illness, he made a short film for the American Cancer Society to warn others about the hazards of smoking.

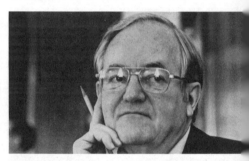

Hubert Humphrey, United States Sena tor from Minnesota and former Vic President, was treated for bladder cance in 1973 and 1976.

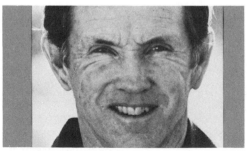

Gene Littler, professional golfer, treated for melanoma in 1972.

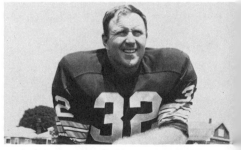

Jack Pardee, professional football playe cured of melanoma in 1965.

Part IV
UNDERSTANDING CANCER

19. Who Gets Cancer?

Cancer is a disease that has been known since ancient times. Evidence of cancer has been found in fossil bones, and descriptions of cancer symptoms appear in the Egyptian papyri dating back to around 1700 B.C. But for the most part, cancer is a disease of modern civilization. In societies where poor housing, nutrition and medical care have kept the lifespan short, cancer is a relatively uncommon disease. But in countries that have achieved a high standard of living—where infection, malnutrition, internal warfare, and other threats to life and health have been largely overcome—cancer is a leading cause of death. It is, in a sense, the price one pays for the opportunity to lead a relatively good, long life.

Cancer is also a democratic disease. It is found in all races and ages of man, in all animals and in many, if not all plants. While the incidence of different types of cancers varies with different population groups, virtually no group is exempt from the threat of cancer. Prince and pauper, saint and sinner, atheist and true believer, black and white, Northerner and Southerner, urbanite, suburbanite, and country folk—all are at risk of developing cancer.

There are differences, however, in cancer rates among these various groups—differences that sometimes give clues to the causes of certain kinds of cancers. For example, cancer is considerably less common among Mormons and Seventh-day Adventists, who adhere to various restrictions in diet and lifestyle, than among their less ascetic compatriots. People like nuns and other women who refrain from sexual activity face little or no risk of developing cancer of the cervix, which, by contrast, is common among promiscuous women. On the other hand, women who do not have children have a greater than usual chance of getting breast cancer. People who live in cities, where the air and water is often heavily polluted with industrial chemicals and vehicular exhaust, have an increased risk of developing a variety of cancer, including lung and bladder cancer, compared to persons living in nearby rural areas.

213

One in four Americans can expect to develop cancer at some point during his lifetime. Ultimately the disease afflicts two in three families. The greatest number of cancer cases occurs around the ages of 65 to 70. Sixty-seven percent of the cancers in man and 63 percent of those in women occur at age 55 or older. The risk of getting cancer more than doubles with each decade of life after age 20. Fifteen of every 100,000 20-year-olds get cancer, compared to 1,000 of every 100,000 60-year-olds. Although cancer is generally considered a disease of old age, it is also the largest cause of death—except for accidents—among Americans between the ages of 1 and 35. It is the leading disease-related cause of death in females up to age 65 and in males between the ages of 5 and 25.

Women generally get cancer at a younger age than men. Between the ages of 20 and 40, cancer occurs three times more often among women than men. But between ages 50 and 80, men have more cancer than women. Overall, cancer occurs more frequently in women than in men, but men have higher cancer death rates. This is largely because the cancer that occurs most frequently in men—lung cancer—is far less curable than the most common cancer in women—breast cancer. But it is also true that, site for site, women are more likely than men to survive cancer. This suggests that certain constitutional factors in women make them more resistant to the effects of cancer than men are. In general, for unknown reasons, married people are less likely to die of cancer than other people their age who are single, widowed or divorced. And people who live in urban areas have higher cancer death rates than rural residents. Leukemia and cancers of the respiratory tract, esophagus, kidney, bladder, mouth and throat are more common in cities.

In advanced societies like the United States, poor people tend to have more cancers and a greater cancer death rate than those who are financially better off. Among the poor, there is a marked excess of cancers of the cervix, esophagus, stomach, mouth, and respiratory tract. But the opposite is true for breast cancer, which occurs more frequently among middle and upper-income women, possibly because they tend to start having children later in life.

Religious factors indirectly influence a person's cancer risk. Cancer of the cervix is relatively rare among Jews. In a Boston study this disease occurred nine times more often among non-Jews. Prostate cancer is also less common in Jews. There is some suggestion that both these facts may be related to a greater tendency toward monogamy among Jews. Seventh-day Adventists have half the cancer rate of the general population. Strict Adventists do not smoke or drink alcoholic beverages, they seldom

ANNUAL NUMBER OF CANCERS BY AGE, RACE, AND SEX: United States (10% sample), 1969-1971 (All sites except skin and carcinoma-in-situ).

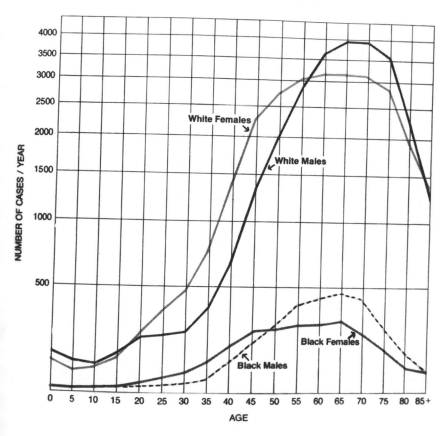

Cancer is primarily a disease of older people, with the vast majority of cases occurring among persons past the age of 50. At all ages, cancer occurs more frequently among whites than among blacks.

drink tea or coffee, often use whole grains and other unrefined foods, and most Adventists do not eat meat or very spicy foods. Cancer rates among Mormons are somewhat higher than those among Adventists, but still considerably lower than the general population. Mormons—members of the Church of Jesus Christ of Latter-Day Saints—prohibit smoking and drinking and use little coffee and tea. Their diet is less restricted than that of Adventists, but they put a great deal of emphasis on physical exercise, sleep, outdoor activities, and family life. Some of these factors, like smoking and alcohol, have been directly linked to an increased cancer risk. Others, like caffeine intake, are being studied to see what, if any, relationship they may have to cancer.

There are also differences in cancer rates among different racial groups. While white Americans of both sexes develop more cancer than nonwhites, cancer incidence and mortality have been increasing faster among American black men than any other group. Cancer death rates in American white men have also been increasing, but not as rapidly. The rapid recorded increase among blacks is in part a statistical artifact due to the fact that blacks now receive better medical care and are thus more likely to get their cancers diagnosed. But it also undoubtedly reflects the greater exposure of black men to cancer-causing agents on their jobs and to industrial and urban pollution, as well as differences in lifestyles, such as greater use of alcohol and tobacco. While cancer death rates have decreased among white women in this country, among American black women they have been holding relatively steady for several decades. In general, blacks are more likely than whites to develop cancer of the esophagus, pancreas, stomach, cervix, prostate and lung. But whites are more susceptible to cancer of the colon and rectum, breast, bladder, uterus, ovary and to leukemia and lymphoma.

The section of the country in which one lives also influences his cancer risk. Cancer death rates are highest in the Northeastern and Middle Atlantic states, lowest in the Rocky Mountain states, the Southwest, and the South (except the Atlantic coastal states and the Mississippi Delta), with intermediate rates along the Pacific Coast, South Atlantic coast and in the West Northcentral states. Cancer mortality in Alaska is less than half that in the New England states. In general, cancer rates are higher in the industrial states, with pockets of especially high cancer mortality in large cities.

In 1975 the National Cancer Institute issued a county-by-county atlas of cancer death rates for the 3,056 counties of the forty-eight contiguous states. The atlas represents more than five million cancer deaths that occurred between 1950 and 1969 for thirty-five cancer sites.

Studying these cancer patterns will help cancer specialists identify causes of cancer and alert them to population groups that may face an especially high risk of developing a particular cancer. This knowledge will make it easier to prevent cancer and detect it at its earliest, most curable stage. A number of cancer "hot spots" showed up on the maps. For example, in the 139 counties where chemical industries are located, rates for cancer of the bladder, lung, liver and certain other sites exceeded the expected rates

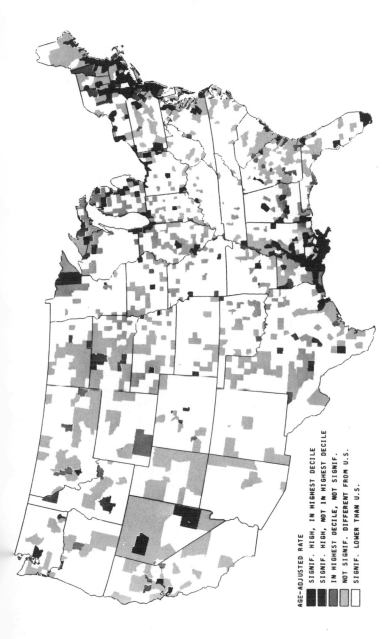

AGE-ADJUSTED RATE

■ SIGNIF. HIGH, IN HIGHEST DECILE
■ SIGNIF. HIGH, NOT IN HIGHEST DECILE
▨ IN HIGHEST DECILE, NOT SIGNIF.
░ NOT SIGNIF. DIFFERENT FROM U.S.
□ SIGNIF. LOWER THAN U.S.

In 1975, the National Cancer Institute compiled and published a series of maps showing cancer patterns throughout the country. The map above, representing all types of cancer occurring in white men in the years 1950 through 1969, shows that the highest cancer death rates were in the heavily industrialized sections. Salem County, New Jersey, the home of many chemical factories, had the highest cancer death rate of any county in the country.

among men. Salem County, New Jersey, where 25 percent of the men work in the chemical industry, had the highest rate of bladder cancer in the country. There were also excessive numbers of bladder cancer deaths in areas of heavy automobile production and increased lung cancer rates near copper, zinc, and lead smelters, possibly the result of arsenic given off by the smelter smokestacks. Surprisingly high death rates from lung cancer were found in the predominantly rural seaport areas along the Gulf Coast from Texas to the Florida Panhandle. The reason for this is as yet unclear.

Cancer of the colon and rectum, which is believed to be related to diet, was found in both men and women at above average rates in the Northeast and in urban areas along the Great Lakes. And breast cancer in women showed a similar pattern, suggesting that it too may have a dietary factor in common with bowel cancer. Stomach cancer was found to occur with unusual frequency in the Northcentral states, possibly reflecting the dietary habits associated with the Scandinavian and German ethnic backgrounds of many residents there.

In 1959 the American Cancer Society, through its elaborate network of volunteers, began a study of one million adult Americans around the country in the hopes of learning more about the factors that influence a person's chances of developing various types of cancers. Persons in the study represented a broad spectrum of socioeconomic and ethnic groups. Each participant completed a 200-item questionnaire that explored everything from family and personal medical history to dietary patterns, habits and exposure to air pollution. The participants were asked their occupational histories, including the names of any chemicals, fumes, or dusts they may have encountered on their jobs; what and how much they drank and smoked; how often they had sexual intercourse; their exercise patterns; use of medications; where they lived at different times of their lives; what kinds of stress they were under and any physical complaints they currently had. The women were quizzed on their reproductive and menstrual histories and whether they had nursed their children and for how long. The one million persons were recontacted annually for six years, and then again in 1971 and 1972. Each time they completed an abbreviated questionnaire, and death certificates were obtained for those who died. The initial contacts and all the subsequent tracing of participants in the study were done by American Cancer Society volunteers.

The findings of this massive study are still being analyzed. One major result thus far has been a detailed description of the relationship of tobacco smoking to lung cancer and other diseases. Dr.

E. Cuyler Hammond, Vice-President for Epidemiology and Statistics at the American Cancer Society and director of the study, was able to determine the precise relationship between the risk of death from various causes and factors such as how many cigarettes smoked, for how long and with what degree of inhalation. He was also able to demonstrate the life-saving value of stopping smoking. Continued analyses of the voluminous data gathered in this study are expected to reveal much more about who gets cancer and why.

20. The Impact of Cancer

Worldwide, between five and six million people get cancer each year, and more than three million eventually succumb to the disease. Cancer death rates are increasing throughout the world, in developed as well as in developing nations. Today in the United States, cancer is the second leading cause of death—after heart disease—among American men and women, white and nonwhite. And for women between the ages of 40 and 45, cancer is the leading cause of death. In the 1950s and 1960s, the cancer death rate among Americans increased six times faster than the death rate for heart disease. In 1935 there were 137,649 cancer deaths reported; in 1971, cancer accounted for 337,398 reported deaths. This increase in the total number of deaths reflects better reporting of cancer deaths and the fact that our population in the 1970s is older as well as larger, and therefore more prone to cancer. It also reflects a true increase in the incidence of cancer at all ages.

The incidence of cancer—that is, the number of new cases diagnosed over a given time period per 100,000 people in the population—increased by about one-third from 1935 to 1960. The rate as well as the number of cancer deaths in the United States has been increasing: the death rate rose from 112 per 100,000 in 1930 to 125 in 1950, to 132.7 in 1975. These figures have been adjusted for the changing age distribution of the population over the years compared. A major factor in the rising death rate is the cigarette smoking-caused epidemic of lung cancer, a cancer which is curable in less than 10 percent of patients.

Cancer survival rates among black Americans are nearly all lower than among whites with the same disease. On the basis of national statistics, Dr. LaSalle D. Leffall, Jr., Professor and Chairman of the Department of Surgery at Howard University College of Medicine, says, "We estimate that the present overall cancer cure rate [the percentage of patients alive with no apparent cancer five years after treatment] is 37 percent for black and 45

220

percent for white cancer patients." The difference in cure rates reflects the fact that cancer in blacks tends to be diagnosed at a later stage of disease than in whites, and, probably, that blacks are less likely to get the most up-to-date treatments. Survival rates are generally lower among black cancer patients even when their disease is diagnosed at a localized stage. Between 1950 and 1967, Dr. Leffall reports, the cancer death rate per 100,000 population for blacks of both sexes increased 20 percent, while it remained unchanged for whites. By 1967 the cancer death rate was 18 percent higher in blacks than in whites, although it was two percent lower in 1950. National statistics show that the most common cancers, including lung, breast, colon, pancreas, prostate, esophagus and bladder, are increasing in frequency faster in blacks than in whites. Several of these—lung, esophagus and pancreas—are associated with very low survival rates. And for cancers that are becoming less common, such as cancer of the stomach and cervix, the decrease is occurring more slowly in blacks than in whites.

If all cancer deaths were eliminated, the average lifespan of Americans would increase by two years. While this may not seem like much, for the person who actually gets cancer, prevention of cancer deaths would mean that an average of sixteen years would be added to his life expectancy. Obviously, the younger the person when cancer strikes, the more significant the elimination of cancer death would be.

Dr. James L. Murray and Lillian M. Axtell of the National Cancer Institute measured the impact of cancer in terms of years of life and work lost because of deaths from various cancers. Their analysis puts a new perspective on the relative importance of the different cancers because it reflects lost potential instead of merely counting deaths of individuals, many of whom were old and would have died shortly of something else had they not died of cancer. All told, based on the 318,495 reported deaths from cancer in the United States in 1968 (the total is considerably higher now), 1.7 million years of work and 5.1 million years of life were lost to cancer. Lung cancer, which is the leading cause of cancer death in American men, resulted in three times more lifetime lost than any other type of cancer in men. After lung cancer came cancer of the colon, lymphoma, leukemia, prostate, pancreas, stomach and brain.

When just the total number of deaths is considered, lymphoma ranks as the sixth leading cause of cancer deaths in American men. But since lymphoma tends to strike at a relatively young age as cancers go, it is number three when calculated as years of lifetime lost. And prostate cancer, the second leading cause of cancer

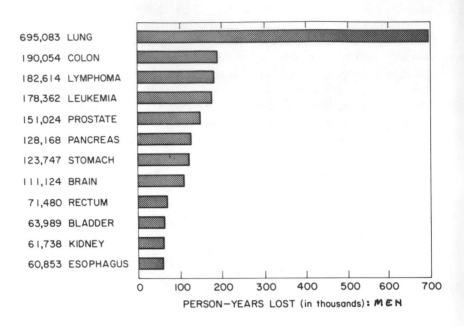

695,083 LUNG
190,054 COLON
182,614 LYMPHOMA
178,362 LEUKEMIA
151,024 PROSTATE
128,168 PANCREAS
123,747 STOMACH
111,124 BRAIN
71,480 RECTUM
63,989 BLADDER
61,738 KIDNEY
60,853 ESOPHAGUS

PERSON—YEARS LOST (in thousands): MEN

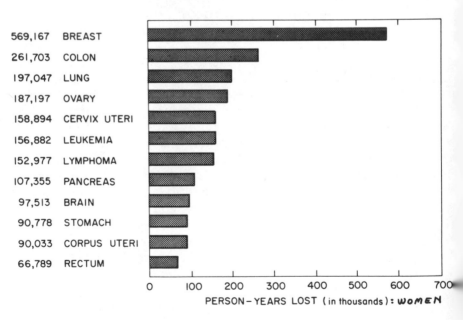

569,167 BREAST
261,703 COLON
197,047 LUNG
187,197 OVARY
158,894 CERVIX UTERI
156,882 LEUKEMIA
152,977 LYMPHOMA
107,355 PANCREAS
97,513 BRAIN
90,778 STOMACH
90,033 CORPUS UTERI
66,789 RECTUM

PERSON—YEARS LOST (in thousands): WOMEN

The impact of cancer can be measured in part in terms of the number of years of life lost as a result of cancer deaths. The charts show the number of "person-years" of life lost from the leading types of cancer in the United States in 1968, for men above, and for women below.

deaths in men when just numbers are counted, becomes the fourth when considering years of lifetime lost, since it is primarily a disease of elderly men.

For women, breast cancer is the leading cancer killer, resulting in more than twice the years of lifetime lost than from any other cancer. After breast cancer come cancers of the colon, lung, ovary, cervix, leukemia and lymphoma. When men and women are considered together, leukemia—which ranks seventh in terms of numbers of deaths among men and ninth among women— becomes second in terms of work years lost because it tends to strike in childhood. Thus, improvements in treatment that lead to cures of some of the more infrequent cancers that occur at an early age can mean a lot more years of life saved than progress toward curing a common disease like prostate cancer.

Indeed, in 1960 few children with acute lymphocytic leukemia survived a year after diagnosis and less than 10 percent of patients with advanced Hodgkin's disease, a lymphoma that usually strikes in the early decades of life, lived for five years. Today, some medical centers report that more than half their young patients with acute leukemia are alive and well five years later and at other centers five-year survival among all patients with advanced Hodgkin's disease has increased to about 80 percent. A substantial proportion of these patients are believed to have been cured of their disease; that is, they can be expected to live out a normal life span. In one leading medical center in 1967, one quarter of all children with cancer survived five years free of disease following treatment; by 1972, half of young patients with cancer could expect to be alive and well five years later. The savings in years of life from this kind of progress against cancer are enormous— greater than if similar progress had been made in the treatment of prostate cancer, which is far more common than leukemia.

Progress in preventing cancer can also result in significant monetary savings. According to a survey by the National Cancer Institute, approximately 1.3 million people in the United States get hospital care for cancer each year. With the average hospital stay lasting sixteen days, the annual cost of in-hospital care for cancer in this country in 1969 was $1.8 billion. If doctors' fees and costs of outpatient care are added to this, the total comes to about $3 billion. In 1975 Institute officials estimated that inflation had increased the total to $4 billion, which they call a highly conservative estimate.

To the medical costs must be added the cost of time lost from work and other disease-related costs, including the need for a housekeeper or at-home nursing care, and the cost of cancer rapidly mounts into the tens of billions of dollars a year. Just in terms of the wages involved in the 1.8 million years of potential working time lost as a result of cancer deaths each year, the disease represents an economic loss nationally of $18.9 billion a year.

In a report to Congress in 1970 that led to the establishment of the National Cancer Program, a panel of expert consultants pointed out that cancer is the Number One health concern of the American people. In a national poll in 1966, 62 percent said that they feared cancer more than any other disease. The panel added, "Cancer often strikes as harshly at human dignity as at human life; and more often than not it represents financial catastrophe for the family in which it strikes." The nation—mainly through the National Cancer Program and the American Cancer Society— is now waging an $800 million-a-year battle against this scourge.

21. What Is Cancer?

Perhaps the most telling fact about cancer is that the more scientists have learned about it, the more complex a disease it is understood to be. When the National Cancer Institute was established by an act of Congress on August 5, 1937 there was a naive optimism among scientists and legislators that the concentration of several hundred thousand dollars a year on the cancer problem would lead to its prompt solution. The institute spent $4 million on cancer research in its first thirty-six years, only to discover that the mystery scientists were trying to unravel was far darker and more entangled then they could ever have dreamed a generation earlier.

The disease cancer was named by ancient Greek physicians for the sea crab, because the earliest known form of cancer, breast cancer, resembled claws extending from a central lump. Cancer might be thought of as a population problem among cells. Cancer cells continue to grow and multiply out of control, irrespective of the needs of normal surrounding cells. In the process cancer cells are greedy consumers of the body's resources, using space and nutrients as if they were in unlimited supply. Cancer cells can grow even if the rest of the body is starving. Since they grow at the expense of the normal cells, cancer cells, if unchecked, eventually destroy the organism that harbors them.

All cancers except leukemia form tumors, but not all tumors are cancer. Most tumors—such as warts, moles, and cysts—are benign. Like cancers, benign tumors also can continue to enlarge, but they rarely kill the host unless they happen to severely compress a vital organ, such as the brain, or cause a hemorrhage.

Cancer cells, however, have another deadly property not found in benign tumors: cancers can invade surrounding tissues and can dispatch small groups of cells to set up colonies of cancer in distant parts of the body. This is called the ability to metastasize—to spread through the blood or lymph system and establish tumors elsewhere. In most cases of cancer, it is the metastases that actually

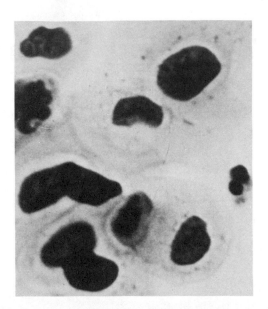

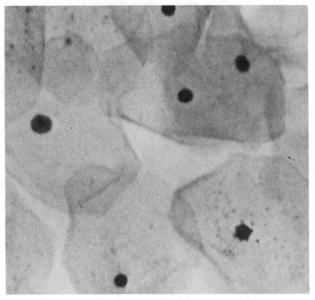

Under a microscope, cancer cells look very different from normal cells. Notice the enlarged nuclei (dark central portions) of the cells, top, which are cancer cells taken from the cervix, compared to normal cells, bottom, from the same organ.

kill the patient. Completely localized cancers can nearly always be cured through surgery, radiation therapy or drug therapy.

Ordinary cells, be they in the liver, heart, muscles, or lungs, are governed by some control mechanism that tells them when to stop multiplying. This control in part involves how a cell responds to its neighbors—a kind of social interaction that dictates the size and shape of cells and how many copies they make of themselves. Cellular "social restraints" keep normal cells in their place. Thus, a normal liver gets so big and no bigger. When some liver cells die, they are replaced by new healthy cells—just enough to maintain the proper size and function of this vital organ. Even in the growing child, the mechanism governing the rate of cell multiplication is finely controlled, so that at each stage of a child's life, his organs are of an appropriate size. But for reasons not completely understood, cancer cells seem to have lost this fine control. They have no respect for the rights of their neighbors and readily invade territory that is already occupied. Either the message telling cancer cells when to stop dividing is not being given out, or it is somehow garbled, or the cancer cells can no longer receive it in a meaningful way. In short, there seems to be a serious communications failure involved in cancer. Scientists throughout the world are working very hard to understand how and why this failure occurs, with the hope that such an understanding will lead to more effective means of detecting and controlling the disease.

Although no single distinguishing biochemical characteristic has yet been found for all cancers, certain important differences between cancerous and normal cells have already been identified. These include differences in cell chemistry, such as the presence or absence of certain enzymes, and differences in immunology— the production of substances by cells that tell the body's natural defense system that a foreign material is present. These differences are being intensively explored for their potential value in providing very early clues to the presence of cancer cells in the body. Such differences have already given scientists several ways of attacking cancer cells while causing little or no harm to normal cells, and additional methods will undoubtedly emerge from continuing research.

Although both may come from the same organ, cancer looks different from normal tissue under a microscope, and it is on the basis of these differences that the pathologist makes a diagnosis of cancer. Cancer cells tend to have different shapes and sizes and take up cell stains in different ways. Cancer cells are arranged differently in relation to one another and sometimes their invasion of surrounding tissues can be seen.

It is not yet known exactly what happens to a cell to make it a cancer cell. Is there an underlying type of derangement common to all cancer cells? Can cancer start from any of a number of different changes in the cell? Are several simultaneous or sequential changes necessary? Opinions abound, but facts are relatively few. Here again, though, the resolution of this question should give medicine a much better handle on controlling the cancer process.

22. How Does Cancer Start?

One thing definitely known about cancer is that many different agents can in some way initiate its growth. The list of known cancer-causing agents—or carcinogens—includes physical things like ultraviolet light, X-rays, and radioactive elements; inorganic substances like asbestos, arsenic, and nickel; organic chemicals like benzidine, tobacco products, and dyes derived from coal tars; natural body substances like estrogens; and poisons like aflatoxin, which is produced by a mold.

Some cancer-causing agents appear to act alone; others need helpers, called cocarcinogens or promoters, to start the cancer process on a lethal course. Certain hormones can sometimes act as promoters of carcinogens. Although it is not known exactly how carcinogens work, many are known to be able to throw a monkey wrench into the genetic material of cells and in the process may disrupt the cell's growth-controlling machinery. Some chemical carcinogens may also act by suppressing the body's ability to recognize and destroy foreign invaders, thus allowing a cancer to grow. Other carcinogens may work by activating a cancer-causing virus, enabling it to change the genetic message of cells.

In animal studies, carcinogens have been shown to cause irreversible changes in cells. Usually, many exposures to a carcinogen are necessary to cause cancer, but it has yet to be demonstrated that there can be a dose of a carcinogen so low that cancer would not result in any exposed individuals. In other words, it has not been possible to determine a "safe" level of any cancer-causing agent, although the lower the level, the less likely it is that cancer will develop during the lifetime of those who come into contact with it. Thus, a two-packs-a-day smoker is more likely to get lung cancer than someone who smokes only half a pack a day. However, the half-a-pack-a-day smoker still is exposed to the cancer-causing effects of cigarette smoke and is more likely to get lung cancer than someone who does not smoke at all.

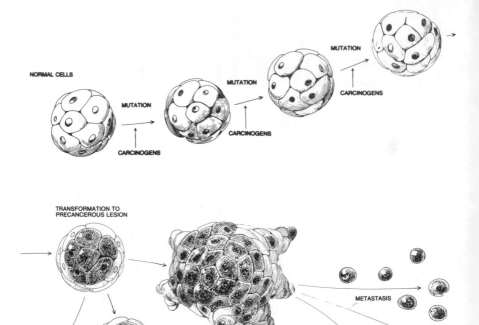

One theory of how cancer starts is that a series of mutations, or changes in the genetic material of cells, must occur in a single line of cells. The mutations (represented as black dots in the nuclei, or center, of the cells) are apparently caused by carcinogenic factors in the environment that reach the cells. After an unknown number of mutations, the cells are transformed into a precancerous lesion, which may then regress back to normalcy, grow very slowly or develop into a rapidly growing malignant tumor that can send offshoots through the blood or lymph system to establish cancer colonies elsewhere in the body. This system of spread, which is the usual cause of death from cancer, is called metastasis. (*Scientific American*)

A further mystery about carcinogens is the fact that, unlike a cold which develops within a few days of exposure to the infectious virus, cancer does not appear until many years after a person has been exposed to the cancer-causing agent. In some cases, like lung cancer induced by cigarette smoking, exposure over a period of many years seems to be necessary to produce the cancer. In others, such as radiation-induced cancers, a brief exposure to the carcinogen followed by many years without any subsequent exposure seems capable of initiating the cancer process. Thus, carcinogens have a "time bomb" effect, and the exact setting of the bomb's clock in any particular case is not known until the bomb goes off—that is, until the cancer becomes clinically apparent. The time between first exposure to the carcinogen and the onset of cancer is called the latent period. For some carcinogens and the cancers they cause, the latent period can be as long as twenty-five, thirty, or even forty years. For others, it may be relatively short—ten or fifteen years. Cancer promoters, such as hormones, can sometimes shorten the latent period. In any case this latency effect makes it all the more difficult to identify agents that cause particular cancers. Not only do people often forget relevant experiences, they also tend to dissociate events that are not closely linked in time. Many cigarette smokers think, "Well, I've been smoking for thirty years and I haven't got cancer yet, so I guess I'm not going to get it." This attitude is not uncommon with respect to other carcinogens as well. And a worker who gets cancer at age 45 is not likely to link it to the job he had for a few years after he left high school.

Exactly what happens during the latent period is not known, but it is likely that a complex progression of events must take place before clinical cancer can develop. A cell may be changed from normal to abnormal (with the potential for being a cancer cell) at the time of initial exposure to the carcinogen. This abnormality may be passed on to daughter cells but remain dormant for many years. With time, however, further changes may occur in the abnormal cells' machinery making them more and more independent of the controls on normal cells. Eventually, the abnormal cells may become totally independent and divide and reproduce in a totally uncontrolled fashion. Whether these events take place or not depends on many factors, including the dose of the carcinogen, how it enters the body, and how long and how often one is exposed to it, as well as characteristics of the individual, such as age, sex, and genetic background. Because this chain of events is long and complex, it may one day be possible to interrupt it before clinical cancer develops. With lung cancer caused by cigarette smoking, this is already possible merely by stopping smoking. The body is somehow able to repair the cellular damage even after decades of exposure to cigarette smoke. The former smoker's risk of lung cancer drops quickly, and ten years after quitting his risk is nearly as low as that of the person who never smoked.

In animals it is well known that certain cancers are caused by viruses. But human cancer viruses, if there are any, have thus far eluded the intensive search of scientists. Several viruses have recently been closely linked with certain human cancers, but proof positive that these viruses were somehow involved in causing the disease is still lacking.

Even if a viral cause for some human cancers is proven, this does not mean that cancer is a contagious disease that can spread from one person to another. Although "clusters" of cases of a few types of cancer have been identified, there is no evidence that cancer is "contagious" in the usual sense of the word. Thus far, cancer virus research has indicated that if viruses can cause cancer in man, they work quite differently from viruses that cause infectious, contagious diseases. Rather than invading and destroying normal cells like an infectious virus does, the cancer virus seems capable of becoming a permanent part of the machinery of a normal cell without killing it. The genes of the cancer virus become incorporated into the genetic material of the normal body cells, subtly subverting them into doing work dictated by the virus genes in addition to the work of the cell's own genes. A cancer virus seems able to remove the normal growth restraints on a cell. Many scientists believe that cancer viruses are only able to do their dirty work if they are in some way activated by another agent, such as a chemical carcinogen or radiation, which allows the information in the viral genes to be expressed.

Despite the widespread presence of cancer-causing agents, relatively few of the people exposed to these agents actually get cancer. Some studies of suspected cancer viruses—for example, the herpes virus that causes a common venereal disease and that has been linked to cancer of the cervix—indicate that cancer viruses may be present in very large numbers of people, but only relatively few of those who have the virus actually get cancer. Only one in ten cigarette smokers eventually contracts lung cancer, although a smoker's chances of getting this disease is ten times higher than it would be if he did not smoke. While many smokers die of other smoking-caused diseases before they have a chance to develop lung cancer, others smoke heavily for decades and live to a ripe old age without getting cancer. Thus, there is something inherent in certain individuals that makes them prone—or resistant—to the effects of cancer-causing substances.

The differences between cancer-prone and cancer-resistant individuals are not yet well understood. Those differences that have been identified or suspected include the lack of certain enzymes, defects in the body's natural immunological defense system, changes in hormone patterns and perhaps psychological states. Sometimes certain types of cancer, such as cancer of the breast or cancer of the colon and rectum, seem to run in families. In these families, a particular genetic characteristic predisposes many of the family members to cancerous or precancerous changes. For example, in families where multiple benign tumors of the lower bowel (polyps) are extremely common—a very rare condition known as familial polyposis—the incidence of colon-rectal cancer is extremely high. In such families, members who develop familial polyposis are advised to have their colons removed as a cancer preventive.

It is also likely that in the course of a person's lifetime, his relative resistance or susceptibility to cancer may vary. Some change in body physiology may temporarily render a person more susceptible to the disease, although the exact reasons for such changes in susceptibility are not fully understood. It is generally believed that tiny colonies of cancer cells arise fairly frequently in most people, but that under ordinary circumstances, the body's immunological system is able to recognize these cancer colonies as "foreign" to the body and can marshal the necessary forces either to hold them in check or wipe them out before they get a firm foothold.

According to this view, it is only the rare cancer colony that manages to escape the body's continual surveillance of all its nooks and crannies for the presence of foreigners. This may result from a breakdown in immunologic surveillance or because the cancer cells acquire a "disguise" that prevents the immune system from recognizing them as foreigners. In doing autopsies on people who died from causes other than cancer, doctors frequently find small "silent" cancers that the body apparently was able to control. For some cancers such silent cases are actually more common than the clinical disease itself. Since it is already known that the immunological capabilities of the body decline with age, this view of how cancer can start is consistent with the fact that most cancers do not strike until middle age and that the disease becomes more and more common as people get older.

An unfortunate episode in the history of modern organ transplants also demonstrates the importance of the immune system in cancer. In the early days of organ transplants, an occasional patient received a seemingly cancer-free organ donated by a person who had cancer elsewhere in the body. In a few cases, however, the transplanted organ apparently contained some cancer cells and the recipient of the organ himself developed cancer. This apparently happened because, in an effort to prevent rejection of the donated organ, the recipient was placed on large doses of drugs that suppress the body's immunological response. When the donor's cancer appeared in the recipient, the immune-suppressing drugs were stopped. In many cases the recipient then rejected not only the donated organ but the cancer as well. Now transplant surgeons are extremely careful in choosing organs for transplants from donors who have no evidence of cancer.

However, transplant recipients and patients with diseases that require treatment with immunosuppressive drugs have been found to face an increased risk of developing their own cancers or recurrences of previous cancers that had not been totally eradicated. In most cases the cancers appear within two years after transplantation, indicating that immune suppression can speed up the development of cancer. In fact, since many of the drugs (and radiation therapy) used to treat cancer also happen to suppress the immunological response, cancer patients who receive prolonged therapy of this sort also seem to face a somewhat higher than normal chance of developing a second cancer. Furthermore, persons who are already suffering from what are called immunological deficiency diseases—that is, their bodies fail to produce all the cells that normally comprise the immune defense system—are far more likely than other people to develop cancer and often at a younger age than would be expected.

Changes in immunological capabilities probably also explain at least some of the rare cases of cancer that seem to disappear on their own, rather than as a result of any definitive therapy. In some cases of "spontaneous regression" of cancer, it appears that the person's immune system got a sudden jolt to wake it up, allowing it to recognize the foreign invader and destroy it. A better understanding of how the body's immune system works or fails to work in cancer could provide important therapeutic tools as well as invaluable aids in early diagnosis of the disease. Immunological therapy of cancer is still in its infancy and more refined methods are needed before it can be widely and most effectively applied, but its promise has already been clearly demonstrated by physicians in several countries.

23. What Causes Cancer?

Although the exact mechanisms of how cancer starts remain a mystery, it has been possible to identify many actual and potential causes of cancer. There is little doubt that prevention is currently our most effective weapon against cancer. If human exposure to known cancer-causing agents could be avoided and if other factors involved in stimulating cancer could be modified, the cancer problem would be reduced to a fraction of its current size.

"The germs of cancer in the year 2000 are in our environment now," says Dr. Irving J. Selikoff, Director of the Environmental Sciences Laboratory at Mount Sinai School of Medicine in New York. "Research into the environmental causes of cancer, followed by application of the findings to protect the public from unnecessary exposure to agents found to be cancer-causing, is essential if we are going to prevent new 'epidemics' of cancer twenty and thirty years from now." Dr. Selikoff points out that such preventive action is necessary to avoid future disasters such as the one that has followed the widespread adoption of cigarette smoking. A generation passed before the cancer-causing effects of cigarette smoking were recognized, and only then after the nation faced an epidemic of smoking-caused cancers.

The first step in any control program must be identification of the "bad actors." Some 20,000 chemicals are currently in wide use, and several thousand new ones are introduced each year. Very few of these substances are tested first for their cancer-causing potential. In a policy statement issued by the Board of Directors in 1976, the American Cancer Society urged "government, industry, and labor to share responsibility for the screening and testing of products and by-products of industry to which large numbers of human beings are, and will be, exposed."

The National Cancer Institute is currently supporting cancer tests in animals of some 450 different chemicals that are both widely used and suspect because they are related to known carcinogens. Included in the tests are drugs, industrial chemicals, pesticides, and other agricultural chemicals, food additives, metallic compounds, and natural plant products. At best, though, animal tests can only suggest—never prove—that a substance is carcinogenic for man. Different animals are susceptible to the effects of different agents. A particular substance may cause cancer in one type of animal and have no effect in several others. Indeed, one kind of mouse may be totally resistant to an agent that causes cancer in large numbers of mice of a different strain. Thus, animal experiments merely raise a red flag for man, and judgments taking many different factors into account must be made in applying the findings of animal tests to man.

Many thousands of substances should ultimately be tested for cancer-causing potential. But since animal tests take a minimum of two years to complete and cost about $75,000 for each substance tested, simpler, faster, and less expensive tests on bacteria have been devised to screen large numbers of substances for possible cancer-causing effects. The bacterial tests indicate whether partic-

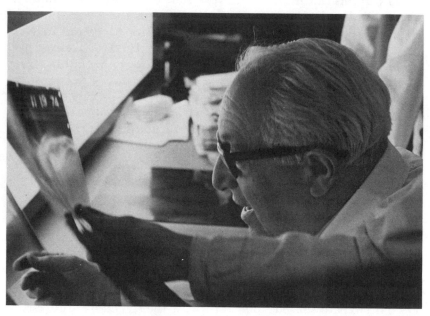

Dr. Irving J. Selikoff, director of the Environmental Sciences Laboratory at Mount Sinai Medical Center in New York, reviews chest X-rays of a worker who is participating in an extensive study to help define causes of cancer. The study of various occupations is being supported by the American Cancer Society.

ular substances can damage the genetic material of cells. Because genetic material is essentially the same type of substance regardless of whether it comes from a microorganism, a mouse, or a man, the bacterial tests can serve as an early warning system and help in the selection of agents that should be examined for cancer-causing ability in animal experiments and in studies of people who have been exposed to the suspected agents. Recently, for example, Dr. Bruce Ames, a biochemist at the University of California in Berkeley who devised the most widely used of these bacterial tests, showed that the vast majority of hair dyes, both permanent and semi-permanent, currently sold in the United States can damage bacterial genes. Since it is known that the dyes can be absorbed into the body through the skin, this finding warrants a much closer look at the possible effects of these substances on man, especially since they are used regularly by an estimated 20 million Americans.

Thus far, the major tool used to identify cancer-causing agents has been man himself—through the study of groups of people who seem to face a much higher than usual chance of getting a certain type of cancer. This is the science of epidemiology, which involves the study of patterns of disease in various populations. Thus, among cigarette smokers, asbestos workers, uranium miners, and others, lung cancer has been found to be unusually common, and studies of such people have helped researchers pinpoint certain causes of lung cancer. Light-skinned people who are out in the sun a lot are especially prone to skin cancer, caused by damage to skin cells by the ultraviolet rays in sunlight. Certain dye workers face an unusually high risk of bladder cancer, and the dyes they work with have been shown to be carcinogenic. In parts of Africa and Asia where liver cancer is extremely common, its likely cause has been traced to a poison called aflatoxin produced by a mold that grows on poorly stored foods.

In other cases, relationships between certain cancers and particular circumstances have been described, but the precise cancer-causing factors have not yet been identified. For example, people living in urban areas are more prone to several kinds of cancer than are people living in rural areas. Exposure to various air pollutants is suspected as one possible causal factor, but this has yet to be proved. Similarly, whereas the Japanese have a very high incidence of stomach cancer and a low incidence of cancer of the colon and rectum, the situation is precisely reversed in the United States. Dietary factors are thought to be involved in these cancers —and a number of plausible suggestions have been made—but the precise causes of these different cancer patterns is still unknown.

If the most effective possible weapon against cancer—prevention—is ever to be widely wielded, it will be necessary to understand the reasons for all such patterns and then take the necessary action to change them. Otherwise, we will always be fighting the cancer battle with one or two strikes against us—after cancer has already developed or after it has spread beyond the site of origin. For the last several years, the American Cancer Society has been sponsoring an extensive epidemiological study of some ten different groups of workers who are exposed to a variety of agents that may play a role in cancer. Included in the study being conducted by Dr. Selikoff of Mount Sinai Medical Center and Dr. Hammond of the Society are typographers, roofers, building tradesmen, insulation workers, printers and pressmen, painters, and chemical workers.

At the request of the workers, usually in cooperation with their union, the Selikoff team sets up what resembles the field hospital in "M*A*S*H*" as hundreds of workers line up for an intensive examination at a makeshift medical clinic. The team ships essential medical equipment from New York—centrifuges, microscopes, machines to measure lung function, blood pressure cuffs, stethoscopes, hundreds of slides, and thousands of test tubes. Conference tables covered with blankets and paper sheets become examining beds; motel ice buckets hold hundreds of tubes of blood; executive offices become medical laboratories.

One by one, the workers file through the examining procedure, starting with a seemingly endless questionnaire exploring their medical, family, and work histories. Then comes a urine sample, blood test, thorough physical, and lung function test. The medical team wants to know how every organ system is working—liver, kidneys, lungs, heart, brain—and attempts to relate any unusual incidence of abnormalities found to exposure to some noxious agent on the job. It may take a week to examine all the workers at one plant and months to analyze the results of all the studies.

Dr. Selikoff explains that workers are being studied not only to determine threats to their health but also because they are like "canaries in a coal mine" for the rest of the population. Because the workers are intensively exposed to many substances that are widespread in the general environment in less concentrated doses, the disease experience of the workers could help to zero in on agents that contribute to cancers in the general population and suggest which substances the public, as well as the workers, should be protected against.

One such substance Dr. Selikoff and his colleagues have found is asbestos, about four million tons of which are produced each year.

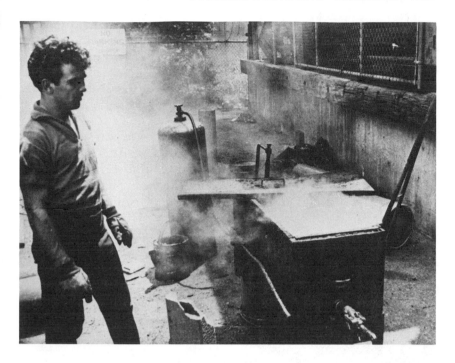

Roofers are exposed to fumes containing several known or suspected cancer-causing agents. Roofers are among the occupational groups being studied by the American Cancer Society to gain a better understanding of the causes of cancer.

A ubiquitous, inexpensive mineral well known for its fire-retardant properties and resistance to wear, asbestos has been used in such wide-ranging items as brake linings, pot holders, fire curtains, water pipes, spackle, floor and ceiling tiles, ironing board covers, insulation for pipes and ducts, paper, and textiles. As many as 3,000 different products in use throughout the world contain some asbestos. Asbestos had long been thought to be biologically inert—that is, with no effect on body tissues. But as the unfortunate experience of workers who mined asbestos and fashioned it into all these miraculous products so painfully demonstrated, asbestos fibers could wreak havoc years—decades—after it entered the body. The tiny, microscopic fibers are readily inhaled and once they enter the lungs or other body tissues (perhaps by swallowing asbestos-laden sputum), they tend to stay put.

Over the last twenty years Dr. Selikoff's careful studies of the death records of workers in a New Jersey asbestos factory showed that their death rate from lung cancer was about seven times what it should be and deaths from cancer of the gastrointestinal tract were three times higher than expected. Interestingly, lung cancer developed only in asbestos workers who smoked cigarettes, but these men faced a nine times greater risk of this disease than other smokers without occupational exposure to asbestos. There seems to be an interaction between asbestos and the carcinogens in cigarette smoke that multiplies the effects of the individual substances. All told, an asbestos worker who smoked was about sixty times more likely to get lung cancer than a nonsmoker who did not work with asbestos. In addition, the asbestos workers, whether they smoked or not, were prone to an otherwise extremely rare—and thus far invariably fatal—cancer called mesothelioma, which affects the lining of the chest or abdominal cavity. Recently, Dr. Selikoff's team found that not only were the workers more likely to get asbestos-related cancers, but so were their families—their wives and children and anyone who may have lived with them when they

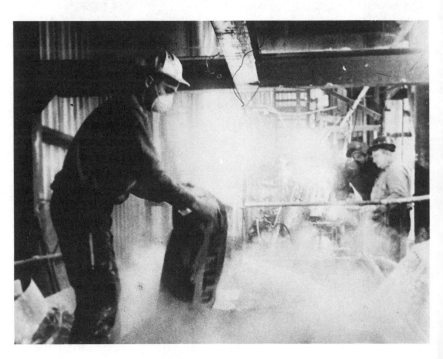

Worker in this asbestos plant was poorly protected from exposure to asbestos fibers, which lodge in the lungs and elsewhere, causing a crippling lung disease and cancers of the lung and gastrointestinal tract. The fate of asbestos workers has been studied intensively by Dr. Irving J. Selikoff of Mount Sinai School of Medicine.

returned home from the dusty factory in clothes covered with the deadly fibers. Some thirty years later, cases of mesothelioma, which almost never occurs without some link to asbestos, have begun to appear among family contacts of the New Jersey workers. Mesotheliomas are also being found among the millions of men and women who worked in shipyards during World War II, where asbestos was used as insulation. Some of the victims were only indirectly exposed to the mineral fibers, merely by working in the environment where asbestos was used. Dr. Selikoff reports that as little as one week of working in the shipyard may have been sufficient to plant the seeds of a cancer that would not become apparent until a generation later.

Why is this important to the average person? Because asbestos fibers contaminate the environment of most of us. The air in urban areas is filled with asbestos fibers, especially at street corners where cars stop and fibers from brake linings wear off. Air samples from sixty American cities showed that all had asbestos particles in the air, and autopsy studies have revealed that the lungs of nearly every New Yorker and other city residents who have been studied contain some asbestos fibers. The fibers have also been found in ovaries and other tissues. In 1973 large amounts of asbestos fibers were discovered in the drinking water of the city of Duluth, Minnesota, and other communities that draw their water from Lake Superior. Although long considered one of the world's purest lakes (so pure that Duluth didn't even bother to filter the water as it came from the lake), the clear blue lake waters were found to be contaminated with asbestos-laden rocky wastes from a mining company fifty miles north of Duluth where iron ore was being extracted from a rock called taconite.

A lengthy court battle raged, Duluth installed a filtration system, and the company which had been dumping into the lake for eighteen years was at last ordered to find an on-land site to get rid of its wastes. But then arguments over what site to use further delayed the court-ordered cleansing of the lake, and in 1976— three years after the original discovery—asbestos continued to enter the lake and large amounts of fibers also continued to enter the air through the company's smokestacks. Even after the dumping stops, the people of Duluth must live with the knowledge that their bodies may contain a cancer time bomb that could go off at any time, in a decade from now or even later.

The Duluth situation led to a check of water supplies in communities throughout the nation and, sure enough, many were found to contain fair amounts of asbestos, although none as much as Duluth's water. The source of the mineral fibers has variously been ascribed to the facts that the natural waterways pass through asbestos-containing rock formations, that asbestos-containing "gravel" is used to sand the roads in winter (running off into streams that feed reservoirs), that the very pipes that carry the water contain a mixture of asbestos and cement. As yet, it is not known whether lifelong exposure to such low levels of asbestos in any way contributes to the development of cancer in the general population. But since the causes of most cases of cancer can not be pinpointed, many doctors suspect that contamination of the general environment with such cancer-causing agents as asbestos increases the risk of cancer in many susceptible persons.

Another recently discovered occupational cancer also highlighted the potential risk to the public created by a substance once considered inert and remarkably safe. This substance is a manufactured organic chemical called vinyl chloride, a gas at room temperatures that is widely used in the plastics industry. Vinyl chloride is polymerized into more than four billion pounds a year of a plastic resin known as polyvinyl chloride, which in turn is fashioned into thousands of consumer products including paints, water pipes, furniture, upholstery, draperies, wall coverings, floor tiles, table cloths, toys, clothing, footwear, food packages, garden hoses, phonograph records, dentures, bottles and pharmaceutical products. More than a decade after exposure to vinyl chloride began, some workers employed in the polymerization plants developed an extremely rare and thus far invariably fatal liver cancer called angiosarcoma. A few cases of the cancer have since turned up among employees who make polyvinyl chloride into finished products and several suspicious cases have been found among residents who lived for many years in the immediate vicinity of a polymerization plant. There are also indications that prolonged exposure to vinyl chloride may cause cancers of the brain, lung, and lymph system.

It is unlikely that people who use products made from polyvinyl chloride could ever be exposed to enough vinyl chloride (tiny amounts of it remain unpolymerized in the plastic) to pose a cancer hazard of any significance. However, it soon came to light that vinyl chloride gas was widely used as a propellant in such household products as hair sprays, room fresheners, and pesticide sprays. An "average" spray in a small bathroom, for example, resulted in a concentration of vinyl chloride in the room air that readily caused cancer in experimental animals who inhaled the gas for prolonged periods. In addition, the Environmental Protection Agency found that vinyl chloride contaminates the air and runoff water around polymerization plants, with a total of 300 million pounds of the cancer-causing chemical entering the general environment each year. And the Food and Drug Administration has found that when polyvinyl chloride is used as food packaging, some vinyl chloride can be found in the foods. There is also some concern now about the potential hazards of a closely related chemical, vinyl bromide, that is widely used as a flame retardant on fabrics.

Although a great deal has been learned about what does and does not cause cancer through the types of studies described above, much undoubtedly remains to be discovered. Research into the causes of cancer has expanded rapidly in the 1970s and will continue to increase in scope and intensity. Cancer specialists realize now more than ever that the best way to prevent cancer deaths is to prevent cancer from starting in the first place, and that only through understanding and controlling the causes of cancer will widespread prevention be possible.

The following sections contain descriptions of what scientists have been able to learn so far about the various substances and factors that influence people's chances of getting cancer. Although the sections have been divided into topics, it must be remembered that probably in the vast majority of cases, two or more factors work together to cause cancer in an individual.

OCCUPATIONAL HAZARDS

The first description of an environmental carcinogen was written 200 years ago by an English surgeon, Percivall Pott, who reported that the chimney sweeps of London had an unusually high rate of cancer of the scrotum. Dr. Pott concluded that these men, who started their jobs as children and worked long hours, seldom washing thoroughly or changing clothes, accumulated deposits of coal soot which remained in contact with the skin for long periods.

Since Dr. Pott's report, the list of occupational cancers has grown tremendously. In recent years, as the episodes with asbestos and vinyl chloride demonstrate, many researchers and Federal agencies have become sensitized to the enormity of the problem and its potential significance to the general population as well as specific workers. Many thousands of workers die each year from occupationally caused cancers, and the same substances may kill equal or greater numbers of people in the general population. But the problems of identifying the causes of cancer in the workplace can be forbidding. Many workers don't even know the names of the chemicals they use, referring to them only by code number. Many work with several different agents, which—like asbestos and cigarette smoke—may act together to cause cancer, but the substances alone may have no such effect. In other cases the cancer-causing agent may produce a relatively small increase—say two-fold—in an otherwise common cancer, such as lung cancer or colon cancer, and it may be decades, if ever, before anyone realizes that the particular group of workers is being affected by an occupational carcinogen. Furthermore, unless a substance is a potent carcinogen and exposure to it is high, it may be decades before the first cancers among exposed workers become apparent.

Despite these difficulties, studies of the cancer experiences of different occupational groups have unveiled many cancer-causing agents. Lung cancer rates, for example, are greatly increased not only among asbestos workers but also among those who work with arsenic, coal tar and pitch, mustard gas, chromates, nickel, isopropyl oil and chloromethyl methyl ether, a substance used in manufacturing other chemicals.

Arsenic is but one example of how widespread the effects of an occupational carcinogen can be. This chemical has been implicated in cancer of the lung and other body sites among copper ore miners, smelters of nickel-cobalt ores, workers in insecticide manufacturing plants, and vineyard workers who apply insecticides. For some occupational carcinogens, dozens of different kinds of workers are exposed to their potential hazards. For example, chromate has been linked to a greatly increased risk of lung and other cancers and various chromium compounds are involved in the work of paper makers, furniture polishers, textile printers, welders and acetylene workers, candle and artificial flower makers, rubber workers, potters, photographic workers, and electroplaters, among many others.

A greatly increased risk of bladder cancer has been found among workers exposed to certain chemical dyes known as aromatic amines. One of these—benzidine—was first recognized by a British factory doctor as a possible cause of bladder cancer as early as 1929, but the exposure of American workers to this substance was not significantly curtailed by government action until 1972. Textile workers, engineering workers, and hairdressers also seem to face a higher than expected risk of bladder cancer, but the precise chemical culprits involved in these cases have not yet been identified. Many, however, work with dyes that are derived from coal tars.

The risk of developing skin cancer is higher than normal among those who work with arsenic, coal tar, petroleum, paraffins, creosote oils, anthracene oils, and carbon black. Workers exposed to benzol are prone to leukemia and various workers, including those involved with wood furniture and leather, have increased rates of cancer of the nasal sinuses.

Many workers are also exposed to the cancer-causing effects of various forms of radiation. In the 1920s women were hired to paint luminous dials on watches, clocks, and other surfaces using radium, a radioactive substance. To make a fine point on the brush the women customarily ran the tip of the brush through their lips. For many of these women, the legacy of this exposure to a radioactive material was cancer of the bone. Workers who mine cobalt and uranium are prone to lung cancer as a result of exposure to radioactive materials in the ores. Great care must be taken by radiologists, X-ray technicians and others who work with X-rays to avoid all unnecessary exposure to radiation. In the past such workers who failed to protect themselves adequately sometimes developed leukemia. Many old time radiologists who were not aware of the danger developed multiple skin cancers. You may have noticed that now when a doctor, dentist, or technician takes an X-ray, he is careful to step into a protected area or even out of the room. However, fishermen, farmers, sailors, and others who work outdoors (particularly in warm climates where little clothing is worn) are often not as careful as they might be about how they expose themselves to the ultraviolet radiation in sunlight, the major cause of superficial skin cancer. Ultraviolet radiation may also cause some cases of melanoma, a more serious and often fatal form of skin cancer.

RADIATION

Radiation has also been linked to cancer among people who were exposed to its damaging effects through ways other than their jobs. The most common cancer in the United States is skin cancer, usually caused by overexposure to the ultraviolet radiation in sunlight. It afflicts an estimated 300,000 to 600,000 Americans each year but is fortunately highly curable if treated early. It most often affects persons with fair, ruddy, or sandy complexions who have relatively little pigment in their skin to absorb the ultraviolet radiation before it damages the skin cells that are sensitive to it.

In addition to sunlight, the once-frequent use of low-dose radiation treatments by dermatologists for a variety of skin disorders and to get rid of excess hair led to the later development of skin cancers in the treated areas. Women who received radiation therapy many years ago for postpartum breast infections face a greatly increased risk of developing breast cancer. Radiation treatment for benign tumors in the uterus (fibroids) later resulted in an unusually large number of cancers of the uterus, cervix, ovary, bladder, and rectum. These treatments have long since been discontinued.

A radioactive material called Thorotrast, which was once used to outline the abdominal organs for diagnostic X-rays, decades later resulted in unexpected cancers of the bone, liver, and kidney. Young patients who received radiation therapy for such conditions as acne, ringworm, inflamed tonsils, or enlargement of the thymus gland, have increased rates of leukemia and cancers of the head and neck regions, including the brain and thyroid.

In 1972 at the age of 25, Andria Reisberg, wife of Allan and mother of a four-year-old son, Kevin, died of cancer of the thyroid. According to a report in the Chicago Sun-Times, Andria had received X-ray treatments for inflamed tonsils twenty-three years earlier when she was two years old. Her former pediatrician who had ordered the treatments explained that in those days "this was the [recognized] therapy for inflamed tonsils. It was well established." Not until years later did the doctors realize that they had unwittingly subjected their young patients to six times the normal risk of developing cancer of the thyroid.

Similarly, in "those days," doctors were unaware of the potential hazards of a then common practice of fluoroscopy, an X-ray procedure in which the area to be studied is viewed directly instead of on a film. Even shoe stores had fluoroscopy machines which they used to see how well a shoe fit, particularly on children who could not be relied upon to determine good fit on their own. Government action led to the elimination of this practice. The old fluoroscopy machines (new versions are still used medically but only for very special reasons) gave off many hundreds of times more radiation than modern X-ray machines do. Since the practice was so routine and widespread, it is virtually impossible to isolate groups for study who received different amounts of radiation from fluoroscopes. Therefore, it is not known to what extent these examinations increased the risk of cancer in people who received them. However, experts point out that radiation has cumulative effects over the years, so that any exposure adds to a person's risk of cancer. Children are five to ten times more sensitive to radiation-induced cancer than adults and the fetus is ten to 150 times more sensitive.

Perhaps the single most dramatic carcinogenic effect of radiation followed the explosion of atomic bombs in Hiroshima and Nagasaki in 1945. There, the survivors—including children in their mothers' wombs at the time of the bombings—have suffered an unusual number of a variety of cancers, including leukemia. Many scientists are concerned that man's increasing use of radioactive materials—in atomic weapons tests, in industry and medicine, and in power plants—is subjecting the general population to greater risks of cancer by contaminating the environment with higher levels of radiation.

While diagnostic X-rays generally deliver extremely low levels of radiation, there is some evidence that the children of women who get diagnostic X rays during pregnancy face a somewhat greater than average chance of developing leukemia or other cancers. Therefore, X-rays during pregnancy should be limited to those circumstances where the benefit of the knowledge to be gained clearly outweighs any possible risk to the unborn child. Wherever possible, when X-rays must be taken during pregnancy, lead shields and careful positioning of the X-ray beam are used to protect the fetus.

CANCER FROM OUR DAILY BREAD

Certain cancers vary greatly in frequency from country to country and within countries, from region to region. Studies of these differences have suggested that various elements of the daily diet can cause cancer in man. The very nourishment on which life depends can—directly or indirectly—steal it away. For example, cancer of the colon and rectum (also called cancer of the bowel) is extremely common in the United States, Scotland, Canada, and other Westernized countries. In fact, if both sexes are considered together, bowel cancer is the most common serious cancer in the United States today, striking nearly 100,000 persons a year. But this disease is relatively rare in countries like Japan, Chile, Portugal, Israel, and among the Bantu of South Africa. Yet, studies of migrants have shown that heredity—a genetic predisposition to the disease—is not the explanation for these differences. For example, when Japanese move to a more Western culture, their chances of developing bowel cancer increase. Japanese living in Hawaii have higher rates of bowel cancer than Japanese living in Japan, and those who emigrated to California are at greater risk of developing the disease than those who settled in Hawaii. As the migrants adopt more and more of the Western way of life, their risk of bowel cancer continues to increase, and first generation

Japanese-Americans have nearly the same rate of bowel cancer as other native Americans.

What could be the reason for these changing rates? Clearly, since the genes don't change when people move, it must be something in their environment. Attention in recent years has focused on a logical possibility—diet. Migrants slowly adopt the dietary habits of the country they live in, and the diet of the next generation is even more like that of the adopted country. What, then, is the critical difference between the diets of persons at high risk of bowel cancer and those at low risk of developing this disease? Certainly, on the surface of things, there is little resemblance between the diets of the Japanese, the Portuguese, and the South African Bantu.

Dr. Denis P. Burkitt, cancer specialist on the Medical Research Council in London, has spent much of his life studying cancer in Africa. He has evolved a theory that is fast gathering support from the findings of other researchers. Dr. Burkitt believes that bowel cancer is more likely to occur among people whose diet is low in fibrous foodstuffs, or "roughage"—like whole grains, beans, fruits, and fresh vegetables—and high in refined carbohydrates, like sugars and processed starches. The theory holds that the higher the fiber content of the diet, the softer the consistency of the stool and the faster it passes through the digestive tract. Therefore, there is less time for the intestinal bacteria to convert substances in the food to chemicals that may be carcinogenic and, thus, there would be less exposure of the colon and rectum to potential cancer-causing agents. Dr. Lauren V. Ackerman, pathologist at the Washington University School of Medicine in St. Louis, points out that unlike Americans, the Bantu are never constipated. In fact, he says, they move their bowels several times a day. They do not develop colon and rectal polyps (benign tumors), which are extremely common among Americans and are associated with an increased risk of developing cancer of the bowel.

Another theory, which in many ways is compatible with Dr. Burkitt's hypothesis, links bowel cancer to a diet high in fats, particularly saturated fats and cholesterol, that are derived from animal products like meat, butter, cheese, and eggs. Dr. Ernst L. Wynder and Dr. Bandaru S. Reddy of the American Health Foundation in New York City have found the same strong correlation between high fat-high cholesterol diet and bowel cancer as has been noted for such a diet and coronary heart disease among the peoples of the world. In one study, Japanese migrants to Hawaii who developed bowel cancer were found to consume more beef than similar persons without the disease.

Several researchers, including Dr. Michael Hill and his coworkers in London, have shown that the feces of people on a high-fat diet contain higher levels of certain substances that may be cancer-causing. Among the substances are derivatives of cholesterol and the bile acids that help to digest cholesterol and fats. Drs. Reddy and Wynder showed that Americans who consume a typical high fat Western-type diet had more of these substances in their feces than American vegetarians and Seventh-day Adventists, most of whom eat no meat and who have a much lower rate of colon and other cancers than average Americans. Further, Dr. Hill's group found that the feces of those on high-fat diets had unusually large numbers of certain bacteria that grow only in the absence of oxygen. These bacteria can convert a substance in the feces, cholic acid, into a chemical that has been shown to cause cancer in laboratory animals. Dr. Hill calculated that living on a high-fat diet for fifty years, 1,300 grams of this chemical would pass through the colon, giving ample exposure to induce cancer.

Dr. Wynder and his colleagues, as well as researchers at Harvard University, have noted that breast cancer patterns in different countries also suggest a link to the consumption of animal fats. The worldwide patterns closely match those of bowel cancer. The highest breast cancer rates are found in the Scandinavian countries, where consumption of animal fats is among the highest in the world. The United States ranks ninth (after several Western European nations) in breast cancer incidence, and Japan, where the traditional diet is very low in animal fat, has the lowest incidence among thirty-nine countries that have been studied. However, when Japanese women migrate to the United States, their risk of developing breast cancer increases. A study of Japanese Americans in the San Francisco Bay area showed that immigrant women had higher rates of breast cancer than Japanese women in Japan, and that the daughters of Japanese immigrants had still higher rates, now approaching the rate of native American women. The link of breast cancer to dietary fats is further supported by the finding that obese women are much more likely to develop the disease than are slender women.

The possible connection between diet and bowel cancer is easy to understand, but how might something a woman eats end up affecting her breasts? As we have seen with other cancers, such as liver cancer caused by vinyl chloride, a carcinogen need not be directly applied to an organ to cause cancer in it. Substances that enter the body through a variety of routes—inhalation, ingestion, even absorption through the skin—can travel through the body to sensitive "target" organs. Or otherwise harmless substances may

be converted by body enzymes or bacteria into potential carcinogens. In the association between breast cancer and dietary fats,
one suggested link is the degradation of the large amounts of
cholesterol found in a fatty diet. Cholesterol can be metabolized,
or converted, in the body to hormone-like compounds. These
compounds act like hormones that are known to have cancer-
inducing effects on breast tissue in animals. An experiment with
mice at Southern Illinois University showed that animals fed a
high-fat diet—similar in fat content to the typical American diet—
developed more breast cancers than mice on a normal low-fat
mouse diet. The high-fat diet seemed to trigger an excessive production of sex hormones in both female and male mice. Further
discussion of the relationship between hormones and other factors
that affect a person's risk of breast cancer appears later in the
sections on "Cancer and Heredity" and "Cancer and Hormones."

The pattern for stomach cancer is in direct contrast to the
incidence of bowel cancer in most countries. Stomach cancer is
very common among the Japanese, where it is that country's leading cancer killer. But it is relatively uncommon and has long been
on the decline in the United States. Unlike the situation with
bowel cancer, when Japanese migrate to this country their stomach cancer rate does not drop until the next generation. This
suggests that the disease is irreversibly triggered by some environmental factor, probably something in the Japanese diet, early
in life. Thus, migrants arrive already prone to the disease. Among
possible causative dietary factors suggested by the results of a National Cancer Institute study were dried, salted fish, pickled
vegetables, and the absence of uncooked Western vegetables.
Another study conducted among stomach cancer patients in Israel
suggested that the disease was more common among people who
consumed a great deal of starchy foods—breads, noodles, cereals,
beans, and nuts. The researchers suggested that longterm consumption of starches may change the gastric juices and render the
stomach lining more susceptible to the action of carcinogens.

Similarly, studies of differing rates of liver cancer in different
parts of the world have pinpointed a dietary factor that is undoubtedly an important cause of this usually fatal disease—a
poison called aflatoxin produced by a fungus that grows on foods
stored under humid conditions. Aflatoxin can be found on moldy
corn, cottonseed, wheat, peanuts, rice, black pepper, wine, and
other commodities that enter the human food supply either directly or through animal feed. As little as one part of aflatoxin per
billion parts of food—currently the lowest detectable level of this
substance—produces cancer when fed to rats. Liver cancer is rela-

tively rare in the United States, but in what was Portuguese East Africa it is probably more common than anywhere in the world. In some areas, the rate is fifty-eight times higher than in the United States.

In the early 1960s an epidemic of liver disease struck poultry farms in England, killing 100,000 young turkeys as well as thousands of ducklings, pheasants, and partridge. The deaths were finally linked to Brazilian peanut meal that had come from one London mill. The meal was found to be contaminated with a common fungus called Aspergillus flavus, which produced aflatoxin. The same substance was linked to the deaths from liver cancer of two brown bears who had been fed moldy bread at the St. Louis Zoo and to an epidemic of liver cancer among rainbow trout on a commercial fish farm.

At high doses, aflatoxin has been shown to destroy liver tissue; at low doses, however, it can cause liver cancer. It is widely believed that this toxin is largely responsible for the high incidence of liver cancer in parts of Africa and Asia. Its effects are most pronounced where the diet is deficient in protein. Whether aflatoxin can cause cancer in organs other than the liver is not known. In the United States, Federal regulations prohibit the presence of aflatoxin in foods consumed by people and limit how much can be in animal feeds. However, periodic seizures of grains by the Food and Drug Administration indicate that these limits are occasionally exceeded.

Cancer of the esophagus is also believed to be associated with dietary factors. In the 1950s, the Bantu living in the Transkei region of South Africa suddenly experienced a dramatic rise in the incidence of esophageal cancer, suggesting the recent introduction of a causative factor, possibly something in their beer. Recently a medical survey of China revealed that in one region southwest of Peking, esophageal cancer is so common that it is the leading cause of death there, whereas in other parts of China it is a rare disease. The survey suggested a possible link to the consumption of pickled vegetables, which are preserved in large earthen jars that are often contaminated by fungi. In France and Switzerland, cancer of the esophagus strikes unusually large numbers of men, but it is rare among the women of those countries. And in the United States, the incidence of this disease has been rising rapidly among black Americans—in fact, it has tripled among blacks in the last generation—but it is relatively uncommon and declining in frequency among white Americans.

The single most important factor associated with cancer of the esophagus in Western nations is alcohol, particularly alcohol and cigarettes together. The risk of developing esophageal cancer is approximately twenty-five times greater for heavy drinkers than for nondrinkers, and in parts of the United States where the per capita consumption of distilled spirits is highest, so is the death rate from esophageal cancer.

Alcohol consumption also increases the chances of developing cancers of the oral cavity (mouth and throat), the larynx, and the liver.

Together, alcohol and cigarette smoking account for about three-fourths of the cancers of the oral cavity in American men. Heavy drinkers face a two- to six-fold increase in risk; heavy smokers have a two- to three-fold greater risk. But heavy drinking and smoking together raise the risk fifteen times, indicating that the cancer-inducing effects of one enhance those of the other. Animal studies indicate, in fact, that alcohol stimulates the activity of cancer-causing agents in tobacco smoke. All told, studies to date suggest that the consumption of alcoholic beverages may increase the cancer death rate in Americans by seven percent in men and two percent in women. In general, heavy drinkers face about a 20 percent greater risk of developing cancer than non-drinkers or moderate drinkers.

A variety of other dietary factors have been associated with cancer causation, although in some cases their role in human cancers is still uncertain. One of the most widely discussed of these agents is a combustion product called benzo(a)pyrene, a member of a class of compounds called polycyclic hydrocarbons, many of which readily cause cancer in animals. Benzo(a)pyrene is found in smoked foods, bread, roasted coffee, and steaks and other foods broiled over charcoal. In animals it is a potent carcinogen. Its very high level in home-smoked foods has been suggested as the cause of the extremely high incidence of stomach cancer in Iceland, where home-smoking is very popular.

Compounds known as nitrosamines are also potent carcinogens in animals. Nitrosamines can be formed in the digestive tract when a common food preservative, nitrite, combines with amines that result from the digestion of proteins. Nitrates, also commonly used to preserve such foods as sausages, bacon, cold cuts, and frankfurters, can be changed into nitrites in the body and may have a similar effect.

The cancer-causing potential of caffeine, the stimulant found in coffee and tea and to a lesser extent in cola and cocoa, has been hotly debated. In a number of tests, caffeine has been shown to enhance the effects of certain known cancer-causing agents, including some tumor viruses. On the other hand, caffeine seems to protect against the effects of other cancer-causing agents. At very high doses—equivalent to the amount found in 300 to 600 cups of coffee—caffeine interferes with the ability of damaged genetic material to repair itself. But caffeine is rapidly metabolized in the body, and at most one-twentieth of this amount has been found in the blood of heavy coffee drinkers. Another constituent of coffee, chlorogenic acid, has been shown to speed the formation of nitrosamines, but it is not known whether this reaction actually can take place in the stomach. If it does, the common breakfast combination of coffee and bacon or sausages, which are preserved with nitrates and nitrites, may lead to significant exposure to one of the most powerful cancer-causing agents known. Ironically, the National Cancer Institute recently discovered that the solvent used to remove caffeine from coffee—trichloroethylene—is a potent carcinogen in animals. The Food and Drug Administration has allowed residues of up to 25 parts per million of the chemical in decaffeinated coffee, but manufacturers have recently substituted another chemical to remove caffeine.

Several potential cancer-causing agents have been banned from the American diet. The first, a food coloring called butter yellow, was found in the 1930s to cause cancer in animals. In 1958 a section called the Delaney Amendment was added to the American Food and Drug laws. It dictates that no substance that has been shown to cause cancer through appropriate tests in animals can be added to foods sold in the United States. Under this rule, safrole, a plant chemical that had been used for decades to flavor root beer and sarsaparilla, was taken off the market after it was shown to cause liver tumors in rats and a related substance, dihydrosafrole, was shown to cause cancer of the esophagus in the animals. A vermouth flavoring was also banned because it caused cancer in test animals. Violet No. 1, a food coloring formerly used by the United States Department of Agriculture to stamp meats, was eliminated after Japanese studies showed it caused cancer in animals. The artificial sweetener sodium cyclamate was banned after rats got bladder cancer when pellets of cyclamates and saccharin were implanted in their bladders. In 1977, a ban of saccharin as a food additive was proposed by the Food and Drug Administration after bladder cancers occurred in a significant number of laboratory rats fed large doses of saccharin. The drug agency proposed to allow the sale of saccharin as an over-the-counter drug to reduce the hardship of a complete ban on persons with diabetes or obesity.

The widely used food coloring Red Dye No. 2, used to tint hundreds of food products, lipsticks, pill coatings, and medicines, was finally banned in 1976 after a long and heated debate over animal tests that indicated the chemical was a weak cancer-causing agent. The Soviet Union had banned the dye in the 1960s and in 1972 the World Health Organization had advised strict limitations on its use. But not until the Food and Drug Administration's own tests in rats showed that high doses of Red Dye No. 2 increased the animals' risk of getting a wide variety of cancers did the agency decide to ban it for American use. In September 1976 the F.D.A. also banned Red No. 4, which has long been used to color maraschino cherries, because it is suspected of causing polyps in the bladder; and carbon black, used in candies, drugs and cosmetics, because there was no way to be sure it does not contain a cancer-causing byproduct.

The courts invalidated a government ban on another agent, diethylstilbestrol, or DES, a synthetic hormone that is used to hasten the fattening of cattle. This substance has caused cancer in both animals and man, and residues of the hormone have periodically been found in meats—particularly liver—sold to consumers.

Also ingested unwittingly by hundreds of millions of people are tiny amounts of cancer-causing pesticides that may remain on treated foods when purchased or that enter the food supply through the food chain. In 1974 two such pesticides—aldrin and dieldrin—were banned because dieldrin (and indirectly aldrin because it readily decomposes into dieldrin) was shown to cause cancer in tests on mice and rats and because residues of the pesticides are widespread in the food supply. Cancer developed when as little as one part of dieldrin per million parts of food was fed to the animals for a brief period. Tests by the Food and Drug Administration revealed "measurable amounts" of dieldrin in 83 percent of all dairy products sampled, in 88 percent of all fruits sampled and in 96 percent of samples of meat, fish and poultry, as well as in lesser percentages of grains, vegetables, fats, and oils. An earlier study showed that nearly all of human fat tissue samples had detectable residues of dieldrin, indicating that the body can store this cancer-causing chemical.

Other carcinogenic pesticides include arsenicals, DDT, aramite, and carbamate. The unexpectedly high death rates from cancer among people living around the Mississippi Delta is believed to be related in part to intensive exposure to carcinogenic agricultural chemicals that drain through the Mississippi and other rivers.

In addition to such direct carcinogenic effects from dietary elements, other factors in the diet seem able to set the stage for cancer while not directly causing the disease themselves. Among them are a variety of dietary deficiencies, including insufficient vitamin A, riboflavin, iodine, protein, and the trace elements molybdenum and selenium. At the other end of the malnutrition spectrum—among the obese, who are also malnourished in the real sense of the word—cancer rates are also higher than expected. Obese women have higher than normal rates of cancer of the uterus, pancreas, gallbladder and breast.

CANCER IN WATER AND AIR

As the story of Duluth and Lake Superior so clearly demonstrates, even the purest water can contain hidden hazards that may contribute to the development of cancer in man. Studies by the Environmental Protection Agency have revealed that, in addition to asbestos, the water supplies in many cities contain such cancer-causing chemicals as arsenic and benzene, as well as several carcinogenic substances—chloroform, carbon tetrachloride, and tetrachloroethylene, among them—that are apparently formed during the very process that is supposed to purify water, chlorination. In a study in New Orleans, these substances were found in the blood of residents as well as in their drinking water. Drinking water may also be contaminated with small amounts of carcinogenic chemicals deposited into waterways as industrial wastes and runoff from agricultural lands.

Air pollution, too, probably contributes to the human cancer burden, although in most cases the carcinogenic culprits in the air we breathe have not been singled out. A recent analysis by the National Cancer Institute of death rates from thirty-five types of cancer in each county of the forty-eight contiguous United States revealed that the residents of communities where copper, lead, or zinc smelters are situated had significantly higher-than-average death rates from lung cancer. Arsenic spewed into the air by the smelting process is considered a likely cause. The study strongly suggested that this increased cancer risk applied not only to workers in smelting plants but also to other people living in the area.

For a wide variety of cancers, including cancer of the lung, the incidence is higher among people living in urban areas than residents of rural communities. The contribution, if any, of air pollution to these cancers is yet unknown. However, studies conducted by government agencies have indicated that city air contains, on the average, sixteen times more carcinogens than rural air. In one experiment mice exposed to the smoke and dust of city air developed nearly five times more lung cancers than mice who breathed filtered "mountain-fresh" air. And a study in the Swiss village of

Netstal revealed that cancer mortality in general was nine times higher among residents living within fifty yards of a heavily traveled highway than among villagers further off the road. When carcinogens in air and water are identified, the Environmental Protection Agency tries to eliminate them through appropriate regulations, legislation, or court proceedings.

CANCER AND HABITS

In Travancore on the southwestern coast of India, people are in the habit of chewing on a mixture of betel nuts, tobacco and lime from crushed sea shells. Seventy-five percent of the oral cancers in that region are attributed to the effects of this habit. Oral cancer also afflicts persons in the southeastern United States who dip snuff and those in South Asia who practice a habit called chutta— smoking cigars with the lighted end in the mouth. And clay pipe smokers of Ireland are prone to cancer of the lip. In Kashmir the natives used to bind small charcoal-burning earthen ovens around their waists for warmth in the cold season. Many developed cancers of the abdominal wall as a result.

But there is no more dramatic example of the cancer-causing effects of a particular custom than in the phenomenon of cigarette smoking. In the United States about 30 percent of the cancer deaths in men—and a much smaller but rapidly increasing percentage of deaths in women—are directly attributable to the carcinogenic effects of cigarette smoking. The leading cancer killer in this country—cancer of the lung, which in 1975 was diagnosed in some 91,000 persons and claimed 81,000 lives—has been shown unequivocally to be caused by cigarette smoking. At least 75 percent of lung cancer cases would not occur if the victims had not smoked. Only 10 percent of lung cancers occur in individuals who never smoked cigarettes, and those are mostly a different type of cancer than the kind related to smoking. The incidence of lung cancer among American men has increased twenty-fold in forty years, and in women the incidence is increasing now more rapidly than in men.

Although the first reports linking use of tobacco to cancer date back to the late 1700s, it was not until the 1930s—approximately twenty-five years after cigarette smoking started to become popular among Americans—that the first public reports appeared linking the habit to the occurrence of lung cancer in the United States and in Germany. The link between smoking and lung cancer has been confirmed in extensive studies in at least four countries—the United States, Canada, Britain, and Japan. In a study sponsored by the American Cancer Society, lung cancer was produced in dogs who "smoked" cigarettes (seven a day for two and a half years) through a tube in their windpipes (animals can not be made to inhale cigarette smoke the way people do). Thus, the claim of some smokers and tobacco industry representatives that the link between smoking and lung cancer "is only a statistical relationship" is neither true nor adequate justification for continuing to smoke. In addition to cancer of the lung, cigarette smokers also face increased risks of dying of cancer of the larynx, oral cavity, esophagus, bladder, kidney, stomach, prostate, and pancreas, not to mention heart and chronic lung diseases. Arthur Godfrey, who smoked for more than three decades and for years advertised Chesterfield cigarettes on his radio and television shows, developed lung cancer at the age of 56. He and John Wayne are among the relatively few persons to have been cured of this disease, which now claims the lives of approximately 90 percent of those who get it. Two other well-known television personalities, commentator Edward R. Murrow and William Talman, who played the prosecuting attorney on the Perry Mason Show, both died of lung cancer long before their careers would have ended. Both had been chain smokers for many years. William Gargan, noted stage and screen actor, lost his larynx—and his natural voice and acting career—to cancer caused by years of cigarette smoking. However, he is alive, well, and free of cancer many years later and actively working with the American Cancer Society to help others escape his predicament.

Cigarettes increased steadily in popularity after World War I. In the early 1920s Americans smoked 600 cigarettes per capita each year; by the mid-1960s the per capita rate had climbed to 4,000. Significant numbers of women did not become regular cigarette smokers until the 1930s, but in the 1960s they nearly closed the gap in cigarette consumption between them and men.

The risk of developing smoking-caused cancer is directly related to the extent of exposure to the carcinogenic agents in cigarette smoke. Thus, the risk increases the longer one smokes and the greater the number of cigarettes smoked daily. Risk is also affected by the extent of inhalation and the amount of "tars" present in the smoke. The use of low-tar filtered cigarettes is associated with a lower cancer risk, although it is still substantially higher than that of nonsmokers.

Heavy pipe and cigar smokers are also more likely than nonsmokers to develop cancer of the lung and cancer of the kidney, but their risk is only about half as high as that for cigarette smokers, probably because few pipe and cigar smokers inhale. However, a recent study indicated that when cigarette smokers who inhaled switch to cigars, they also tend to inhale the cigars, which exposes them to as bad or worse doses of carcinogens.

Extensive studies have been done to identify the cancer-inducing agents in cigarette smoke and to determine how smoke damages the respiratory organs. It is hoped that the results of such studies may lead to ways of developing safer cigarettes and of interrupting the cancer process before it is too late. But most researchers believe it will never be possible to develop a truly safe cigarette. As long as it is burned, cancer-inducing combustion products will be produced. More than 1,200 components have been identified in tobacco smoke, 95 percent of them in the "tar" or smoke condensate. Many of these components are known carcinogens, cocarcinogens (those that act in conjunction with some other substance to cause cancer), and tumor promoters. Included are benzo(a)pyrene, the major carcinogen in coal tar, chrysene and methylchrysenes, terpenes, catechol, and the radioactive element polonium 210.

In addition to exposing the respiratory tract to such cancer-causing agents, cigarette smoke also produces several effects that enhance the action of these agents. The first of these is impairment or destruction of the cilia, or hairs, that line the respiratory tract. These hairs normally serve as the body's defensive barrier to inhaled agents. The cilia both protect underlying cells from exposure to harmful substances and help to "sweep" particles out of the respiratory tract by stimulating the flow of mucus that traps harmful substances and moves them up and out of the lungs. But with the cilia paralyzed or destroyed, up to 90 percent of the particles inhaled in tobacco smoke may remain in the lungs. Smoke from a nonfiltered cigarette contains 50,000 more particles than the same volume of polluted urban air. What's more, the size of the particles in tobacco smoke (which affects their likelihood of entering and remaining in the lungs) is similar to that of other inhaled substances that are known to be capable of damaging the lungs.

The cell damage wreaked by tobacco smoke has been documented in detailed studies of human lung tissue removed at autopsy from patients who died at various institutions, including the Veterans Administration Hospital in East Orange, New Jersey. There, Dr. Oscar Auerbach, a pathologist who did the smoking dog study, showed that cigarette smokers have unusually extensive hyperplasia, or an increase in the number of cells, in the lining of the respiratory tract. This is a usual response to any type of chronic irritation. The frequency and amount of hyperplasia was directly related to how much the person smoked. Another effect Dr. Auerbach found was the loss of ciliated cells and a flattening and enlargement of the remaining lining cells. Again, this effect was related to the amount smoked. A third effect he found involved changes in the nuclei of cells, where the genetic material is housed. Such cells with abnormal nuclei, also found much more often in smokers, are called cancer in situ (that is, noninvasive cancer still in its original place). This can progress to invasive cancer, which can spread throughout the lungs and to other parts of the body. These, then, appear to be the crucial stages leading toward smoking-induced lung cancer.

More recently, Dr. Auerbach studied persons who had stopped smoking five or more years before they died and he found that the body could repair the smoke-caused damage that leads to cancer. Former smokers had less hyperplasia and fewer cells with abnormal nuclei than persons who had smoked for the same number of years but who were still smoking at the time of death.

CANCER AND HEREDITY

It has often been said that one cannot escape his heritage. It is the same with cancer. A person's biological inheritance in many ways can influence his susceptibility to the effects of cancer-causing factors, and, consequently, his chances of developing one or another type of cancer. This genetic "predisposition" to cancer may be determined by such things as inherited immunological defects, hormonal patterns, enzyme deficiencies, bone abnormalities, or a tendency to develop certain benign growths or cysts, as in the colon, breasts or ovaries.

A survey of 4,515 persons in Nebraska showed that when one parent or a brother or sister had cancer, 8.9 percent of the persons checked also had had cancer. In families where two immediate relatives had cancer, the risk to others in the immediate family rose to 16.3 percent, and it increased to 27.4 percent (more than one in five) for persons with three or more close relatives who had cancer. But several cases of a particular kind of cancer—or a whole variety of cancers—in a single family does not mean that one person somehow "caught" the disease from another. Rather, it indicates that since the genetic traits of blood relatives have many similarities, more than one member of a family may have inherited a predisposition to cancer, usually of a particular type.

Although common exposure to an environmental carcinogen

may contribute to some cases of familial cancers, studies indicate that inherited factors play the more important role, sometimes by increasing susceptibility to a carcinogen. Virtually every form of cancer that has been studied in the laboratory has shown an increased frequency in some species or strain of animal whose members share very similar genes, and it is likely that this is also true for man. Various studies of cancers among family members have indicated that there is an increased familial risk associated with cancer of the breast, colon and rectum, endometrium (the lining of the uterus), lung, prostate, and possibly ovary. In studies of childhood cancers, Dr. Joseph Fraumeni of the National Cancer Institute reports that brothers and sisters of youngsters with leukemia, brain tumors, and sarcomas seem to face a somewhat greater than expected risk of developing these cancers themselves. In studies of identical twins, it was shown that if one twin develops leukemia, the other has a one in five chance of also developing the disease within two years. In the general population, the annual risk for children developing leukemia is approximately one in 20,000.

Breast cancer, in particular, has been carefully studied in this regard. Since it is the leading cancer killer of women in the United States, knowing which women may face an unusually high risk can help in efforts to detect the disease early and hence cure it. Women in general in the United States have a five to seven percent chance of developing breast cancer sometime during their lifetimes. However, it has been shown that on the average, close blood relatives of breast cancer patients—daughters, sisters, maternal aunts, and nieces—are two to three times more likely to get breast cancer than women whose families are free of this disease.

Closer scrutiny of these relationships has revealed that for relatives of some breast cancer patients, the risk of developing the disease themselves can be as high as one in two. Dr. David E. Anderson, geneticist at the M. D. Anderson Hospital and Tumor Institute in Houston, has studied the families of several hundred breast cancer patients. He found that if the original patient had cancer in only one breast, the risk to her relatives is only slightly higher than that faced by women in the general population. However, if the cancer affected both breasts (called bilateral cancer), the relatives' risk is five-and-a-half times higher than it would otherwise be. And if the cancer was both bilateral and occurred before the patient reached menopause, her relatives' risk is nine times higher than expected—giving them nearly a 50 percent chance of developing breast cancer themselves. The greatest risk of all—forty-seven times the average—is faced by women under the age of 40 whose sister and mother both had breast cancer before menopause, Dr. Anderson found. It is hoped that further studies of such patients to see how they may differ biochemically and hormonally from women who do not get the disease may yield clues to the causes of breast cancer, as well as more refined methods of detecting the disease before it is clinically obvious or identifying just who is and who is not at high risk of developing it.

Dr. Fraumeni reports that breast cancer in men—a relatively rare event—also seems to run in families and may be associated with hormone abnormalities. Dr. Anderson found that the daughters of men who come from breast cancer families also have a higher than expected risk of the disease, indicating that the hereditary tendency can be transmitted through the male as well as the female line.

Another genetics study at M. D. Anderson Hospital showed that about nine percent of the population inherits an ability to produce high levels of an enzyme that seems to increase susceptibility to the cancer-causing agents in cigarette smoke. The rest of the population is divided between low and moderate levels of the enzyme. Those with low levels of this enzyme, called aryl hydrocarbon hydroxylase (AHH), appear to be relatively resistant to lung cancer, Drs. Gottfried Kellerman, Mieke Luyten-Kellerman and Charles R. Shaw reported. The enzyme, which is released when smoke reaches the lungs, interacts with the hydrocarbons in the smoke and converts them to active forms that can induce cancerous growths. However, the importance of the role that AHH plays in a person's chances of developing lung cancer is not yet clear. Dr. Shaw has cautioned that a person found to have low levels of AHH cannot assume that he is safe in smoking all he pleases, especially since smoking is also associated with an increased chance of developing a wide range of other diseases in which AHH plays no role at all. But if further studies confirm the predictive value of high AHH levels, a test for this enzyme might be used to identify persons with an inherited susceptibility to lung cancer and then more intensive stop-smoking efforts might be focused on them.

Another potential test for inherited cancer susceptibility currently under study involves the sensitivity of a person's skin cells to the cancer-causing effects of a virus called SV-40. Thus far, family studies indicate that persons whose cells are highly sensitive to the effects of SV-40 in a laboratory test seem to be unusually likely to develop leukemia. However, many further studies are needed to establish the usefulness of this test.

A number of relatively rare inherited conditions have been definitely shown to greatly enhance a person's risk of cancer. One of these is a precancerous condition called familial polyposis of the colon, in which approximately half of blood relatives inherit the tendency to form multiple polyps, or benign growths, in the large bowel. Eventually, all who inherit this condition develop colon cancer. But even in the absence of this rare condition, there is some inherited susceptibility to colon cancer. In general, the immediate relatives of colon cancer patients face a two to three times greater than expected risk of developing colon cancer themselves.

Retinoblastoma, a rare form of eye cancer, is caused by a genetic abnormality, and the siblings or children of retinoblastoma victims would have a 50 percent chance of getting the disease. The risk of leukemia is increased among persons with mongolism, a disorder in which the cells contain an extra piece of genetic material, as well as among persons with Bloom's syndrome and Fanconi's anemia, inherited conditions in which the gene-bearing chromosomes tend to break. Another usually fatal genetic disorder called xeroderma pigmentosum, which involves an abnormality in the pigment-forming cells of the skin, predisposes its victims to sunlight-induced skin cancer because their bodies lack the ability to repair the genetic damage to skin cells caused by ultraviolet radiation.

Doctors at the Mayo Clinic in Rochester, Minnesota, have studied nine families in which members have inherited a strong likelihood of developing a rare type of thyroid cancer called medullary carcinoma. In one family, headed by Cyril Tholkes of Minneota, Minnesota, four children and two grandchildren have thus far been struck by the disease. According to a report in the Minneapolis *Tribune*, in 1972 Mr. Tholkes went to the Mayo Clinic because of eye troubles and doctors there found his cancer. Knowing of isolated reports that this type of cancer might be hereditary, the doctors asked to examine his seven sons and daughters. Four were found to have the cancer (one died of the disease following two operations). The five-year-old daughter and two-year-old son of one of Mr. Tholkes' sons also had to have cancers removed. The Mayo doctors concluded that each member of this family had a fifty-fifty chance of inheriting the genetic trait that led to this cancer. Early recognition of this genetic factor led to lifesaving surgery for all but one of its victims.

In addition to such rare genetic disorders that predispose to particular cancers, there are some families in which, for reasons not yet known, many members develop cancers of different types.

In such "cancer families" the disease tends to develop at a younger age than in the general population. For example, in Miami, Florida, three sons of Raymond Sutherland have been struck with three different kinds of cancer. One died of leukemia at the age of four, a second was treated for an extremely rare cancer of the nerve lining called malignant Schwannoma, and a third is being treated for bone cancer in his leg.

Among cancer families studied by Dr. Henry T. Lynch of Creighton University in Omaha, Nebraska, in one family eight of nineteen members through three generations developed cancer, including colon cancer, uterine cancer, and lymphosarcoma. Two sisters in the family each developed several different cancers. In another family Dr. Lynch studied, eighteen of sixty-four members in three generations developed cancers, including cancers of the colon, uterus, ovary, pancreas, and lip.

Dr. Lynch emphasizes, however, that just as a person's genetic inheritance may confer a particular susceptibility to cancer, it may also result in a relative resistance to this disease. He has also studied families in which cancer is extremely uncommon. Intensive investigation of such families—including studies of their enzyme and hormone patterns and immune systems—may further reveal how heredity and environment interact to cause cancer in man.

CANCER AND HORMONES

There is little question that hormones, particularly sex hormones, can influence the growth of cancers in man as well as in experimental animals. However, with a few exceptions, the precise nature of this influence and its relative importance in human cancer is still unclear and under intensive study.

Do some hormones act as carcinogens directly or set the stage on which other carcinogens can act? Do other hormones inhibit cancers from starting or growing? Do different levels of the same hormone have different effects with regard to cancer? And does it matter when in life the hormone exposure or lack of exposure occurs? The answers to such questions are all the more important today because millions of young women throughout the world are now swallowing a hormone pill nearly every day for contraception. Hormones are being used as "morning after" birth control methods, they are taken to control the symptoms of menopause, and they are under study as contraceptives for men as well as new birth control methods for women. Hormones are also used to fatten farm animals, with residues often remaining in the edible meat.

In experimental animals changing the hormone environment, such as by removing the hormone-producing glands, by administering hormones or by changing natural hormone production through pregnancy, can greatly increase or decrease the spontaneous development of cancers or the induction of tumors by carcinogens. In animals researchers have succeeded in using hormones to cause, accelerate, prevent and sometimes even cure cancer. Hormones given to animals have induced cancers of the breast, prostate, uterus and cervix, ovary, testis, bone, kidney, liver, bladder, and other organs.

The possible roles played by hormones in cancer include directly (or indirectly through a metabolic product) changing normal cells into cancer cells; activating another agent, such as a chemical or virus, to behave as a carcinogen, or changing the cells of a target organ in such a way as to make them susceptible to the effects of a carcinogen. Hormones may also act indirectly to change the immune response, allowing an incipient cancer to grow.

In humans there is evidence that different levels of naturally produced hormones can affect the chances of developing certain cancers and that some administered hormones can cause cancer in certain circumstances. In addition, for some cancers, among them cancers of the breast and prostate, hormone therapy in the form of removing or adding particular hormones can often lead to shrinkage or temporary disappearance of the tumor.

One of the most dramatic effects of a hormone on cancer yet demonstrated has been the finding that DES (diethystilbestrol), a synthetic substance that mimics the action of the female sex hormone estrogen, can cause a rare cancer of the vagina and cervix called clear-cell adenocarcinoma in young women who were exposed to the drug while still in their mothers' wombs. Ten, fifteen, or twenty years after birth, such cancers have developed in the daughters of some of the thousands of women who had been given DES during pregnancy to avert a threatened miscarriage. Ironically, DES therapy for threatened miscarriage was later abandoned because it was found to be only possibly effective. Dr. Arthur Herbst and his colleagues at the Massachusetts General Hospital in Boston, who first noticed the association between prenatal DES exposure and the rare cancer in seven young women, have since uncovered more than 200 similar cases around the world. Many more women exposed to DES have been found to have benign growths or peculiar ridges in the vagina which are not thought to be related to cancer. However, repeated examination of these women to detect a possible early vaginal or cervical cancer is strongly advised.

The doctors believe that DES can change the way in which cells of the vagina develop during fetal life, initiating abnormal growth patterns and possibly the start of the cancer process. The vast majority of the DES-caused cancers appear after puberty, indicating that sex hormones from the ovaries may act upon sensitized vaginal cells to produce the cancer. The doctors emphasize, however, that this prenatally caused cancer is still quite rare, occurring in probably no more than one of every 1,000 exposed, and most daughters of women who took DES during pregnancy seem to be perfectly healthy.

But the problem of human exposure to DES is far from resolved. This synthetic hormone has been approved by the Food and Drug Administration for use as a "morning-after" contraceptive pill taken for five days after mid-cycle intercourse, the presumed time of ovulation. It is supposed to be used only in "emergency" situations, such as rape or inadvertent misuse of a contraceptive, and not as a regular means of birth control. However, morning-after contraception has proved to be quite popular, particularly on college campuses, and a controversy rages over the wisdom of allowing the cancer-causing drug DES on the market for this purpose. DES had also been widely used for years as implants and feed additives to stimulate growth in cattle, but in 1973 this use was prohibited by the F.D.A. because of the chemical's relationship to cancer and the finding of DES residues in meat. However, the ban was overturned in court on a technicality and farmers are once again free to use it. In mice DES has produced breast cancers at the dose ranges used in women. The chemical has also been linked to the development of breast cancer in two male transvestites who took it to stimulate more feminine breast growth. And several cases of cancer of the endometrium, the lining of the uterus, have developed in girls who were given DES because their sex organs failed to develop properly.

In 1975 two medical research teams reported that women who take estrogen hormones to alleviate the symptoms and aftereffects of menopause face a five to fourteen-fold increased risk of developing cancer of the endometrium, a cancer that is usually curable with surgery and radiation therapy. The studies by these researchers suggest, but do not prove, that the hormones can cause cancer. These hormones, which are most commonly prescribed under the brand name of Premarin, are used by millions of women, sometimes for just a few months or years but often starting at menopause and continuing for the rest of the woman's life. The use of estrogens during and after menopause has increased greatly in the last decade, and several state cancer registries report that endometrial cancer is also now rising rapidly in frequency. The risk of the cancer developing in women who use the estrogens for longer than a few months has been estimated at four to eight per 1,000. At the same time, doctors in Denver have been collecting cases of young women who developed cancer of the endometrium and who were taking oral contraceptives. The cases, which are apparently quite rare, were nearly all associated with the use of sequential oral contraceptives, where the estrogen is taken for fifteen days of the month, followed by a progestin pill for five days. These pills had represented only six percent of the oral contraceptives sold, and the Food and Drug Administration has since taken them off the market.

Two large studies showed no relationship between postmenopausal use of estrogens and breast cancer, and one study indicated that the risk of breast cancer may actually be decreased by the drug. However, a study of 1,891 women published in 1976 indicated that a decade or more after women begin using postmenopausal estrogens, the risk of breast cancer may increase. For the women generally, estrogen use was associated with 30 percent more breast cancer cases than expected, and fifteen years after beginning estrogen therapy, breast cancer developed at twice the expected rate. Doctors generally recommend that postmenopausal hormone therapy be avoided by women who already have a high risk of developing breast cancer. This might include women with a strong family history of the disease, women who have benign breast disease (chronic cystic mastitis), women who already have had cancer in one breast, and women with abnormal or suspicious findings on a breast X-ray.

Similarly, such women have been urged not to take oral contraceptives, although there is as yet no firm evidence that the pill increases the breast cancer risk. The pill contains synthetic versions of the hormones estrogen and progesterone, and studies in mice, rats, and dogs have suggested that estrogens (and some of the synthetic contraceptive progesterones that are not currently in use) can cause or promote the development of breast cancer. However, thus far no such effect has been found in monkeys or women. One large study in San Francisco did find that women who used the pill for two to four years—but not for shorter or longer periods—may have an increased risk of breast cancer, but the meaning of this relationship is as yet unclear.

The World Health Organization's International Agency for Research on Cancer points out that the studies in women have not been large enough nor has enough time elapsed since oral contraceptives came into wide use to determine if a small increase in breast cancer risk might be associated with their use. In fact, the bulk of evidence thus far suggests a protective effect of the pill, since women on the pill are less likely to develop benign breast disease and, possibly, ovarian cysts, both of which are associated with an increased cancer risk.

Controversy also surrounds the possible relationship of the pill to cancer of the uterine cervix. Although one large study found that women on the pill were three times more likely than women using a diaphragm to develop precancer of the cervix, the study did not single out the pill as the culprit. This is because the diaphragm (since it covers the cervix) may protect against this condition, because women on the pill tend to be more active sexually (a factor known to be associated with an increased risk of cervical cancer), and because in another study women who chose the pill were found to have more abnormalities of the cervix at the outset (before even starting the contraceptive) than women who chose other methods.

The pill has been linked to the development of rare and usually benign—but sometimes fatal—liver tumors. More than one hundred cases of the tumors among women who have taken the pill have been reported in the medical literature. But the frequency with which these tumors occur among women who do not take the pill is unknown. Therefore, it cannot be said yet that there is a causal relationship between the pill and the tumors or, if such a relationship exists, whether it includes malignant as well as benign liver tumors. The National Cancer Institute is now exploring these questions, as well as ways to diagnose and treat the liver abnormalities.

While it is uncertain whether administered hormones encourage the development of breast cancer, there is little doubt that the natural hormones produced by a woman's body are extremely important both in initiating the disease and often in promoting its growth. Approximately one-third of breast cancer patients with metastatic disease are benefited by the surgical removal of their ovaries and adrenal glands, which are sources of hormones that stimulate the growth of these women's cancers.

A less direct demonstration of the importance of hormones comes from extensive studies of many thousands of women with different risks of developing breast cancer. Certain hormone-related characteristics seem to protect women from developing breast cancer; others increase risk of this disease. These factors have been summarized by Dr. Brian MacMahon and his colleagues at Harvard University School of Medicine as follows:

● In general, women who have borne children have a lower risk than women who remain childless, and the younger in life a woman has her first child, the lower her risk of breast cancer. Nuns have one of the highest breast cancer rates. Women who give birth to their first child before the age of 18 have about one-third the breast cancer risk of women whose first delivery occurs at age 35 or older. However, the protective effect of pregnancy occurs only prior to age 30. In fact, women older than 30 at first birth have a greater breast cancer risk than those who have no children. And the pregnancy, to be protective, must be full term. An aborted pregnancy, no matter when in life it occurs, has no protective effect.

● Contrary to popular belief, the fact that a woman breast feeds her children does not seem to reduce her breast cancer risk. However, some researchers have suggested that perhaps in the United States few women nurse children long enough to make a difference, and in other countries it is possible that prolonged breast feeding confers some protection.

● The fewer years that the woman's ovaries are actively producing sex hormones, the lower her risk of breast cancer. Women whose menstrual periods started at a relatively late age and whose menopause began relatively early have a lower than expected risk. Women whose natural menopause occurs after age 55 have twice the risk as women whose menopause starts before age 45. Surgical removal of the ovaries prior to menopause has an even greater protective effect, with a 70 percent reduction in breast cancer risk if surgical menopause occurs before age 35.

To Dr. MacMahon, these findings indicate that early in a woman's life—probably during the teen years and the 20's—there is a hormonal "priming" effect that either increases or decreases her chances of later developing breast cancer. Once the cancer develops, natural hormones may stimulate its growth. The Harvard team has also found evidence that while certain natural estrogens seem to promote the development of breast cancer, others may actually confer protection against the disease. Of a woman's three main estrogens, two—estrone and estradiol—have been shown repeatedly to produce breast cancer in rats. But the third main estrogen, estriol, has generally failed to promote animal breast cancers and seems to be able to impede the activity of the other two estrogens.

Compared to Western women, among whom breast cancer is common, Asian women, who have a much lower risk of the disease, have been found to produce more estriol in relation to estrone and estradiol. In fact, among Japanese migrants to the United States and their descendants, the estriol ratio becomes closer to that of native Americans, just as the Japanese-American risk of breast cancer does. (See the earlier section, "Cancer from Our Daily Bread.") If further study bears out this relationship, it may be possible to favorably alter the hormone ratio by drugs.

Greater breast cancer risk has also been associated with the production of a less than normal amount of androgen (a male sex hormone produced by women's adrenal glands), as measured by androgen metabolites excreted in the urine. It is not known if the androgens directly affect breast cancer risk or if they are merely an index of other more pertinent hormone factors. But if the initial findings are borne out, they could form the basis for a simple screening test for increased risk of breast cancer.

Recently, yet another hormone—prolactin, produced by the pituitary gland—has been singled out as important to the growth of breast cancers. Prolactin's best known role is to stimulate the development of breast tissue in preparation for milk production. It is produced in large amounts at the end of pregnancy. In rats, prolactin enhances the effects of carcinogens that cause breast cancer, and removal of the pituitary gland impedes the cancer's development. In women, removal of the pituitary leads to a remission (shrinkage or temporary disappearance) of breast cancer in about 30 percent of patients with metastatic disease. Even with the pituitary intact, the use of drugs, such as l-DOPA, which block prolaction secretion inhibits the growth of breast cancer in rats. In animals, if prolactin secretion is increased before exposure to a carcinogen, it seems to confer protection against breast cancer (this observation could possibly account for the protective effect of an early pregnancy), but when a tumor is already present prolactin enhances its growth. But Dr. Brian Henderson of the University of Southern California in Los Angeles has suggested that breast cancer may result from an indirect effect of an excess of prolactin and other pituitary hormones. These hormones can stimulate the ovaries to produce estrone and estradiol, the two estrogens that have been linked to an increased breast cancer risk. Because the body's hormone-producing glands operate on a finely tuned feedback system, (releasing more or less hormone depending upon how much is already circulating in the blood), Dr.

Henderson believes that the taking of hormone pills, such as oral contraceptives, can shut off the body's own production of breast-stimulating hormones and thereby reduce the risk of breast cancer.

Prolactin production can also be stimulated by a drug called reserpine that is commonly used to treat high blood pressure. Reserpine can stimulate the production of prolactin, and several studies have suggested that women who take reserpine have approximately a three-fold greater risk of developing breast cancer. However, one study showed no such relationship and the matter is still in question. Thus far, the evidence suggests that reserpine may stimulate the development of breast cancer from cells that had already undergone precancerous changes. It has also been suggested that thyroid hormone may play a role in breast cancer by influencing the effects of prolactin on breast tissue. The theory holds that the more thyroid hormone produced, the less the breast cancer risk. However, a study published in 1976 showed that breast cancer was twice as common among women who received thyroid hormone supplements as among women the same age who did not take the additional hormones. Among those who received the supplements, the risk of breast cancer increased with increasing years of use of the hormones.

Men, too, can develop cancers that are affected by hormones. Dr. Charles B. Huggins of the University of Chicago received a Nobel Prize for his discovery that cancer of the prostate could be dramatically reversed, although not cured, in about 80 percent of cases by removing the patient's testes, his source of male sex hormones, and by administering estrogen.

CANCER AND DRUGS

As the story of DES (described in the preceding section) so clearly demonstrates, sometimes the very drugs used to treat other medical problems may result in one that is worse—cancer. In all cases where the cancer-causing potential of a drug is recognized, the decision to give it to patients must involve an evaluation of benefit versus risk. Obviously, a drug that might cause cancer should not be used to treat a minor and self-limited illness or a disorder where there are plenty of other safer drugs that would take care of it. By the same token, however, a drug with carcinogenic potential may be more than justified in treating a life-threatening illness for which no equally effective therapy is available.

Among therapeutic substances that have been linked to cancer in man are the potent antibiotic, chloramphenicol, which depresses the bone marrow and may result ultimately in leukemia; medicinal arsenic, which can produce cancers of the lung and liver; the immunosuppressive drugs used in transplant patients, which increase the risk of lymphomas thirty-five times, the risk of lip and skin cancers four times, and the risk of several other cancers two and a half times; reserpine for treating high blood pressure, linked in four studies (but not in a fifth) to an increased breast cancer risk; phenacetin in pain-relieving tablets, which can increase the risk of kidney cancer; amphetamines used for weight reduction, which in one study was linked to a six-fold increase in the risk of Hodgkin's disease, and iron dextran, used to treat severe cases of iron-deficiency anemia, which causes cancer in animals and has been reported to have produced some cancers in man at the site of injection.

In addition, cancer has been produced in animals exposed to synthetic female sex hormones, such as are in oral contraceptives (see the preceding section, "Cancer and Hormones"); isoniazid, used to treat tuberculosis; chloroform, found in many cough syrups and throat lozenges; and Flagyl, used to treat common vaginal infections caused by Trichomonas vaginalis. The significance of these findings to man is not yet known. Other drugs are suspect because of secondary actions that can occur in the body. The antibiotic, oxytetracycline, and the sedative, chlorpromazine, may result in the formation of carcinogenic nitrosamines when they mix with nitrites in the stomach. Also, chlorpromazine and other sedatives in the phenothiazine class of drugs are potent stimulators of prolactin, which has been shown to enhance the growth of breast cancer in some cases.

CANCER AND STRESS

Emma G., a phlegmatic, hard-working Wisconsin farm wife, had devoted twenty years to caring for a mentally retarded daughter. She accepted the child's inevitable early death with tight-lipped stoicism. A few months later, another of Emma's daughters married against her parents' wishes and cut herself off from the family. Later that year, Emma suddenly became severely ill, collapsed, and within a month died of widespread breast cancer. Was Emma's cancer and rapid death attributable in some way—as family folk wisdom held—to her stubborn refusal to discuss her losses and express the emotions that must have surrounded them? Or was the close association between the events in her life and the onset of her illness merely coincidental? This kind of question has been debated by doctors for decades, but the debate has intensified in recent years as new evidence has begun to accumulate documenting the ability of the mind to control "automatic" body functions like blood pressure, heart rate, and digestive secretions. For example, psychological stress is known to change the output of hormones from the adrenal glands. These hormones, in turn, affect the immunological responses to various disease-causing agents, including bacteria and viruses. At the same time, doctors are gaining a clearer understanding of the subtle interactions between changes in various body functions and the onset of disease.

It has long been recognized that a person's mental attitude can significantly alter the course of an illness, with people who "give up hope" or wallow in depression often dying sooner or remaining sick longer than people who are optimistic about their chances for recovery. Voodoo deaths, in which perfectly healthy—at least physically healthy—individuals die because they believe in the power of a curse, have been reported in the medical literature. In addition, a host of so-called psychosomatic illnesses—in which emotional factors so distort body physiology that a disorder like peptic ulcers or high blood pressure can result—are well-recognized by physicians generally to have psychological as well as physical causes. Many doctors speak freely of an "ulcer personality" or a "hypertensive personality" or an "arthritis personality." But is there such a thing as a "cancer personality"—people who because of their emotional responses, the way they cope with life's stresses, become especially prone to developing cancer?

The notion is far from being generally accepted at this time, but experts in psychosomatic medicine have gathered a fair amount of data that suggest there may be an association between certain emotional characteristics and susceptibility to cancer. The case for this relationship, however, has not yet been proved.

What is needed, among other things, to confirm or refute this idea is a series of studies that evaluate the emotional lives of thousands of healthy persons who are then followed for many years to see which ones get cancer, under what kinds of circumstances and in relation to what sorts of emotional responses. Also needed is a clearer understanding of the precise disturbances in body physiology and chemistry caused by particular psychological factors, disturbances that may in turn set the stage for the development of cancer.

Before the birth of modern scientific medicine in the nineteenth century, the notion was widely held that personality and emotions were important factors in causing illness, including cancer. But this idea was spurned by many physicians when infectious organisms and other physical factors were isolated as direct causes of various illnesses. Only now is the subtle interplay between physical and psychological factors coming to be recognized and appreciated by the mainstream of modern medicine.

In 1931 Dr. E. Foque, a French physician, reported his belief that "sad emotions" could work through the central nervous system and affect metabolism and hormone-producing glands in such a way as to make cells vulnerable to the effects of physical cancer-causing agents like X-rays, chemicals or viruses. Dr. Foque wrote, "How many times have I heard—with variation due to different social statuses—the same litany, 'Since the death of my child, doctor, I am not the same. I do not recognize myself. I cannot find my equilibrium, and that certainly is the beginning of my illness because before, nothing like this had come to my attention.' " Although skeptical at first, Dr. Foque took a closer look at his patients with cancer and found that many had experienced "great crises, grave depressive afflictions, profound mourning, and all the sad emotions which have prolonged repercussions . . . You can see in the patients prolonged and silent sorrow without the release of sobs and tears." Often the patients themselves had related these feelings to the onset of their cancers.

Is this mere coincidence? Does the existence of sadness and depression simply serve to turn a person's thoughts inward on himself and make him more aware of physical symptoms that he had not noticed or had ignored when his life was more pleasant? Or is there a real connection between mental state and the onset of physical illness, in this case, cancer?

More systematic studies since Dr. Foque's time have tended to support his observations. Among the dozens of studies completed, Dr. William A. Greene, physician at the University of Rochester, found in interviews with more than 100 patients with leukemia or lymphoma that these diseases are likely to arise when the person is reacting to a loss or separation with feelings of sadness, anxiety, helplessness or hopelessness. In another Rochester study, doctors were able to predict with 75 percent accuracy on the basis of psychiatric interviews alone which of 51 women who had entered the hospital for a biopsy would turn out to have cancer.

The late Dr. David M. Kissen and his colleagues at the University of Glasgow in Scotland made a psychological comparison of 200 lung cancer patients with 200 patients suffering from other chest diseases and found that the cancer patients were less emotionally reactive and lacking in outlets for emotional release.

Intensive psychological interviews conducted by Lawrence LeShan, a New York psychotherapist, with 500 cancer patients and 500 persons with no known physical illness indicated that the cancer patients' lives were far more often characterized by early losses that brought pain and feelings of desertion, loneliness, and often guilt and self-condemnation. The cancer patients frequently had lost something or someone of extreme emotional significance to them and had been unable to find a satisfactory substitute relationship. The cancer patients also were less able to express hostile feelings and other strong emotions.

A study was done in London recently among women who were scheduled to have a biopsy for possible breast cancer. The women were given personality tests prior to their biopsies. Sixty-eight percent of the women whose biopsies turned out to be positive for cancer were people with an abnormal tendency to suppress anger and other emotions, whereas only 25 percent of those with negative biopsies had this personality trait.

In the only study in which individuals' personalities and backgrounds were studied years before they developed cancer it was found that those who got cancer tended to be low-keyed, quiet, emotionally self-contained and lonely people who were not close to their parents as children. In this study, Dr. Caroline Bedell Thomas of Johns Hopkins University Medical School followed 1,337 medical students who were first interviewed and tested between 1948 and 1964 when they entered medical school. The forty-three doctors who years later developed cancer were found to have personalities very much like those who became mentally ill or committed suicide.

Dr. Claus Bahne Bahnson of Eastern Pennsylvania Psychiatric Institute in Philadelphia studied cancer patients, patients with other diseases and healthy persons and found that, unlike the others, the cancer patients characteristically were "closed-up" and defensive people who operate with high levels of internal conflict, or stress, and attempt to cope with these conflicts by denying or repressing their existence. The cancer patients typically denied feelings and attitudes that were not socially acceptable and repressed all unpleasant emotions—anxiety, depression, hostility, guilt and the like—to a much greater extent than the other persons studied. The cancer patients also had great difficulty dealing with and expressing anger. They tended to live formal and common-sensical social and family lives, all the while ignoring the basic needs for affection, warmth and personal creativity. Dr.

Bahnson also found that, as the probable cause for this repressed emotional life, the cancer patients typically had ungratifying, cold relationships with their parents—particularly their mothers—who were "there" physically but not emotionally. As a result, the children learned to deny their emotions rather than discharge them. When such persons experience a loss, instead of going through a typical cathartic mourning process, they tend, like Emma G., the Wisconsin farm wife, to deny the loss, adopt a Pollyanna attitude that says "Everything is fine" and keep on with their activities as if nothing had happened. Dr. Bahnson believes that when such intense emotions are not expressed as external behavior, they are internalized and expressed instead as changes in the body's central nervous system, which in turn can upset the hormone balance or immunological response and interfere with resistance to cancer.

Experiments with laboratory animals that have been subjected to various kinds of stress lend some support to this belief. A study of laboratory rats at Stanford University showed that those animals who were separated from their mothers early in infancy and thus deprived of their mothers' "love" were less resistant to cancer later in life than those animals who received a normal amount of mothering. Early life experiences seem to alter the immunological responses in adulthood, with animals that received attention during infancy being more resistant to infections than those who had "deprived" childhoods. In another study in which mice were subjected to the stress of an anticipated mild electric shock, the stressed animals succumbed much more rapidly to the effects of a tumor-causing virus than animals that were not stressed. Chickens are susceptible to a virus-caused tumor called Marek's disease. An experiment at Virginia Polytechnic Institute in which chickens were repeatedly moved from cage to cage, forcing them each time to adjust their position in the social pecking order, showed that the birds subjected to this stress were much more likely to develop Marek's disease.

But all experiments have not yielded consistent results. A psychologist at Kent State University in Ohio found that when rats were subjected to the stresses of overcrowding or electric shock, the development of induced breast cancer in the animals was slowed down and in some cases stopped.

What, if any, significance can be attached to such a collection of findings in animals and man will depend largely on the extent to which scientists are able to decipher the precise biochemical effects of stress and personality patterns. If it can be shown that persons who respond to stress in certain ways suffer metabolic, hormonal or immunological upsets that diminish their resistance to cancer, the belief that stress and personality are somehow related to this disease will gain much wider acceptance in the medical community.

CANCER AND VIRUSES

In 1908 Danish scientists Wilhelm Ellerman and Bernard Bang pointed out that a blood cancer in chickens called malignant leukosis seemed to be transmitted from one animal to another just like an infectious disease. Three years later Dr. Francis Peyton Rous of the Rockefeller Institute (now Rockefeller University in New York) demonstrated that the mysterious agent that caused this disease could pass through a filter, or strainer, so microscopically fine that it did not allow bacteria through. He called the agent a "filterable virus." Some years later he showed that this virus could cause solid tumors when injected into the muscle tissue of chickens. Dr. Rous, who thus discovered the first cancer-causing virus, was not duly recognized for his achievement until fifty-five years later when, at the age of 86, he was awarded a long-overdue Nobel Prize. It was often said that the long wait Dr. Rous had for due recognition reflected not on his scientific competence, which was unquestioned, but on the long-prevailing skepticism in science and medicine about the relationship of viruses to cancer in man, which in turn created doubt about the significance of Dr. Rous's discovery. More than 100 different viruses have since been shown to cause cancers in animals, but sixty-five years after Dr. Rous's finding of the avian leukosis virus, science still is uncertain that any human cancers are caused by viruses. Nonetheless, a great deal of evidence has accumulated—at a logarithmic rate in the last decade—indicating that viruses play an important role in the development of at least some human cancers.

By now, viruses have been shown to cause cancer in such animals as mice, rats, rabbits, frogs, birds, cattle, cats, dogs, and monkeys. How different an animal can man be that he should not be on this list? In all likelihood, at some future time, virologists will establish beyond scientific doubt that man is also the victim of virus-induced cancers. Several agents are already in the running to be established as the first-discovered human cancer virus. Perhaps the most talked about is herpes hominis type 2, which has been closely linked to cancer of the cervix. This cancer behaves remarkably like a venereal disease—that is, one that is transmitted through sexual intercourse—and like other venereal diseases, its cause is thought to be an infectious agent, in this case, a virus.

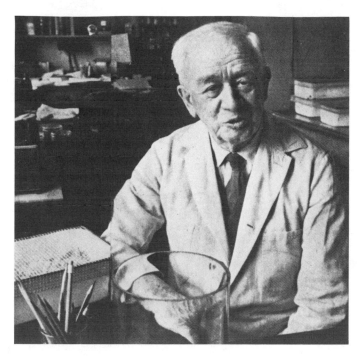

At the age of 86, Dr. Francis Peyton Rous of Rockefeller University, was finally awarded a Nobel Prize for his discovery 55 years earlier of the first cancer-causing virus. The organism, known as the Rous sarcoma virus, infects chickens.

Cancer of the cervix occurs most frequently among women who first had intercourse at an early age (during their teens) and who had many sexual partners. It is also more common among women who are poor, nonwhite, or divorced, as well as women who live in cities and who rarely attend church. But cervical cancer is almost unknown among nuns and nonclerical virgins. It is extremely rare in women from strict religious groups that insist on chastity before marriage and sexual fidelity afterward.

Herpes hominis type 2, also known as genital herpes virus, causes the second most common venereal disease (after gonorrhea) in the three countries where it has been studied, the United States, England, and Sweden. Genital herpes is a first cousin to herpes simplex, the virus that causes unsightly, painful cold sores (fever blisters) on the mouth. Genital herpes virus causes similar sores on the genital organs—on the penis in men and on the vulva and the cervix in women. In men the infection is obvious. But in four out of five infected women, the sores are hidden and the women are unaware of their infection. But traces of a herpes virus infection sometime in the past remain in the blood for years in the form of antibodies to the virus. By studying herpes virus antibodies, doctors have been able to demonstrate that prior herpes infection is far more common among women who develop cervical cancer. In fact, 95 percent of women with the cancer have evidence of a past herpes infection, compared to 25 percent of women with similar backgrounds but free of the cancer. Evidence of herpes infection is also more commonly found in women with early cancer (carcinoma in situ) of the cervix and women with cervical dysplasia, an irregularity in the cells of the cervix which sometimes leads to cancer. Indeed, the relationship between the virus and cervical cancer is so strong that some doctors are convinced it must be causal.

But proof that a virus causes cancer in man can not be obtained in the same way that the disease-causing role of other infectious agents is established. The rules of proof, called Koch's postulates, can not be applied to suspected human cancer viruses. These postulates state that the agent in question first must be isolated from a sick individual; when injected into a healthy individual it should cause the same disease, and then the same agent should be able to be re-isolated from the second case.

First, it has not been possible to isolate from people with cancer a whole, intact, infectious agent. Cancer viruses, if they exist in man, seem to become a permanent part of the genetic material of cells, and only part of the virus is believed to be involved. Second, it is clearly unethical to inject such an agent, if one were found, into another person to see if he gets the same disease. At best, the tests would have to be done in animals, which may not have the same response as man. Therefore, scientists seeking to prove viral causation in certain human cancers rely on more circumstantial evidence. In the case of herpes virus and cervical cancer, for example, large groups of women—some of whom had herpes infections and others who did not—are being followed for many years to see which ones develop cervical cancer. Thus far it appears that women with herpes type 2 antibodies are four to five times more likely to develop the cancer.

The virus is also being studied in the laboratory. It has been shown to be able to "transform" normal cells into cells that are potentially malignant. All told, herpes type 2 and its cousin herpes simplex (also called herpes virus type 1) have been associated with fourteen different human cancers, mainly those involving the mouth area and the genitourinary tract.

But these are not the only herpes viruses suspected of causing cancer in man. Another candidate is a herpes virus known as EB (Epstein-Barr) virus, already proved to be the cause of infectious mononucleosis. In mononucleosis, a large excess of one type of white blood cell is produced and the disease is often described as a self-limiting leukemia. EB virus has been closely linked to Burkitt's lymphoma, a common cancer among young children in tropical Africa, and to cancer of the nasopharynx (nose and throat). EB virus has been grown out of the white blood cells of Burkitt's patients, and 100 percent of African children with the tumor have very large amounts of antibody to this virus in their blood, compared to 50 percent of children without the cancer. Similar antibody levels were found in patients with nasopharyngeal cancer. The virus may also play a role in Hodgkin's disease, chronic lymphocytic leukemia and cancer of the prostate.

In 1938 Dr. John Bittner described the "milk factor" in mice, a virus isolated from animals with breast cancer. The mouse milk factor is passed from mother to offspring through suckling. Traces of this virus, known as the mouse mammary tumor virus, have been found in women with breast cancer and in the breast milk of women at high risk of developing breast cancer. In 1971 two research groups found in human milk samples particles of the same size and structure as mouse mammary tumor virus. In addition, the genes of the virus were found to match the genes in two-thirds of human breast cancer tissue samples, but in none of the tissue samples from healthy women or women with noncancerous breast diseases. This indicates that genetic information from the virus is "hiding" in the cancer cells. Even when the virus cannot be seen, its genetic "footprints" can be detected.

In the mouse the mammary tumor virus depends on female hormones to help it to cause cancer, and there is good reason to believe that if a virus is involved in human breast cancer, hormones act to "promote" its cancer-causing ability. One thing known about the suggested human breast cancer virus is that, unlike its role in the mouse, in women it is not transmitted as a cancer-causing agent through the milk. No increased risk of breast cancer has been found in women who were breast fed in infancy.

Another form of human cancer that has been linked to an animal cancer virus is leukemia. The genes of the Rauscher mouse leukemia virus have been shown to match those contained in the white blood cells of leukemic patients in 89 percent of cases. In 1975 virologists at the National Cancer Institute isolated from a patient with acute myelogenous leukemia a virus which closely resembles the viruses that produce leukemia in nonhuman primates. It is not certain that the virus is of human origin or that it caused the leukemia, but for various biological reasons, this virus is widely thought to be the best candidate for the first human cancer virus. Similar viruses, all of which are known as C-type viruses, have also been linked to human sarcomas, which are cancers of the bone, fat or connective tissue, and lymphomas, cancers of the lymph-producing system.

In 1951 Dr. Ludwik Gross of the Veterans Administration Hospital in the Bronx demonstrated that mouse leukemia was caused by a transmissible virus. Six years later virologists at M. D. Anderson Hospital and Tumor Institute in Houston found particles resembling mouse leukemia virus in human leukemic tissues. C-type viruses have since been established as causes of leukemia, lymphoma and sarcomas in mice, rats, hamsters, cats and nonhuman primates.

It is also now known that many of these viruses are "defective" and need a helper virus in order to cause malignant changes in normal cells. In fact, the evidence on most proposed cancer viruses points to the probability that the virus alone is unable to cause cancer, but needs some sort of a boost—a triggering factor—to enable it to do its dirty work. These triggers may include other viruses, hormones (as in the case of the mammary tumor virus), chemical carcinogens or radiation (both of which enhance the cancer-causing effect of the mouse leukemia virus), or some deficiency or derangement of the immunological system (suspected in the case of Burkitt's lymphoma). Without the triggering factor, the cancer would never appear.

Dr. Fred Rapp, noted virologist at Hershey Medical Center in Hershey, Pennsylvania, believes, as do many others in his field, that there is no "magic" cancer virus for man, no unusual virus that causes cancer and nothing else. Rather, the evidence indicates that cancer viruses are very common viruses and that infection with them is a common event. Many people harbor these viruses, but rarely does the virus cause cancer. Dr. Rapp likens the situation to polio virus. Before polio vaccines, virtually every child became infected with the polio virus, but most developed no outward signs of infection or only very mild symptoms. The rare child, however, developed paralytic polio. In the case of a cancer virus, all or part of the virus seems to become incorporated into the genetic structure of cells, transforming them into potential cancer cells. But there they remain quiescent for years until and unless something activates them. Once activated (presumably by one of the triggers mentioned above), the transformed cells can make many copies of themselves and produce a cancer.

Another theory holds that in some cases the genetic information of a cancer virus can be inherited from one's parents and thus is present in the cells from birth onward. But if nothing "switches" the virus information on, the cancer it can cause never develops. If this theory turns out to be true for some cancers, then preventing those cancers will probably have to involve controlling exposure to whatever factors might trigger the expression of the virus. In such cases a vaccine against the virus would probably not be practical, since vaccines prevent viruses from infecting cells and these cells already have the virus within them.

When speaking of cancer viruses, the question of possible contagion—or spread from one person to another—logically arises in peoples' minds. There is no consistent or convincing evidence that any form of human cancer can be spread from person to person like a cold or the flu. Although "clusters" of certain cancers—namely, Hodgkin's disease and leukemia—have been identified among individuals who had direct or indirect contact with one another, there is no proof that these relationships were anything more than chance occurrences. But even if the existence of a real cluster, beyond the realm of chance, were established, it would not necessarily mean that an infectious agent (that is, a virus) was what the individuals transmitted to one another. They may have all been exposed to the same triggering factor.

In any case with regard to EB virus, the cause of mononucleosis and the suspect agent in Hodgkin's disease, 75 percent of American children already have been infected with the virus by the time they reach adolescence. It seems that in young children, EB virus causes no symptoms or only very mild symptoms indistinguishable from a cold or mild flu, and therefore an EB virus infection is not diagnosed. It is only when infection first occurs in the teen years or later that the more severe symptoms of mononucleosis occur. There is some suggestive evidence that persons with a history of mononucleosis have a greater than expected risk of developing Hodgkin's disease, which most commonly strikes young adults between the ages of 20 and 40.

Because many animal cancers are known to be caused by viruses, another question often raised is whether people can "catch" cancer viruses that infect animals, particularly household pets. Here again, there is no consistent or convincing evidence that this can occur, although certain animal tumor viruses are able to infect the cells of other animal species in the test tube. The cat leukemia virus can be transmitted from cat to cat just like any other viral infection might be, but there is no proof of human infection by cat leukemia virus and no evidence of an increase in human cancer in households where the animals developed cancer (although one study found a high cancer rate in households where there were "sick" cats—with no disease specified—and there are occasional reports of human and animal tumors appearing coincidentally in the same household). The virus that causes a cancer in chickens called Marek's disease does not seem to be transmissible to man, not even to poultry farmers who have close and prolonged contact with infected animals. However, virus-containing milk from a herd of cattle that had a high incidence of leukemia produced leukemia-like illness when fed to newborn chimpanzees.

Viruses are not the only infectious agents suspected of causing cancer in man. Various parasitic infestations are also thought to set the stage for certain human cancers. Severe malaria infestation has been linked to an increased risk of Burkitt's lymphoma in Africa, and it is possible that the malaria parasite directly or indirectly triggers the EB virus to cause the tumor (perhaps by disturbing the immune response). In Egypt and other parts of Africa a relationship has been noted between schistosomiasis, an infestation by blood flukes, and bladder cancer. The belief is that the parasite causes a chronic irritation of the bladder tissue, perhaps producing a toxin, that sets the stage for cancer to develop. Similarly, infection by the oriental liver fluke through consumption of infested raw fish has been linked to liver cancer in Asian countries.

If viruses are eventually proved to cause some cancers in man, a variety of approaches to prevention are possible, including vaccines to prevent the initial virus infection or drugs that prevent the virus from infecting cells or that prevent the viral genes already in cells from being switched on. If triggering mechanisms are involved, exposure to them might be avoidable.

WHAT CANCER IS NOT CAUSED BY

For all the things that do cause cancer, there are a number of factors popularly thought to be related to cancer which have no foundation in fact. One such popular myth is the notion that cancer represents the wages exacted by sin, a punishment for some wrongdoing, real or imagined. There is absolutely no evidence to support the idea that cancer is the penance people pay for moral lapses, evil thoughts or criminal acts. Even cancer of the cervix, which is more common among prostitutes and promiscuous women, is not "just desserts" for moral turpitude; rather, it is associated with sexual activity, which most of us engage in from time to time. The attitude that cancer is somehow sinful has spawned secrecy and shame, attempts to "cover up" the fact of cancer to protect the family name, too often with the unfortunate consequence that treatment and detection of cancer in other family members is delayed beyond medical help.

Another popular misconception is that cancer is caused by an injury or irritation. If that were the case, we should all have cancer of the knees, probably the most frequently injured part of the body, or cancer of the hands and feet, undoubtedly the most "irritated" parts of the body. Fractures, for example, are extremely common, but primary bone cancers are rare. The only part of the body where chronic irritation seems to sometimes cause precancerous lesions is in the mouth.

The idea that chronic irritation could cause cancer evolved partly as a result of early attempts to induce cancer in animals. Scientists would administer an agent daily to animal skin and after a while, a tumor would appear at the site. What the scientists did not realize at the time was that the tumor resulted because the substance they applied was a carcinogen, not because the skin became overly irritated. Thus far, with the exception of mouth lesions, everyone who has tried to prove the idea that irritation, in the ordinary sense of the word, can cause cancer has come up with something else as the actual cause.

Sometimes women think that breast cancer results from being bumped or bruised on the breast or from sexual stimulation and manipulation of the breast and nipples. Since breast cancer is the most common cancer in women and since getting bumped or bruised on a protruding part of the body is extremely common, these two phenomena are more than likely to happen to the same woman. But that does not mean one caused the other. There is no evidence to even suggest that injuring the breast or manipulation during sexual activity increases the risk of breast cancer.

Injury has also been said, without any factual evidence, to increase risk of bone cancer. This cancer most commonly develops in young people in the long bones of the leg, often near the knee, where injuries frequently occur. What child has not hurt his leg? What child, in fact, does not hurt his leg at least once every few months? Thus, should bone cancer develop, it would not be unusual for there to have been an injury near the cancerous bone at some time in the past. More often, when injury is associated with the development of cancer, it is likely that the discomfort or the X-rays taken as a result of the injury called attention to a preexisting cancer, rather than caused it.

For decades groups opposed to the fluoridation of water supplies, a public health measure that has reduced the incidence of tooth decay in children by two-thirds, have been promoting the notion that fluoridation can cause cancer. Claims have included the charge that cities where the water is fluoridated have higher cancer rates than cities without fluoridation. The National Cancer Institute has taken a close look at the cancer rates in different cities and has found no consistent relationship between cancer and fluoridation. In some cases, fluoridated cities do have higher than expected cancer rates, but in most instances this is due to an excess of lung cancer cases, probably related to the heavy industrial pollution in the area. In other instances, the city had high cancer rates long before fluoridation was introduced. Fluoridation opponents often capitalize on the idea that the element fluorine is highly reactive and can combine with organic matter in drinking water to form potential carcinogens. However, it is not *flourine* that is added to fluoridated water, but rather *fluorides*—sodium fluoride, sodium silicofluoride and fluorosilicic acid—which break up into minute inert particles that cannot combine with organic compounds and thus have no cancer-causing potential.

Other myths about causes of cancer can be rapidly dispelled. There is no evidence that cancer results from the use of aluminum pots and pans, or from vaccinations for smallpox, or any other immunizations. And while certain vitamin deficiencies may increase an individual's susceptibility to certain kinds of cancer, there is no convincing evidence that megadoses of vitamins, beyond the amounts needed to prevent common deficiency symptoms, or frequent consumption of large amounts of any particular food can prevent cancer.

24. The Future of Cancer Control

Nothing would please me more than if I could end this book with a prediction that five, ten, twenty or even fifty years from now medical science will have devised a simple way to prevent the scourge of cancer or the deaths it causes. But no such prediction can be made by anyone familiar with the complexities of the cancer problem. It cannot be said with any degree of certainty that a key to controlling cancer will be found within our lifetime, or that a single key will ever be found. Even if scientists can finally understand exactly how a cell changes from normal to malignant, it may not be possible to devise a widely applicable means of interrupting that chain of events. All of this is not to say, however, that many new and life-saving measures designed to interfere with the development and growth of cancer won't be devised in the coming years. Scientists throughout the world are pursuing exciting research findings that promise to lead to new methods of preventing cancer, detecting it in its microscopic stages when the chances for cure are nearly 100 percent, stopping the growth of cancer before it can invade other tissues, and curing cancer that has already become well-established.

Following is a brief description of a few such leads. This is by no means intended to represent a complete list of the most promising avenues of cancer research. It is merely to give you a flavor of what the foreseeable future may hold, as well as a fuller appreciation for the fact that, for many years to come, preventing cancer deaths will continue to depend on the methods described in Part II of this book.

● In 1970 Dr. Howard M. Temin, an oncologist (cancer specialist) at the University of Wisconsin, and Dr. David Baltimore, a microbiologist at the Massachusetts Institute of Technology, discovered an enzyme that enables certain animal cancer viruses to reprogram the genes of normal cells. This enzyme, which in effect would allow the virus to convert a healthy cell to a cancer cell, is being used to study the possible relationship of viruses to human cancers. With this enzyme Dr. Sol Spiegelman of Columbia University has found evidence to suggest that childhood leukemia may be caused by a virus. In 1975 Drs. Temin and Baltimore, both of whom are American Cancer Society Research Professors, received the Nobel Prize in physiology or medicine for their work.

● An ideal test to screen ostensibly healthy people for the presence of cancer would have to be harmless, inexpensive, specific for cancer, and capable of detecting any type of cancer anywhere in the body. Although scientists are still a long way from developing such a test, a number of tests are now being studied which may ultimately prove useful, particularly when two or more are used together, for screening high-risk populations or examining patients who have ill-defined symptoms. These tests capitalize on the facts that persons with cancer tend to have deficiencies in their immune systems and that cancers tend to produce immunological factors that are different from those produced by normal tissues. One or more of these tests may also be a useful guide to treatment planning; the tests could be used to monitor the effectiveness of cancer therapy and to detect the beginning of the spread of cancer. Tests are underway in animals of an approach to cancer detection using radioactive antibodies that recognize and react with the immunological factors produced by cancer cells.

● Other tests are being developed that may help to determine which individuals in the population are unusually susceptible to the development of cancer. One such test for ferreting out high-risk persons uses a monkey virus called SV40. In the test, a very small piece of the person's skin is grown with the virus and then assessed for the degree to which the virus has transformed the cells into potentially malignant cells. Other possible future ways of detecting persons who have a high cancer risk include tests for the presence of certain enzymes or levels of hormones in the blood.

● On a more basic level, scientists like Dr. Robert A. Good, President of the Sloan-Kettering Institute for Cancer Research in New York, are exploring the precise relationships between the state of the immune system and the development of cancer. What part of the immune system is responsible for detecting and destroying cancer cells that might arise and why does it fail sometimes? The answers to such questions will undoubtedly provide new tools for cancer treatment that involve giving a specific boost to the flagging part of the immune system. One such approach that is being explored experimentally in cancer patients involves injections of white blood cells called macrophages that have been "activated" to find and destroy tumor cells. The use of other promising immunological weapons against cancer was discussed in the section on treatment.

● Other basic studies are investigating the changes in the surface, or membrane, of cells that seem to occur in malignant cells but not in normal cells. Just what happens to a cell when it becomes free of the normal restraints on growth? How does it change to get more food so that it can divide endlessly? As Dr. Good put it, "We are especially concerned with the cell surface and surface-to-nucleus signals which actually define what a cell is, what it relates to, where it goes, how its development is controlled, and its replication initiated and stopped." If these mechanisms can be understood, perhaps a way can be found to interrupt or reverse them in cancer cells.

● In 1971 a Harvard University surgeon, Dr. M. Judah Folkman, discovered that the growth of most cancers was dependent on a protein substance without which the tumors remained in a dormant, harmless state. The substance, called tumor angiogenesis factor (T.A.F.), appears to be critical to the ability of a solid tumor to establish the blood supply it needs to nourish it and allow it to grow and spread. Without T.A.F. the tumor becomes trapped in its own wastes and cannot grow beyond the size of a pinhead. Dr. Folkman and his colleagues are trying to develop a means of inhibiting T.A.F. If this is possible without harming normal blood vessels, an entirely new approach to cancer therapy—that of forcing tumors into indefinite hibernation—may become available.

● Other researchers are looking for novel ways to apply already established methods of cancer treatment. One of these approaches is the use of microscopic "guided missiles" that can deliver anti-cancer drugs right to the cancer cells, and thus give the cancer cells a higher dose of poison and reduce damage to normal cells. These "missiles" are called liposomes. They are fatty capsules that can be targeted to attach only to cancer cells, at which time they would deliver their "warhead" of drugs.

● Several groups of scientists are trying to capitalize on the observation that vitamin A and its chemical relatives seem able to prevent the transformation of normal cells to malignant cells after the cells have been exposed to a cancer-causing agent, such as those in cigarette smoke. Because vitamin A by itself is highly toxic, the success of this approach to cancer prevention will depend on the ability to find related active substances that lack the poisonous qualities of large doses of vitamin A. The researchers warn that self-medication with vitamin A, beyond the recommended daily requirements, is very dangerous. Vitamin A analogues, called retinoids, are thought to be needed for the proper functioning of the epithelial cells that line body organs, where 70 percent of human cancers arise.

It is quite possible that only a few—or none—of the above research prospects will pay off in life-saving ways. Most cancer scientists have long ago learned the bitter lesson that it is unwise to make promises about the ultimate value of cancer research. Premature predictions based on the early results of small studies have too often fallen through. The cancer detection test that looks great after tests on 200 people turns out to detect everything from hepatitis to pregnancy, as well as cancer, when tried on thousands. The microorganism that seems to be a cause of cancer in one or more people initially examined is found to be a freeloader that infected the individuals after they got cancer.

A great deal of time, effort, talent, and money has gone into research to crack the mysteries of cancer, and doubtless many times more research will be needed before the final answers become known. The American Cancer Society, the nation's largest voluntary health organization, spends 30 percent of its $100-million annual budget—and the National Cancer Institute 80 percent of its $700-million-a-year budget—on cancer research, ranging from studies of basic cell mechanisms to the development of new approaches to treatment.

The nation's current "war on cancer" is not like the Manhattan Project to build an atomic bomb or the Apollo program to reach the moon. In those cases, the scientific knowledge needed to achieve the goals was in hand. All that was needed was a concentration of resources, talent, and effort to put the knowledge into effective technological form. In the case of cancer much fundamental knowledge still needs to be attained before a directed project to "conquer cancer" can be effectively launched. Indeed, a few cancer experts, including Dr. Lewis Thomas, President of Memorial Sloan-Kettering Cancer Center, believe that something entirely unexpected and unknown at this time could turn out to be the ultimate key to solving the cancer problem. As Dr. Thomas put it, "None of us can say which of the several lines that are presently being pursued will turn out to be right. I am quite prepared for the eventuality that the cause of cancer is something no one has yet thought of. In fact, I would not be surprised to learn that we are all wrong at the present time." Dr. Frank J. Rauscher, Jr., who directed the National Cancer Program, has pointed out that "the conquest of cancer is a long-term objective. We are still exploring vast, uncharted areas of biology and medicine ... It will probably take years to achieve dramatic results."

Lest these sound like depressing and discouraging viewpoints, it is important to keep in mind the message that Dr. Justin J. Stein, then President of the American Cancer Society, delivered to the Society's annual seminar for science writers in 1974; "Much is known to permit us now to make a greater effort toward saving the lives of those who die needlessly every year. We do not need to know *why* the normal cell is susceptible to malignant transformation to accomplish this goal. What we need to know is *what, when,* and *where,* and most of these facts already exist or can be obtained."

As described in the section on preventing cancer, medical scientists already know how to reduce greatly the incidence of some cancers, including the nation's leading cancer killer, lung cancer. Cancer prevention will necessarily involve some changes in lifestyles. Americans will have to learn to forego some of the harmful so-called pleasures this affluent society provides if a serious dent is to be made in the incidence of cancer. But the fact remains that we already have many of the tools for preventing cancer.

Rapid progress is also being made in identifying persons who are at high risk of developing one or another type of cancer. This knowledge can be life-saving if such persons are subjected to periodic screening procedures that can detect early, curable cancers. At the same time, doctors are becoming better equipped to recognize and treat cancer. Growing numbers of physicians' groups are developing subspecialties in oncology. Radiologists, internists, obstetrician-gynecologists, and pediatricians already have such a subspeciality. Many surgeons are becoming identified as specialists in surgical oncology. The medical oncologist can function as the effective leader of a team that plans the most appropriate treatment for each patient. To provide chemotherapy to more cancer patients, medical oncologists who were trained at major cancer centers are setting up practices in communities, and some of them are affiliated with a good many hospitals in their geographic area. Similarly, community hospitals throughout the country are upgrading the quality of radiation therapy they can provide by getting new equipment and training physicians in the latest techniques for providing the optimal radiation dose to the cancer while sparing the normal tissue.

More and more, cancer treatment is becoming a multidisciplinary effort, using combinations of therapies to wipe out cancers that individual treatment approaches would be unable to cure. It is difficult to put into words the almost tangible excitement that is apparent today among physicians using the new combination therapies. As described in the section on treatment, these new approaches have completely turned around the prognosis for a number of once-hopeless cancers, and they now show promise for long term control in patients with relatively advanced forms of the common cancer killers and for preventing recurrences of these diseases.

Some critics have charged that the leaders of the "war on cancer" have made unjustifiable claims about the advances in cancer treatment achieved under the National Cancer Program. The critics cite the most recent available national cancer survival statistics and say that little if anything has been accomplished. What these critics fail to realize is that these statistics reflect the outcome in patients treated for cancer no later than 1969. But the National Cancer Act did not become law until 1971 and the National Cancer Program was not fully operational until 1973. Treatment advances that were put into effect in 1973 cannot even begin to be reflected in survival figures until 1978, because survival is measured as the chance of being alive five years after treatment of cancer. Dr. Rauscher points out that testing the effectiveness of new treatment methods takes a minimum of three to five years, and usually more. Once a new treatment has been evaluated, the information must then be widely disseminated to the medical profession so that it can be applied to cancer patients throughout the country. Then another five years must elapse before the overall effects of this change in treatment are reflected in national survival figures. He explains that "new treatment methods necessarily require ten or more years to be reflected in overall survival figures."

The public is used to far more rapid effects of advances in medicine. When the polio vaccine was developed, it took but one summer to prove it was effective; the next year millions of people were immunized and polio epidemics became a thing of the past nearly overnight. But a test of a new cancer treatment is a far more time-consuming process. A new therapy must first be tried on a handful of patients at a few medical centers. If it appears more effective than current treatments (an assessment which may itself take five years), then it must be tested more widely—on hundreds of patients in half a dozen or more hospitals—with the results of these tests not known for another five years. All told, cancer experts estimate that it takes at least fourteen years to accumulate satisfactory evidence that a new treatment method is indeed better than the one that doctors had been using. Only then will the new method become widely used and begin to change the outlook for cancer patients in general.

So you can see that it is unwise to take a cavalier or head-in-the-sand attitude toward cancer—to think, for example, that it is all right to smoke because you're young and by the time you get lung cancer medical science will have found a way to cure it, or to avoid thinking about cancer at all because you believe there is really nothing you can do about it anyway. For many, if not most, persons, the weapons to fight cancer and win are already available. Those people who are now suffering from cancer can take advantage of the most effective forms of treatment known. Those who suspect they might have cancer can see a physician without delay to have the diagnosis confirmed or denied. And the vast majority of people who are currently healthy and without any suspicious symptoms can begin now the battle to stay healthy by becoming aware of the known causes of cancer and avoiding those hazards wherever possible, and by taking advantage of routine detection methods that can find hidden cancers while they are still virtually 100 percent curable.

The answer to cancer is in your hands.

APPENDIX
CANCER SERVICES

The following organizations can help you or your physician obtain information about the services related to cancer—its causes and prevention, detection and diagnosis, treatment and rehabilitation.

I. The American and Canadian Cancer Societies: Chartered Divisions by State and Province

The American and Canadian Cancer Societies, their divisions, units and all their activities, are supported by public contributions and volunteered services. Contacts for services and information are best made through divisions and units. The addresses of the Societies' national headquarters are:

The American Cancer Society, Inc.
777 Third Avenue
New York, New York 10017
(212) 371-2900

Canadian Cancer Society
Administrative Offices, Suite 401
77 Bloor Street West
Toronto, Ontario M5S 2V7
(416) 961-7223

CHARTERED DIVISIONS: BY STATE

Alabama Division, Inc.
2926 Central Avenue
Birmingham, Alabama
35209
(205) 879-2242

Alaska Division, Inc.
1343 G Street
Anchorage, Alaska 99501
(907) 277-8696

Arizona Division, Inc.
634 West Indian School
Road
Phoenix, Arizona 85011
(602) 264-5861

Arkansas Division, Inc.
5520 West Markham
Street
Little Rock, Arkansas
72203
(501) 664-3480-1-2

California Division, Inc.
731 Market Street
San Francisco, California
94103
(415) 777-1800

Colorado Division, Inc.
1809 East 18th Avenue
Denver, Colorado 80218
(303) 321-2464

Connecticut Division, Inc.
Professional Center
270 Amity Road
Woodbridge, Connecticut
06525
(203) 389-4571

Delaware Division, Inc.
Academy of Medicine
Bldg.
1925 Lovering Avenue
Wilmington, Delaware
19806
(302) 654-6267

District of Columbia Division, Inc.
Universal Building, South

1825 Connecticut Avenue, N.W.
Washington, D.C. 20009
(202) 483-2600

Florida Division, Inc.
1001 South MacDill
Avenue
Tampa, Florida 33609
(813) 253-0541

Georgia Division, Inc.
2025 Peachtree Road,
N.E.
Suite 14
Atlanta, Georgia 30309
(404) 351-3650-1-2

Hawaii Division, Inc.
Community Services
Center Bldg.
200 North Vineyard
Boulevard
Honolulu, Hawaii 96817
(808) 531-1662-3-4-5

Idaho Division, Inc.
P.O. Box 5386
1609 Abbs Street
Boise, Idaho 83705
(208) 343-4609

Illinois Division, Inc.
37 South Wabash Avenue
Chicago, Illinois 60603
(312) 372-0472

Indiana Division, Inc.
2702 East 55th Place
Indianapolis, Indiana
46220
(317) 257-5326

Iowa Division, Inc.
P.O. Box 980
Mason City, Iowa 50401
(515) 423-0712

Kansas Division, Inc.
3003 Van Buren
Topeka, Kansas 66611
(913) 267-0131

Kentucky Division, Inc.
Medical Arts Bldg.
1169 Eastern Parkway
Louisville, Kentucky
40217
(502) 452-2676

Louisiana Division, Inc.
Masonic Temple Bldg.,
Room 810
333 St. Charles Avenue
New Orleans, Louisiana
70130
(504) 523-2029

Maine Division, Inc.
Federal and Greene
Streets
Brunswick, Maine 04011
(207) 729-3339

Maryland Division, Inc.
200 East Joppa Road
Towson, Maryland 21204
(301) 828-8890

Massachusetts Division,
Inc.
247 Commonwealth
Avenue
Boston, Massachusetts
02116
(617) 267-2650

Michigan Division, Inc.
1205 East Saginaw Street
Lansing, Michigan 48906
(517) 371-2920

Minnesota Division, Inc.
2750 Park Avenue
Minneapolis, Minnesota
55407
(612) 871-2111

Mississippi Division, Inc.
345 North Mart Plaza
Jackson, Mississippi
39206
(601) 362-8874

Missouri Division, Inc.
P.O. Box 1066
715 Jefferson Street
Jefferson City, Missouri
65101
(314) 636-3195

Montana Division, Inc.
2115 Second Avenue
North
Billings, Montana 59101
(406) 252-7111

Nebraska Division, Inc.
6910 Pacific Street,
Suite 210
Omaha, Nebraska 68106
(402) 551-2422

Nevada Division, Inc.
4220 Maryland Parkway
Suite 105
Las Vegas, Nevada 89109
(702) 736-2999

New Hampshire
Division, Inc.
22 Bridge Street
Manchester, New Hampshire 03101
(603) 669-3270

New Jersey Division,
Inc.
2700 Route 22, P.O.
Box 1220
Union, New Jersey 07083
(201) 687-2100

New Mexico Division,
Inc.
205 San Pedro, N.E.
Albuquerque, New
Mexico 87108
(505) 268-4501

New York State Division, Inc.
6725 Lyons Street
East Syracuse, New York
13057
(315) 437-7025

☐ Long Island Division
Inc.
535 Broad Hollow
Road
(Route 110)
Melville, New York
11746
(516) 420-1111

☐ New York City
Division, Inc.
19 West 56th St.
New York, New York
10019
(212) 586-8700

☐ Queens Division, Inc.
111-15 Queens
Boulevard

Forest Hills, New York
11375
(212) 263-2224

☐ Westchester Division,
Inc.
107 Lake Avenue
Tuckahoe, New York
10707
(914) 793-3100

North Carolina Division
Inc.
P.O. Box 27624
222 North Person Street
Raleigh, North Carolina
27611
(919) 834-8463

North Dakota Division
Inc.
P.O. Box 426
Hotel Graver Annex
Bldg.
115 Roberts Street
Fargo, North Dakota
58102
(701) 232-1385

Ohio Division, Inc.
453 Lincoln Bldg.
1367 East Sixth Street
Cleveland, Ohio 44114
(216) 771-6700

Oklahoma Division, Inc.
1312 Northwest 24th
Street
Oklahoma City,
Oklahoma 73106
(405) 525-3515

Oregon Division, Inc.
1530 S.W. Taylor Street
Portland, Oregon 97205
(503) 228-8331

Pennsylvania Division,
Inc.
P.O. Box 4175
Harrisburg, Pennsylvania
17111
(717) 545-4215

☐ Philadelphia Division,
Inc.
21 South 12th Street
Philadelphia, Pennsyl-
vania 19107
(215) 567-0559

Puerto Rico Division,
Inc.
GPO Box 6004
San Juan, Puerto Rico
00936
(809) 764-2295

Rhode Island Division,
Inc.
333 Grotto Avenue
Providence, Rhode Island
02906
(401) 831-6970

South Carolina Division,
Inc.
4482 Fort Jackson
Boulevard
Columbia, South
Carolina 29209
(803) 787-5624

South Dakota Division,
Inc.
700 South 4th Avenue
Sioux Falls, South Dakota
57104
(605) 336-0897

Tennessee Division, Inc.
2519 White Avenue
Nashville, Tennessee
37204
(615) 383-1710

Texas Division, Inc.
P.O. Box 9863
Austin, Texas 78766
(512) 345-4560

Utah Division, Inc.
610 East South Temple
Salt Lake City, Utah
84102
(801) 322-0431

Vermont Division, Inc.
13 Loomis Street,
Drawer C
Montpelier, Vermont
05602
(802) 223-2348

Virginia Division, Inc.
3218 West Cary Street
P.O. Box 7288
Richmond, Virginia
23221
(804) 359-0208

Washington Division,
Inc.
323 First Avenue West
Seattle, Washington 98119
(206) 284-8390

West Virginia Division,
Inc.
325 Professional Building
Charleston, West Virginia
25301
(304) 344-3611

Wisconsin Division, Inc.
P.O. Box 1626
Madison, Wisconsin
53701
(608) 249-0487

☐ Milwaukee Division,
Inc.
6401 West Capitol
Drive
Milwaukee, Wisconsin
53216
(414) 461-1100

Wyoming Division, Inc.
1118 Logan Avenue
Cheyenne, Wyoming
82001
(307) 638-3331

Affilliate of the Ameri-
can Cancer Society
Canal Zone Cancer
Committee
Drawer "A"
Balboa Heights,
Canal Zone

BY PROVINCE

Quebec Division
Canadian Cancer Society
1118 St. Catherine Street West
Montréal, Quebec
(514) 866-2613

Manitoba Division
Canadian Cancer Society
960 Portage Avenue
Winnipeg, Manitoba R3G 0R4
(204) 775-4449

British Columbia & Yukon Division
Canadian Cancer Society
1926 West Broadway
Vancouver, British Columbia V6J 1Z2
(604) 736-1211

New Brunswick Division
Canadian Cancer Society
(61 Union Street, E2L 1A2 — parcels)
Post Office Box 2089
Saint John, New Brunswick E2L 3T5
(506) 652-7600

Nova Scotia Division
Canadian Cancer Society
1485 South Park Street
Halifax, Nova Scotia B3J 2L1
(902) 423-6550

Newfoundland Division
Canadian Cancer Society
3rd Floor, Philip Place
St. John's, Newfoundland A1A 2Y4
(709) 753-6520

Ontario Division
Administrative offices
suite 401 — 77Bloor Street West
Toronto, Ontario M5S 2V7
(416) 961-7223

Canadian Cancer Society
185 Bloor Street East, 6th Floor
Toronto, Ontario M4W 3G5
(416) 923-7474

Alberta Division
Canadian Cancer Society
Main Floor, 1134 — 8th Avenue South
West
Calgary, Alberta T2P 1J5
(403) 263-3120

Saskatchewan Division
Canadian Cancer Society
1501 — 11th Avenue
Regina, Saskatchewan
S4P 0H3
(306) 522-6320

Prince Edward Island Division
Canadian Cancer Society
51 University Avenue, 3rd Floor
Charlottetown, Prince Edward Island
(709) 753-6520

In addition to the 58 chartered divisions, there are 2,792 local units of the American Cancer Society, usually at the county or town level. Contact your state division or check your area telephone directory (under "American Cancer Society" or "Cancer") for the unit nearest you.

II. The National Cancer Institute

The National Cancer Institute, a federally supported organization that sponsors cancer research and patient services throughout the country, provides public information and educational materials through the following office:

Office of Cancer Communications
National Cancer Institute
Building 31, Room 10 A 30
Bethesda, Maryland 20014
(301) 496-6631

A. COMPREHENSIVE CANCER CENTERS.

The National Cancer Institute has designated 18 medical institutions as "comprehensive cancer centers," capable of providing up-to-date information and care for all major types of cancer. In addition to these 18 centers, there are other medical institutions around the country that also provide excellent care. Most are affiliated with medical schools and some are called "cancer centers." In the list of comprehensive cancer centers below, the first item is the name and telephone number of the center director and the second item is the address and telephone number of the director of public and professional information. Ten of the centers operate toll-free cancer information services; an 800 area code indicates this service.

ALABAMA
University of Alabama Hospitals and Clinics
619 South 19th Street
Birmingham 35233
1. John R. Durant, M.D.
   Director, Cancer Research and Training Center
   (205) 934-5077
2. Director, Cancer Communications Office
   205 Mortimer Jordan Hall

University of Alabama in Birmingham
Birmingham 35294
(205) 934-2651 or 934-2671

CALIFORNIA

Los Angeles County–University of Southern California
Cancer Center School of Medicine
2025 Zonal Avenue
Los Angeles 90033
1. G. Denman Hammond, M.D.
   Associate Dean and Director
   (213) 226-2008
2. Director, Office of Cancer Communications
Los Angeles County–University of Southern California
Cancer Center
   1721 Griffin Avenue
   Los Angeles 90031
   (213) 226-4043 or 226-4044

COLORADO

Colorado Regional Cancer Center, Inc.
165 Cook Street
Denver 80206
1. Ernest Borek, Ph.D.
   Acting Director
   (303) 320-5921
2. Director of Education and Information
   Colorado Regional Cancer Center, Inc.
   165 Cook Street
   Denver 80206
   (303) 320-5921
   (800) 332-1850

CONNECTICUT

Yale Comprehensive Cancer Center
Yale University School of Medicine
333 Cedar Street
New Haven 06510
1. Jack W. Cole, M.D.
   Director
   (203) 432-4122
2. Communications Program Manager
   Yale Comprehensive Cancer Center
   Yale University School of Medicine
   333 Cedar Street, Room IHR-E19
   New Haven 06510

(203) 436-3779 or 436-0517
(800) 922-0824

DISTRICT OF COLUMBIA

Howard University with Georgetown University
1. Jack E. White, M.D.
   Director, Cancer Research Center
   Howard University Hospital
   Department of Oncology
   2041 Georgia Avenue, N.W.
   Washington, D.C. 20060
   (202) 745-1406 or 462-8488

   John F. Potter, M.D.
   Director, Lombardi Cancer Research Center
   Georgetown University
   3800 Reservoir Rd., N.W.
   Washington, D.C. 20007
   (202) 625-7066
2. Communications Officer
   Cancer Communications for Metropolitan Washington
   Suite 218
   1825 Connecticut Avenue N.W.
   Washington, D.C. 20009
   (202) 797-8876 or 797-8893

FLORIDA

Comprehensive Cancer Center for the State of Florida
University of Miami School of Medicine
Jackson Memorial Medical Center
P.O. Box 520875
Biscayne Annex
Miami 33152
1. C. Gordon Zubrod, M.D.
   Professor and Chairman
   Department of Oncology
   (305) 547-6096
2. Cancer Information Service
   Comprehensive Cancer Center for the State of Florida
   2 S.E. 13th Street
   Miami 33131
   (305) 547-6920
   (800) 432-5953

ILLINOIS

Illinois Cancer Council
37 S. Wabash

Chicago 60603
1. Samuel G. Taylor, III, M.D.
   Director
   (312) 942-6028
2. Communications Specialist
   Illinois Cancer Council
   37 S. Wabash
   Suite 507
   Chicago 60603
   (312) 346-9813
   (800) 972-0586

MARYLAND

The Johns Hopkins Medical Institutions
Baltimore 21205
1. Albert H. Owens, Jr., M.D.
   Director, Oncology Center
   The Johns Hopkins Medical Institutions
   601 N. Broadway
   Baltimore 21205
   (301) 955-3300
2. Communications Director
   Johns Hopkins Cancer Center
   550 N. Broadway
   Suite 303
   Baltimore 21205
   (301) 955-3636

MASSACHUSETTS

Sidney Farber Cancer Center
44 Binney Street
Boston 02115
1. Emil Frei, III, M.D.
   Director and Physician-in-Chief
   (617) 739-1100, ext. 3140 or 3149
2. Communications Officer
   Cancer Control Program
   35 Binney Street
   Boston 02115
   (617) 734-7950
   (800) 952-7420

MINNESOTA

Mayo Comprehensive Cancer Center
Mayo Clinic
Rochester 55901
1. Charles G. Moertel, M.D.

    Director
    (507) 282-2511, ext. 3261
  2. Communications Specialist
    (507) 282-2511, ext. 8377
    (800) 582-5262

NEW YORK CITY

Memorial Sloan-Kettering Cancer Center
1275 York Avenue
New York 10021
  1. Lewis Thomas, M.D.
    President
    (212) 794-7646
  2. Director of Cancer Communications
    (212) 794-7982

NEW YORK STATE

Roswell Park Memorial Institute
666 Elm Street
Buffalo 14263
  1. Gerald P. Murphy, M.D.
    Director
    (716) 845-5770
  2. Cancer Control Communications Officer
    Roswell Park Memorial Institute Research Study Center
    666 Elm Street
    Buffalo 14263
    (716) 845-4402

NORTH CAROLINA

Duke University
Comprehensive Cancer Center
Duke University Medical Center
Box 3814
Durham 27710
  1. William W. Shingleton, M.D.
    Director
    (919) 684-2282
  2. Coordinator, Cancer Information Services
    200 Atlas Street
    Durham 27705
    (919) 286-2214
    (800) 672-0943

OHIO

Ohio State University Cancer Research Center
1580 Cannon Drive
Columbus 43210
1. David S. Yohn, Ph.D.
   Director
   (614) 422-5602
2. Communications Office
   Ohio State University Cancer Research Center
   1580 Cannon Drive
   Columbus 43210
   (614) 422-5022

PENNSYLVANIA

Fox Chase and University of Pennsylvania Cancer Center Program
7701 Burholme Avenue—Fox Chase
Philadelphia 19111
1. Timothy R. Talbot, M.D.
   President, Fox Chase Cancer Center
   (215) 342-1000, ext. 402
2. Communications Coordinator
   (215) 342-1000, ext. 498
   (800) 822-3963

TEXAS

The University of Texas System Cancer Center
M. D. Anderson Hospital and Tumor Institute
6723 Bertner Avenue
Houston 77030
1. R. Lee Clark, M.D.
   President
   (713) 792-3000
2. Program Administrator
   (713) 792-3363
   (800) 392-2040

WASHINGTON

Fred Hutchinson Cancer Research Center
1124 Columbia Street
Seattle 98104
1. William B. Hutchinson, M.D.
   Director
   (206) 292-2930
2. Communications Director
   Fred Hutchinson Cancer Research Center
   1124 Columbia Street, Room 176
   Seattle 98104
   (206) 292-6301

WISCONSIN

University of Wisconsin
Clinical Cancer Center
701C University Hospitals
1300 University Avenue
Madison 53706
1. Harold P. Rusch, M.D.
   Director
   (608) 262-1686 or 263-2553
2. Public Affairs Coordinator
   1900 University Avenue
   Madison 53705
   (608) 262-0046
   (800) 362-8038

B. CANCER CLINICAL COOPERATIVE GROUPS.

Following is a list of the chairmen of groups of medical institutions that cooperate in studying and applying the latest methods of treatment for various types of cancers. The research, in which more than 20,0000 patients participate annually, is sponsored by the National Cancer Institute, and in many cases, patients in the study groups may obtain part of their care free. Immediately following the list of cooperative groups is a "Tumor Types Index"—a guide to the types of cancers treated by the different groups. A patient's physician may contact the chairman of the appropriate group for guidance or referral.

COOPERATIVE GROUP CHAIRMEN

Acute Leukemia Cooperative
Group B
James F. Holland, M.D.
Mount Sinai Hospital
100th Street and Fifth Avenue
New York, New York 10029
Phone: (212) 650-6364

Brain Tumor Chemotherapy Study
Group
Michael D. Walker, M.D.
Baltimore Cancer Research Center
3100 Wyman Park Drive
Baltimore, Maryland 21211
Phone: (301) 528-7516

Central Oncology Group
Robert O. Johnson, M.D.
Headquarters Office
University of Wisconsin
   Medical School
1300 University Avenue
Madison, Wisconsin 53706
Phone: (608) 262-1626

Children's Cancer Study Group
Denman Hammond, M.D.
Operations Office
University of Southern California
1721 North Griffin Avenue
Los Angeles, California 90031
Phone: (213) 226-2008

Cooperative Breast Cancer Group
  Albert Segaloff, M.D.
  Alton Ochsner Medical
    Foundation
  1514 Jefferson Highway
  New Orleans, Louisiana 70121
  Phone: (504) 837-3000 or 834-7070

Eastern Cooperative Oncology Group
  Paul P. Carbone, M.D.
  University Hospitals
  1300 University Avenue
  Madison, Wisconsin 53706
  Phone: (608) 262-9703

Gynecologic Oncology Group
  George Lewis, M.D.
  Thomas Jefferson Medical College
  Room 300
  1025 Walnut Street
  Philadelphia, Pennsylvania 19107
  Phone: (215) 829-6507

Malignant Melanoma Clinical
  Cooperative Group
  Thomas B. Fitzpatric, M.D., Ph.D.
  Massachusetts General Hospital
  Fruit Street
  Boston, Massachusetts 02114
  Phone: (617) 726-3990

Polycythemia Vera Study Group
  Louis R. Wasserman, M.D.
  Mount Sinai Hospital
  100th Street and Fifth Avenue
  New York, New York 10029
  Phone: (212) 650-6191

Primary Breast Cancer Therapy
  Group
  Bernard Fisher, M.D.
  University of Pittsburgh
  School of Medicine
  3550 Terrace Street
  Pittsburgh, Pennsylvania 15261
  Phone: (412) 624-2666

Radiation Therapy Oncology Group
  Simon Kramer, M.D.
  Thomas Jefferson University
    Hospital

Department of Radiation Therapy
    and Nuclear Medicine
  1025 Walnut Street
  Philadelphia, Pennsylvania 19107
  Phone: (215) 829-6702

Radiotherapy Hodgkin's Disease
  Group
  James J. Nickson, M.D.
  University of Tennessee
  Radiation Oncology Division
  Chandler Building–B106
  Memphis, Tennessee 38103
  Phone: (901) 523-2471

Southeastern Cancer Study Group
  John Durant, M.D.
  University of Alabama Hospitals
    and Clinics
  619 S. 19th Street
  Birmingham, Alabama 35233
  Phone: (205) 934-5077

Southwest Oncology Group
  Barth Hoogstraten, M.D.
  Operations Office
  Suite 201
  3500 Rainbow Boulevard
  Kansas City, Kansas 66103
  Phone: (913) 831-5996

Veterans Administration Cooperative
  Urological Research Group
  George T. Mellinger, M.D.
  Veterans Administration Hospital
  5500 E. Kellogg Avenue
  Wichita, Kansas 67218
  Phone: (316) 658-2282

Veterans Administration Cooperative
  Urology Radiotherapy Research
  Group
  David F. Paulson, M.D.
  P.O. Box 2977
  Duke University Medical Center
  Durham, North Carolina 27710
  Phone: (919) 684-5057

Veterans Administration Lung
  Cancer Study Group
  Julius Wolf, M.D.

Veterans Administration
  Hospital
130 West Kingsbridge Road
Bronx, New York 10468
Phone: (212) 584-9604

*Veterans Administration Surgical
Adjuvant Cancer Chemotherapy
Study Group*
George A. Higgins, M.D.
Veterans Administration
  Hospital
50 Irving Street, N.W.
Washington, D.C. 20422
Phone: (202) 483-6666, ext. 266

Western Cancer Study Group
Joseph R. Bateman, M.D.
University of Southern California
John Wesley Hospital
2825 South Hope Street
Los Angeles, California 90007
Phone: (213) 748-3111 ext. 331

Wilms's Tumor Study Group
Giulio J. D'Angio, M.D.
Director, Cancer Center
Children's Hospital of Philadelphia
1 Children's Center
3400 Civic Center Boulevard
Philadelphia, Pennsylvania
Phone: (215) 387-5518

TUMOR TYPES: INDEX BY SPECIALITY GROUPS

ACUTE LEUKEMIA
Acute Leukemia Cooperative
  Group B
Children's Cancer Study Group
Eastern Cooperative Oncology
  Group
Southeastern Cancer Study
  Group
Southwest Oncology Group
Western Cancer Study Group

BLADDER CANCER
Radiation Therapy Oncology
  Group
Southeastern Cancer Study
  Group
Veterans Administration
  Cooperative Urological
  Research Group

BREAST CANCER
Acute Leukemia Cooperative
  Group B
Central Oncology Group
Cooperative Breast Cancer
  Group

Eastern Cooperative Oncology
  Group
Primary Breast Cancer Therapy
  Group
Southeastern Cancer Study
  Group
Southwest Oncology Group—
  Adult Division
Western Cancer Study Group

CERVICAL CANCER
Gynecologic Oncology Group
Radiation Therapy Oncology
  Group

CENTRAL NERVOUS
SYSTEM TUMORS
Acute Leukemia Cooperative
  Group B
Children's Cancer Study Group
Eastern Cooperative Oncology
  Group
Radiation Therapy Oncology
  Group
Southwest Oncology Group—
  Adult Division
Western Cancer Study Group

CHRONIC LEUKEMIA
Acute Leukemia Cooperative
Group B
Central Oncology Group
Eastern Cooperative Oncology
Group
Southeastern Cancer Study
Group
Southwest Oncology Group—
Adult Division
Western Cancer Study Group

COLON-RECTAL CANCER
Central Oncology Group
Eastern Cooperative Oncology
Group
Radiation Therapy Oncology
Group

ESOPHAGEAL CANCER
Eastern Cooperative Oncology
Group

GASTROINTESTINAL
CANCER
Southwest Oncology Group—
Adult Division

GYNECOLOGIC AND
GENITOURINARY CANCER
Southwest Oncology Group—
Adult Division

HEAD AND NECK CANCER
Central Oncology Group
Eastern Cooperative Oncology
Group
Radiation Therapy Oncology
Group
Southwest Oncology Group—
Adult Division
Western Cancer Study Group

HISTIOCYTOSIS
Southwest Oncology Group—
Pediatric Division

LUNG CANCER
Acute Leukemia Cooperative
Group B
Central Oncology Group
Eastern Cooperative Oncology
Group
Radiation Therapy Oncology
Group
Southeastern Cancer Study
Group
Southwest Oncology Group—
Adult Division

LYMPHOSARCOMA AND
HODGKIN'S DISEASE
Acute Leukemia Cooperative
Group B
Eastern Cooperative Oncology
Group
Radiation Therapy Oncology
Group
Southeastern Cancer Study
Group
Southwest Oncology Group—
Adult Division
Western Cancer Study Group

MELANOMA
Central Oncology Group
Eastern Cooperative Oncology
Group
Southeastern Cancer Study
Group
Southwest Oncology Group—
Adult Division
Western Cancer Study Group

MULTIPLE MYELOMA
Acute Leukemia Cooperative
Group B
Eastern Cooperative Oncology
Group
Southeastern Cancer Study
Group
Southwest Oncology Group—
Adult Division
Western Cancer Study Group

OVARIAN CANCER
Eastern Cooperative Oncology
Group
Gynecologic Oncology Group
Western Cancer Study Group

PANCREATIC AND
HEPATOBILIARY (LIVER)
CANCER
Central Oncology Group
Eastern Cooperative Oncology
Group
Southeastern Cancer Study
Group

POLYCYTHEMIA VERA
Polycythemia Vera Study
Group

PROSTATIC AND
TESTICULAR CANCER
Cooperative Breast Cancer
Group
Eastern Cooperative Oncology
Group
Southeastern Cancer Study
Group
Veterans Administration
Cooperative Urological
Research Group
Veterans Administration
Cooperative Urology
Radiotherapy Research
Group

RENAL CELL (KIDNEY)
CANCER
Cooperative Breast Cancer
Group

Eastern Cooperative Oncology
Group

RETICULOENDOTHELIOSIS
(HISTIOCYTOSIS X)
Children's Cancer Study Group

SARCOMAS
Acute Leukemia Cooperative
Group B
Children's Cancer Study Group
Southwest Oncology Group

SOLID TUMORS
Acute Leukemia Cooperative
Group B
Central Oncology Group
Children's Cancer Study Group
Eastern Cooperative Oncology
Group
Radiation Therapy Oncology
Group
Southeastern Cancer Study
Group
Southwest Oncology Group—
Pediatric Division
Western Cancer Study Group

UTERINE CANCER
Gynecologic Oncology Group

WILMS'S TUMOR
Acute Leukemia Cooperative
Group B
Children's Cancer Study Group
Southwest Oncology Group—
Pediatric Division
Wilms's Tumor Study Group

III. Approved Hospital Cancer Programs

As of January 1, 1976, the cancer programs at 757 hospitals and medical centers throughout the country had been approved by the American College of Surgeons. Approval is given for 3 years except for those institutions marked with an asterisk, which have been given provisional approval subject to the correction of certain deficiencies within an 18-month period. Inquiries about the current status of an institution's cancer program should be addressed to: Andrew Jayer, M.D., F.A.C.S., Assistant Director, Professional Activities (Cancer); American College of Surgeons; 55 E. Erie Street; Chicago, Illinois 60611. The approval program is funded by the American Cancer Society and the National Cancer Institute.

Key to the categorical code following the name of each institution:

I: Full facilities and personnel within the institution for diagnosis and treatment of cancer in all major sites, or consultation from and referral to another institution within the same community for a few types of cancer or for certain special diagnostic tests or therapies. The institution conducts research and physician training programs in cancer. Three hundred or more new patients are treated annually.

II: Facilities and personnel for diagnosis and treatment of cancer, except for some major sites, with consultation from and referral to another institution. Training programs and research are optional. Three hundred or more new patients treated annually.

III: Facilities and personnel for diagnosis and treatment of cancer, except for some major sites, with consultation from and referral to another institution. Training programs and research are optional. Less than three hundred new patients treated annually.

S: Institutions having full facilities and personnel, excluding megavoltage radiation therapy, for diagnosis and treatment of special types of cancers or special groups of patients; hospitals that treat special diseases other than cancer but which have consultation from and referral to another institution for the diagnosis and treatment of cancer, and clinics (nonhospital medical institutions) that are certified by their county or state medical societies.

ALABAMA
Birmingham
* University of Alabama Medical
Center I
Veterans Administration
Hospital II
Tuskegee
* Veterans Administration
Hospital III

ALASKA
Anchorage
Anchorage Community
Hospital III
U.S.P.H.S. Alaska Native
Medical Center III

ARIZONA
Mesa
Mesa Tempe Cancer Program
Mesa Lutheran Hospital III
Desert Samaritan Hospital and
Health Center III

Phoenix
Good Samaritan Hospital II
Maricopa County General
Hospital I
Memorial Hospital II
* Veterans Administration
Hospital III
Tucson
Tucson Medical Center II
* Veterans Administration
Hospital III

ARKANSAS
Fayetteville
* Washington General
Hospital III
Harrison
Northwest Arkansas Tumor
Clinic Boone County
Hospital III
Little Rock
* University of Arkansas Medical
Center Hospital I
* Veterans Administration
Hospital II
Texarkana
St. Michael Hospital III

CALIFORNIA
Bakersfield
Kern Medical Center III
Berkeley
* Herrick Memorial Hospital III
Camarillo
Camarillo State Hospital S
Camp Pendleton
* Naval Regional Medical
Center III
Concord
* Mount Diablo Hospital Medical
Center II
Duarte
City of Hope National Medical
Center S
Fontana
* Kaiser Foundation Hospital II
Imola
Napa State Hospital S
Inglewood
Centinela Hospital II
La Jolla
Scripps Memorial Hospital II
La Mesa
Grossmont District Hospital II
Loma Linda
Loma Linda University Medical
Center I
Long Beach
Naval Regional Medical
Center III
Los Angeles
* California Hospital Medical
Center II
Cedars-Sinai Medical Center
Cedars of Lebanon Hospital
Division I
Mount Sinai Hospital
Division II
Children's Hospital of Los
Angeles S
* Hollywood Presbyterian Medical
Center II
Hospital of the Good Samaritan
Medical Center II
Kaiser Foundation Hospital I
* Los Angeles County-U.S.C.
Medical Center I
Orthopaedic Hospital Medical
Center III
Queen of Angels Hospital II

* St. Vincent's Medical Center   II
* Temple Hospital   III
  UCLA Hospital   I
  White Memorial Medical
    Center   I
Martinez
  Veterans Administration
    Hospital   II
Oakland
  Highland General Hospital   III
  Naval Medical Center   III
  Samuel Merritt Hospital   II
Orange
  Orange County Medical
    Center   I
  St. Joseph Hospital   II
Oxnard
  St. John's Hospital   III
Palm Springs
  Desert Hospital   II
Riverside
  Riverside General Hospital—
    University Medical Center   III
Sacramento
  Mercy General Hospital   II
  Sacramento Medical Center   I
  Sutter Community Hospitals of
    Sacramento   II
San Bernardino
  San Bernardino County General
    Hospital   III
San Diego
 * Mercy Hospital and Medical
    Center   II
  Naval Regional Medical
    Center   I
San Francisco
  Children's Hospital of San
    Francisco   II
  Ralph K. Davies Medical
    Center—Franklin Hospital   II
 * Letterman Army Medical
    Center   I
  Mount Zion Hospital and
    Medical Center   I
  St. Francis Memorial
    Hospital   II
 * St. Joseph's Hospital   III
  St. Luke's Hospital   II
  St. Mary's Hospital and Medical
    Center   II

San Francisco General
  Hospital   III
U.S. Public Health Service
  Hospital   III
University of California Medical
  Center   I
San Gabriel
  Community Hospital   II
Santa Monica
  The Santa Monica Hospital
    Medical Center   II
Stanford
 * Stanford University Hospital   I
Torrance
  Los Angeles County Harbor
    General Hospital   I
Travis Air Force Base
  David Grant U.S. Air Force
    Medical Center   III
Visalia
  Kaweah Delta District
    Hospital   III

COLORADO
Colorado Springs
  Colorado Springs Medical
    Center   S
Denver
  American Medical Center   III
  Fitzsimons Army Medical
    Center   I
  General Rose Memorial
    Hospital   III
  Presbyterian Medical Center   II
  St. Joseph Hospital   I
  St. Luke's Hospital   II
  Veterans Administration
    Hospital   III
Fort Carson
  U.S. Army Hospital   III
Fort Collins
  Poudre Valley Memorial
    Hospital   III
Greeley
  Weld County General
    Hospital   III
La Junta
  La Junta Medical Center   III
Pueblo
  Colorado State Hospital   S
  St. Mary-Corwin Hospital   II

U.S. Air Force Academy
　　U.S. Air Force Academy
　　　Hospital   III

CONNECTICUT
Bridgeport
　　Bridgeport Hospital   I
　　Park City Hospital   III
　　St. Vincent's Hospital   I
Greenwich
　　Greenwich Hospital
　　　Association   II
Hartford
　　Hartford Hospital   I
　　St. Francis Hospital   II
Meriden
　　Meriden-Wallingford
　　　Hospital   III
Middletown
　　Middlesex Memorial
　　　Hospital   II
New Haven
　　Hospital of St. Raphael   II
　　* Yale-New Haven Hospital   I
Norwalk
　　Norwalk Hospital   II
Norwich
　　William W. Backus Hospital   III
Putnam
　　Day Kimball Hospital   III
Stamford
　　Stamford Hospital   II
Torrington
　　Charlotte Hungerford
　　　Hospital   III
Waterbury
　　St. Mary's Hospital   II
　　Waterbury Hospital   II

DELAWARE
Lewes
　　Beebe Hospital of Sussex
　　　County   III
Wilmington
　　Wilmington Medical Center
　　　Inc.   I

DISTRICT OF COLUMBIA
Washington
　　Children's Hospital National
　　　Medical Center   S

* Columbia Hospital for
　　Women   S
　Doctors Hospital   II
　Freedmen's Hospital   I
　Georgetown University Medical
　　Center   I
　George Washington University
　　Medical Center   I
　Greater Southeast Community
　　Hospital   II
　Malcolm Grow U.S.A.F. Medical
　　Center   III
* Providence Hospital   III
　Walter Reed Army Medical
　　Center   I
* Washington Hospital Center   I

FLORIDA
Daytona Beach
　　Halifax Hospital Medical
　　　Center   II
Gainesville
　　Shands Teaching Hospital and
　　　Clinic   I
Jacksonville
　　St. Vincent's Medical Center   II
　　University Hospital of
　　　Jacksonville   I
Miami
　　* James M. Jackson Memorial
　　　Hospital   I
Miami Beach
　　* Mount Sinai Medical Center of
　　　Greater Miami   I
Pensacola
　　Naval Aerospace Medical
　　　Center   III
Sarasota
　　* Memorial Hospital   II
Tallahassee
　　Tallahassee Memorial
　　　Hospital   II
Tampa
　　Tampa General Hospital   I

GEORGIA
Albany
　　Phoebe Putney Memorial
　　　Hospital   III
Americus
　　Americus and Sumter County
　　　Hospital   III

Atlanta
* Crawford W. Long Memorial
    Hospital   II
  Georgia Baptist Hospital   II
  Grady Memorial Hospital   I
  St. Joseph's Infirmary   III
Augusta
* Medical College of Georgia
    Hospital and Clinics   I
* University Hospital   II
Columbus
  Medical Center   II
Dalton
* Hamilton Memorial
    Hospital   III
Decatur
  De Kalb General Hospital   II
  Veterans Administration
    Hospital Atlanta   II
Fort Benning
  Martin Army Hospital   III
Fort Gordon
  U.S. Army Medical Center   III
Gainesville
  Hall County Hospital   II
La Grange
  City-County Hospital   III
Macon
* Medical Center of Central
    Georgia   II
Rome
* Floyd County Hospital   II
Savannah
  Memorial Medical Center   I

HAWAII
Honolulu
  Kapiolani Hospital   S
  Kuakini Hospital   III
  Queen's Medical Center   II
  St. Francis Hospital   III
  Tripler Army Medical
    Center   III

IDAHO
Boise
  St. Luke's Hospital   II
Nampa
  Mercy Medical Center   III
Twin Falls
* Magic Valley Hospital   III

ILLINOIS
Arlington Heights
  Northwest Community
    Hospital   II
Belleville
  St. Elizabeth Hospital   III
Canton
  Graham Hospital   III
Carbondale
  Doctors Memorial Hospital   III
Centralia
* St. Mary's Hospital   III
Chicago
* Augustana Hospital and Health
    Care Center   III
  Central Community
    Hospital   III
* Children's Memorial Hospital   S
* Columbus Hospital   I
  Cook County Hospital   I
  Edgewater Hospital   III
  Franklin Boulevard Community
    Hospital   III
  Illinois Masonic Medical
    Center   I
  Louis A. Weiss Memorial
    Hospital   II
  Mercy Hospital & Medical
    Center   I
  Mount Sinai Hospital Medical
    Center   I
  Northwestern University
    McGraw Medical Center
    * Northwestern Memorial
      Hospital   I
  Ravenswood Hospital   II
  Rush-Presbyterian-St Luke's
    Medical Center   I
  St. Elizabeth Hospital   III
  St. Joseph Hospital   II
* St. Mary of Nazareth Hospital
    Center   III
  University of Chicago Hospitals
    and Clinics   I
  University of Illinois Hospital   I
  Veterans Administration West
    Side Hospital   II
Elmhurst
  Memorial Hospital of DuPage
    County   II
Evanston
  Evanston Hospital   I

St. Francis Hospital of
Evanston I
Evergreen Park
  * Little Company of Mary
    Hospital II
Great Lakes
  Naval Regional Medical
    Center III
Harvey
  Ingalls Memorial Hospital III
Hines
  Veterans Administration
    Hospital II
Hinsdale
  * Hinsdale Sanitarium and
    Hospital II
Hoopeston
  * Hoopeston Community
    Memorial Hospital III
Kankakee
  St. Mary's Hospital III
McHenry
  McHenry Hospital III
Oak Park
  West Suburban Hospital II
Peoria
  * Methodist Hospital of Central
    Illinois III
  St. Francis Hospital I
Quincy
  Blessing Hospital II
  St. Mary Hospital III
Rockford
  Rockford Memorial Hospital I
  St. Anthony Hospital III
Sterling
  Community General
    Hospital III
Streator
  St. Mary's Hospital III
Urbana
  Carle Foundation Hospital II

INDIANA
Bluffton
  Clinic Hospital III
Evansville
  * St. Mary's Hospital II
Gary
  Methodist Hospital of Gary II
Hammond
  St. Margaret Hospital II

Indianapolis
  Indiana University Medical
    Center I
  Methodist Hospital I
  St. Vincent Hospital II
Lafayette
  St. Elizabeth Hospital Medical
    Center II
Terre Haute
  Union Hospital II

IOWA
Des Moines
  Mercy Hospital II
  Veterans Administration
    Hospital III
Dubuque
  Finley Hospital III
  Mercy Medical Center III
  Xarier Hospital III
Iowa City
  University of Iowa Hospitals and
    Clinics I
Waterloo
  * Schoitz Memorial Hospital II

KANSAS
Halstead
  Halstead Hospital III
Hays
  Hadley Regional Medical
    Center III
  * St. Anthony Hospital III
Kansas City
  Bethany Medical Center II
  University of Kansas Medical
    Center I
Manhattan
  The St. Mary Hospital III
Newton
  * Bethel Deaconess Hospital III
Topeka
  * Veterans Administration
    Hospital S
Wichita
  * St. Francis Hospital II
  Veterans Administration
    Hospital III

* Wesley Medical Center   I
KENTUCKY
Fort Campbell
United States Army
Hospital   III
Harlan
Harlan Appalachian Regional
Hospital   III
Lexington
* St. Joseph Hospital   II
* University Hospital   I
Louisville
Louisville General Hospital   II
Norton Children's Hospitals,
Inc. Children's Unit   S
Norton Unit   II
St. Joseph Infirmary   II
Veterans Administration
Hospital   III

LOUISIANA
Alexandria
Alexandria Tumor Registry
Program
Rapides General
Hospital   III
St. Francis Cabrini
Hospital   III
Lake Charles
* St. Patrick's Hospital   II
New Orleans
Charity Hospital of
Louisiana   I
Louisiana State University
Cancer Service
Tulane University Cancer
Service
Touro Infirmary   II
U.S. Public Health Service
Hospital   III
Veterans Administration
Hospital   II
Shreveport
Confederate Memorial Medical
Center   II
Veterans Administration
Hospital   III

MAINE
Augusta
Augusta General Hospital   III

Bangor
Eastern Maine Medical
Center   II
Lewiston
Central Maine General
Hospital   III
St. Mary's General Hospital   III
Portland
Maine Medical Center   II
Presque Isle
* Arthur Gould Memorial
Hospital   III
Rockland
* Knox County General
Hospital   III
Togus
Veterans Administration
Center   III
Waterville
Mid-Maine Medical Center,
Thayer Unit   III

MARYLAND
Baltimore
Greater Baltimore Medical
Center   II
Johns Hopkins Hospital   I
Union Memorial Hospital   II
U.S. Public Health Service
Hospital   III
University of Maryland
Hospital   I
Bethesda
Naval Medical Center   I
Salisbury
Peninsula General Hospital   III

MASSACHUSETTS
Beverly
Beverly Hospital   III
Boston
Beth Israel Hospital   II
Boston City Hospital   II
Children's Hospital Medical
Center   S
Children's Cancer Research
Foundation
Faulkner Hospital, *Jamaica
Plain*   III'
Lahey Clinic Foundation   S
Lemuel Shattuck Hospital,
Jamaica Plain   III

* Massachusetts General
  Hospital   I
Peter Bent Brigham Hospital   I
* St. Elizabeth's Hospital of
  Boston, *Brighton*   II
* U.S. Public Health Service
  Hospital, *Brighton*   III
University Hospital   II
Veterans Administration
  Hospital, *Jamaica Plain*   III
Brockton
  Brockton Hospital   II
Cambridge
* Cambridge Hospital   III
Chelsea
  Lawrence F. Quigley Memorial
  Hospital, Soldier's Home   III
Concord
  Emerson Hospital   III
Danvers
  Hunt Memorial Hospital   III
Lowell
  Lowell Cancer Clinic Program
  Lowell General Hospital   III
  * St. Joseph's Hospital   III
Lynn
  Lynn Hospital   II
Newton Lower Falls
* Newton-Wellesley Hospital   II
North Adams
  North Adams Regional
  Hospital   III
Salem
* Salem Hospital   III
Springfield
  Mercy Hospital   II
  Springfield Hospital Medical
  Center   II
  Wesson Memorial Hospital   II
Walpole
  Pondville Hospital   I
Worcester
  The Memorial Hospital   II
  St. Vincent Hospital   II
  Worcester City Hospital   II

MICHIGAN
Allen Park
  Veterans Administration
  Hospital   III
Ann Arbor
* St. Joseph Mercy Hospital   I

* University Hospital   I
Battle Creek
  Calhoun County Medical Society
  Cancer Program
  Battle Creek Sanitarium and
  Hospital   III
  Community Hospital   III
  Leila Y. Post Montgomery
  Hospital   III
Dearborn
  Oakwood Hospital   I
Detroit
* Detroit-Macomb Hospital
  Association   II
  Henry Ford Hospital   I
* Hutzel Hospital   II
Flint
  Hurley Hospital   I
Grand Rapids
  Blodgett Memorial Hospital   I
  Butterworth Hospital   I
  Ferguson-Droste-Ferguson
  Hospital   S
  St. Mary's Hospital   II
Menominee
  Menominee County-Lloyd
  Hospital   III
Muskegon
  Hackley Hospital   II
Pontiac
  St. Joseph Mercy Hospital   I
Rochester
* Crittenton Hospital   III
Royal Oak
* William Beaumont Hospital   I

MINNESOTA
Crookston
  Riverview Hospital   III
Fergus Falls
  Lake Region Hospital   III
Grand Rapids
* Itasca Memorial Hospital   III
Hibbing
  Hibbing General Hospital   III
Minneapolis
  Metropolitan Medical Center   II
  St. Mary's Hospital   II
* University of Minnesota
  Hospitals   I
  Veterans Administration
  Hospital   II

Rochester
Mayo Clinic   I

MISSISSIPPI
Biloxi
* Howard Memorial Hospital   III
Gulfport
* Memorial Hospital at
Gulfport   III
Hattiesburg
Forrest County General
Hospital   II
Jackson
University Hospital   I
Veterans Administration
Center   II
Vicksburg
Mercy Regional Medical
Center   III

MISSOURI
Cape Girardeau
St. Francis Hospital   III
Columbia
Ellis Fischel State Cancer
Hospital   I
* University of Missouri Medical
Center   I
Kansas City
* Baptist Memorial Hospital   II
Kansas City General Hospital
and Medical Center   III
* Menorah Medical Center   I
St. Luke's Hospital   I
Poplar Bluff
Doctors Hospital   III
St. Louis
Deaconess Hospital   II
* Homer G. Phillips Hospital   III
Lutheran Hospital Medical
Center   II
* Max Starkloff Memorial
Hospital   II
St. Anthony Hospital of St.
Louis   II
* St. Louis County Hospital,
Clayton   II
St. Louis Little Rock
Hospital   III
St. Mary's Health Center   I

MONTANA
Butte
St. James Community
Hospital   III
Mary Swift Memorial Tumor
Clinic
Missoula
* Blegen-Honeycutt Memorial
Tumor Foundation   S

NEBRASKA
Lincoln
Bryan Memorial Hospital   III
Lincoln General Hospital   II
* St. Elizabeth Community Health
Center   III
Veterans Administration
Hospital   III
Omaha
Bishop Clarkson Memorial
Hospital   III
Immanuel Medical Center   III
Nebraska Methodist Hospital   II
University of Nebraska Medical
Center   I
Veterans Administration
Hospital   III

NEVADA
Henderson
* St. Rose de Lima Hospital   III
Las Vegas
* Southern Nevada Memorial
Hospital   II

NEW HAMPSHIRE
Claremont
* Claremont General Hospital   III
Hanover
Mary Hitchcock Memorial
Hospital   I
Keene
Cheshire Hospital   III

NEW JERSEY
Atlantic City
Atlantic City Medical Center   II
Belleville
Clara Maass Memorial
Hospital   II
Camden
* Cooper Hospital   II

West Jersey Hospital—Northern
    Division   II
Denville
    St. Clare's Hospital   III
East Orange
    * Veterans Administration
        Hospital   II
Elizabeth
    Elizabeth General Hospital and
        Dispensary   II
    Wuester Clinic
Englewood
    Englewood Hospital   II
Hackensack
    Hackensack Hospital   II
Livingston
    St. Barnabas Medical Center   I
Long Branch
    Monmouth Medical Center   I
Montclair
    * Mountainside Hospital   II
Morristown
    Morristown Memorial
        Hospital   II
Mount Holly
    Burlington County Memorial
        Hospital   II
Newark
    * Harrison S. Martland
        Hospital   III
    * Newark Beth Israel Medical
        Center   I
    United Hospitals of Newark   II
Paterson
    Barnert Memorial Hospital
        Center   III
    St. Joseph's Hospital and
        Medical Center   II
Phillipsburg
    Warren Hospital   III
Plainfield
    * Muhlenberg Hospital   II
Princeton
    The Medical Center at
        Princeton   II
Somerville
    The Somerset Hospital   II
Trenton
    St. Francis Medical Center   II
Woodbury
    Underwood Memorial
        Hospital   II

NEW MEXICO
Albuquerque
    Lovelace-Bataan Medical
        Center   II
    Veterans Administration
        Hospital   II
Kirkland Air Force Base
    U.S. Air Force Hospital   III

NEW YORK
Albany
    * St. Peter's Hospital   II
    Veterans Administration
        Hospital   II
Amityville
    Brunswick Hospital Center   II
Batavia
    Veterans Administration
        Hospital   III
Binghamton
    Our Lady of Lourdes Memorial
        Hospital   II
Buffalo
    Deaconess Hospital of Buffalo   II
    Edward J. Meyer Memorial
        Hospital   II
    Roswell Park Memorial
        Institute   I
    Veterans Administration
        Hospital   II
Castle Point
    Veterans Administration
        Hospital   III
Cooperstown
    Mary Imogene Bassett
        Hospital   III
East Meadow
    Nassau County Medical
        Center   I
Elmira
    Arnot-Ogden Memorial
        Hospital   III
Glen Cove
    Community Hospital at Glen
        Cove   II
Johnson City
    Charles S. Wilson Memorial
        Hospital   III
Kenmore
    Kenmore Mercy Hospital   II

Manhasset
   North Shore University
      Hospital   I
Mineola
   Nassau Hospital   I
Mount Kisco
   Northern Westchester
      Hospital   II
Mount Vernon
   Mount Vernon Hospital   III
New Hyde Park
   Long Island Jewish Medical
      Center   I
New Rochelle
   * New Rochelle Hospital   II
New York City
   Bronx *(Mailing address: Bronx)*
      * Bronx-Lebanon Hospital
         Center   I
      * Bronx Muncipal Hospital
         Center   I
      Albert Einstein College of
         Medicine
      Misericordia & Fordham
         Hospitals   I
      * Montefiore Hospital and
         Medical Center   I
      Veterans Administration
         Hospital   II
   Brooklyn *(Mailing address:*
   Brooklyn)
      Brooklyn-Cumberland
         Medical Center   I
      * Caledonian Hospital   II
      * Jewish Hospital and Medical
         Center of Brooklyn   I
      Kingsbrook Jewish Medical
         Center   II
      Long Island College
         Hospital   I
      Lutheran Medical
         Center   III
      Methodist Hospital of
         Brooklyn   I
      St. John's Episcopal
         Hospital   III
      State University of New
         York Downstate Medical
         Center
      Kings County Hospital
         Center   I

   Wyckoff Heights
      Hospital   II
Manhattan, *Mailing address:*
   New York)
   Beekman-Downtown
      Hospital   III
   Beth Israel Hospital   II
   * Columbus Hospital
      Division—Cabrini Health
      Care Center   II
   French Hospital, Division of
      French & Polyclinic
      Medical School and
      Health Center   II
   Harlem Hospital Center   I
   Jewish Memorial
      Hospital   III
   Manhattan Eye, Ear and
      Throat Hospital   S
   Memorial Sloan-Kettering
      Cancer Center   I
   * Mount Sinai Hospital   I
   New York Hospital   I
   * New York Infirmary   II
   New York Medical College
      Flower and Fifth Avenue
         Hospitals   I
   New York Polyclinic Medical
      School and Hospital   II
   New York University Medical
      Center University
      Hospital   I
   * Roosevelt Hospital   I
   St. Luke's Hospital
      Center   I
   St. Vincent's Hospital and
      Medical Center   I
   * Veterans Administration
      Hospital   II
Queens *(Mailing addresses:*
   Astoria, Edgemere, Elmhurst,
   Far Rockaway, Flushing,
   Forest Hills, Glen Oaks,
   Hollis, Jackson Heights,
   Jamaica, Kew Gardens,
   Little Neck, Long Island City,
   Queens Village, St. Albans,
   and Whitestone)
   Flushing Hospital and
      Medical Center,
      Flushing   II

Jamaica Hospital,
 Jamaica II
Mary Immaculate Hospital,
 Division of the Catholic
 Medical Center,
 Jamaica II
Queens Hospital Center,
 Jamaica I
St. John's Queens Hospital,
 Division of the Catholic
 Medical Center,
 Elmhurst II
Richmond (*Mailing address:*
 Staten Island)
 Doctors' Hospital of Staten
 Island III
 St. Vincent's Medical Center
 of Richmond III
 Staten Island Hospital III
 * U.S. Public Health Service
 Hospital III
North Tarrytown
 * Phelps Memorial Hospital III
Oceanside
 South Nassau Communities
 Hospital II
Poughkeepsie
 Vassar Brothers Hospital II
Rochester
 Highland Hospital of
 Rochester II
 St. Mary's Hospital of the Sisters
 of Charity II
Rockville Centre
 * Mercy Hospital II
Suffern
 Good Samaritan Hospital II
Syracuse
 Crouse Irving-Memorial
 Hospital I
 University Hospital of Upstate
 Medical Center I
 Veterans Administration
 Hospital III
Walton
 Delaware Valley Hospital III
White Plains
 * St. Agnes Hospital III
Yonkers
 * St. John's Riverside Hospital III
 * Yonkers General Hospital III

NORTH CAROLINA
Asheville
 Veterans Administration
 Hospital III
Camp Le Jeune
 * Naval Regional Medical
 Center III
Chapel Hill
 North Carolina Memorial
 Hospital I
Durham
 * Duke University Medical
 Center I
 Veterans Administration
 Hospital II
 Watts Hospital III
Valdese
 Valdese General Hospital III
Winston-Salem
 Forsyth Memorial Hospital II
 * North Carolina Baptist
 Hospital I
 Bowman-Gray School of
 Medicine

NORTH DAKOTA
Fargo
 St. Luke's Hospital-Fargo
 Clinic II
 * Veterans Administration
 Center III
Grand Forks
 Grand Forks Clinic S
Rugby
 Good Samaritan Hospital III
Williston
 Mercy Hospital III

OHIO
Akron
 Akron City Hospital I
Cincinnati
 Cincinnati General Hospital I
 * Good Samaritan Hospital II
 * Jewish Hospital of
 Cincinnati II
Cleveland
 * Cleveland Clinic Hospital I

Cleveland Metropolitan General
Hospital I
Deaconess Hospital of
Cleveland III
Fairview General Hospital II
Huron Road Hospital II
* Lutheran Medical Center II
* Mount Sinai Hospital I
St. Alexis Hospital II
St. Luke's Hospital of the United
Methodist Church II
* University Hospitals of
Cleveland I
* Veterans Administration
Hospital II
Columbus
Children's Hospital S
Mount Carmel Medical
Center II
Ohio State University
Hospitals I
Dayton
Miami Valley Hospital I
Montgomery County Medical
Society
Good Samaritan Hospital II
St. Elizabeth Medical
Center II
Veterans Administration
Hospital III
Dover
* Union Hospital III
Elyria
* Elyria Memorial Hospital II
Gallipolis
* Holzer Medical Center III
Mayfield Heights
Hillcrest Hospital III
Painesville
Lake County Memorial
Hospitals II
Sandusky
Good Samaritan Hospital III
Toledo
Medical College of Ohio
Hospital III
St. Vincent Hospital and Medical
Center II
* Toledo Hospital II
Wright-Patterson Air Force Base
U.S. Air Force Medical
Center III

Youngstown
Youngstown Hospital
Association II

OKLAHOMA
Ada
Valley View Hospital III
Ardmore
Memorial Hospital of Southern
Oklahoma III
Chickasha
Grady Memorial Hospital III
Oklahoma City
Baptist Medical Center of
Oklahoma II
Mercy Health Center II
Tulsa
Hillcrest Medical Center II
St. Francis Hospital II
St. John's Hospital II

OREGON
Bend
St. Charles Memorial
Hospital III
Corvallis
Good Samaritan Hospital II
Eugene
Sacred Heart General
Hospital II
Medford
Medford Tumor Clinic
* Providence Hospital III
Rogue Valley Memorial
Hospital II
Oregon City
Willamette Falls Community
Hospital and Oregon City
Hospital III
Pendleton
St. Anthony Hospital III
Portland
Emanuel Hospital I
* Good Samaritan Hospital and
Medical Center II
Kaiser Foundation Hospitals,
Oregon Region II
* Physicians and Surgeons
Hospital III
Portland Adventist Hospital III

Providence Hospital   II
St. Vincent Hospital and Medical
    Center   II
University of Oregon Medical
    School Hospital   I
Veterans Administration
    Hospital   II
Roseburg
  * Veterans Administration
    Hospital   S
Salem
  * Salem Hospital   II

PENNSYLVANIA
Allentown
    Allentown Hospital   II
Altoona
    Altoona Hospital   II
Bethlehem
    St. Luke's Hospital   II
Bryn Mawr
    Bryn Mawr Hospital   II
Coatesville
    Veterans Administration
        Hospital   III
Danville
    Geisinger Medical Center   I
Doylestown
    Doylestown Hospital   III
Drexel Hill
    Delaware County Memorial
        Hospital   II
Easton
  * Easton Hospital   II
Gettysburg
  * Annie M. Warner Hospital   III
Harrisburg
  * Harrisburg Polyclinic
        Hospital   II
Hazleton
  * Hazleton State General
        Hospital   III
Johnstown
    Conemaugh Valley Memorial
        Hospital   II
Lancaster
  * Lancaster General Hospital   II
  * St. Joseph Hospital   III
Lebanon
    Veterans Administration
        Hospital   III

Lewistown
    Lewistown Hospital   III
McKeesport
    McKeesport Hospital   II
Natrona Heights
    Allegheny Valley Hospital   II
Norristown
    Montgomery Hospital   III
  * Sacred Heart Hospital   III
Philadelphia
    Albert Einstein Medical Center—
        Northern Division   I
    American Oncologic Hospital   II
        and Jeanes Hospital   III
    Children's Hospital of
        Philadelphia   S
    Episcopal Hospital   I
  * Graduate Hospital of the
        University of Pennsylvania   I
    Hahnemann Medical College
        and Hospital   I
    Hospital of the Medical College
        of Pennsylvania   III
    Hospital of the University of
        Pennsylvania   I
    Lankenau Hospital   II
    Mercy Catholic Medical
        Center   I
    Naval Regional Medical
        Center   II
  * Pennsylvania Hospital   I
    Philadelphia General
        Hospital   I
  * Presbyterian-University of
        Pennsylvania Medical
        Center   I
    Temple University Hospital   I
    Thomas Jefferson University
        Hospital   I
Pittsburgh
    Children's Hospital of
        Pittsburgh   S
    Magee-Women's Hospital   II
    Mercy Hospital   I
    St. Francis General Hospital   I
    St. Margaret Memorial
        Hospital   III
    Veterans Administration
        Hospital   II
        (University Drive)
    Western Pennsylvania
        Hospital   I

Pottsville
  Pottsville Hospital and Warne
    Clinic   III
Reading
  Community General
    Hospital   III
Sayre
  * Robert Packer Hospital   II
Sewickley
  Sewickley Valley Hospital   III
Sharon
  * Sharon General Hospital   III
West Chester
  Chester County Hospital   III
Wilkes-Barre
  Veterans Administration
    Hospital   III
  Wilkes-Barre General
    Hospital   II
York
  * York Hospital   II

RHODE ISLAND
Newport
  Naval Hospital   III
Pawtucket
  * Memorial Hospital   III
Providence
  * Rhode Island Hospital   I
  * Veterans Administration
    Hospital   III

SOUTH CAROLINA
Anderson
  Anderson Memorial Hospital   II
Beaufort
  Naval Hospital   III
Charleston
  Medical University of South
    Carolina Hospital   I
  Naval Regional Medical
    Center   III
Columbia
  Richland Memorial Hospital   II
  South Carolina Baptist
    Hospital   II
  Veterans Administration
    Hospital   III
Florence
  McLeod Memorial Hospital   II
Fort Jackson
  Moncrief Army Hospital   III

Greenville
  Greenville General Hospital   II
Greenwood
  Self Memorial Hospital   III
Orangeburg
  Orangeburg Regional
    Hospital   III
Spartanburg
  Spartanburg General
    Hospital   II
Sumter
  Tuomey Hospital   III

SOUTH DAKOTA
Watertown
  Watertown Memorial
    Hospital   III
Yankton
  Sacred Heart Hospital   III

TENNESSEE
Bristol
  Bristol Memorial Hospital   III
Chattanooga
  Chattanooga Tumor Clinic,
    Inc.   S
Johnson City
  Memorial Hospital   II
Memphis
  Methodist Hospital   I
  West Tennessee Cancer
    Clinic   S
Millington
  Naval Hospital Memphis   III
Nashville
  George W. Hubbard Hospital of
    Meharry Medical College   III
  Nashville Metropolitan General
    Hospital   III
  Vanderbilt University
    Hospital   I

TEXAS
Amarillo
  Panhandle Regional Tumor
    Clinic and Registry
    High Plains Baptist
    Hospital   III
    Northwest Texas
    Hospital   III

St. Anthony's Hospital III
Big Spring
Malone Hogan Hospitals,
Inc. III
Veterans Administration
Hospital III
Corpus Christi
Memorial Medical Center II
Naval Hospital III
Spohn Hospital II
Dallas
Baylor University Medical
Center I
Methodist Hospital of
Dallas I
St. Paul Hospital I
El Paso
R.E. Thomason General
Hospital III
William Beaumont Army Medical
Center III
Fort Sam Houston
Brooke Army Medical Center I
Fort Worth
John Peter Smith Hospital III
Galveston
University of Texas Medical
Branch Hospitals I
Houston
Ben Taub General Hospital I
* Hermann Hospital I
M.D. Anderson Hospital and
Tumor Institute I
St. Elizabeth's Hospital III
St. Joseph Hospital I
St. Luke's Episcopal Hospital I
Veterans Administration
Hospital II
Jacksonville
Nan Travis Memorial
Hospital III
Kerrville
Veterans Administration
Hospital III
Lackland Air Force Base
Wilford Hall USAF Medical
Center I
Lubbock
Methodist Hospital II
Midland
Midland Memorial
Hospital III

Plainview
* Central Plains General
Hospital III
San Antonio
Bexar Country Hospital—
University of Texas Medical
School II
Santa Rosa Medical Center II
Stephenville
Stephenville Hospital III
Temple
King's Daughters Hospital III
Scott and White Memorial
Hospital I
Veterans Administration
Center II
Texarkana
St. Michael's Hospital III
Wharton
Gulf Coast Medical Center III

UTAH
Ogden
McKay-Dee Hospital Center II
St. Benedict's Hospital III
Provo
* Utah Valley Latter-Day Saints
Hospital III
Salt Lake City
Holy Cross Hospital III
Latter-Day Saints Hospital I
St. Mark's Hospital III
* University of Utah Hospital I
* Veterans Administration
Hospital III

VERMONT
Burlington
Medical Center Hospital of
Vermont I
Newport
North Country Hospital and
Health Center III
Randolph
Gifford Memorial Hospital,
Inc. III

VIRGINIA
Alexandria
* Alexandria Hospital II

Charlottesville
  University of Virginia
    Hospital I
Clifton Forge
  * Emmett Memorial Hospital III
Danville
  Memorial Hospital II
Falls Church
  Fairfax Hospital II
Hampton
  Veterans Administration
    Center III
Harrisonburg
  Rockingham Memorial
    Hospital III
Lynchburg
  Virginia Baptist Hospital III
  Lynchburg General-Marshall
    Lodge Hospital II
Norfolk
  * Norfolk General Hospital I
Portsmouth
  Naval Hospital II
Richmond
  Medical College of Virginia
    Hospital I
  St. Mary's Hospital II
Roanoke
  Community Hospital of Roanoke
    Valley II
Salem
  Lewis-Gale Hospital III
  Veterans Administration
    Hospital III
Winchester
  Winchester Memorial
    Hospital II

WASHINGTON
Bellevue
  Overlake Memorial Hospital III
Bremerton
  * Naval Regional Medical
    Center III
Mount Vernon
  Skagit Valley Hospital III
Olympia
  St. Peter Hospital II
Seattle
  Children's Orthopedic Hospital
    and Medical Center S
  Group Health Hospital II

* Harborview Medical Center III
  Northwest Hospital III
  Providence Medical Center II
  Swedish Hospital Medical
    Center I
  Virginia Mason Hospital I
Sedro Woolley
  United General Hospital III
Spokane
  Deaconess Hospital II
  Sacred Heart Hospital I
Tacoma
  * Madigan General Hospital II
  Tacoma General Hospital II
Wenatchee
  Wenatchee Valley Clinic S

WEST VIRGINIA
Beckley
  Appalachian Regional
    Hospital III
  * Beckley Hospital, Inc. III
Charleston
  * Charleston Area Medical
    Center, Inc.
      General Division II
      Memorial Division II
Clarksburg
  Veterans Administration
    Hospital III
Elkins
  Davis Memorial Hospital III
  Memorial General Hospital III
Huntington
  Cabell Huntington Hospital III
  Doctors Memorial Hospital III
  Veterans Administration
    Hospital III
Kingwood
  Preston Memorial Hospital III
Man
  Man Appalachian Regional
    Hospital III
Montgomery
  * Montgomery General
    Hospital III
Morgantown
  * West Viriginia University
    Hospital I
Parkersburg
  St. Joseph's Hospital III

Philippi
* Broaddus Hospital   III
Williamson
   Williamson Appalachian
      Regional Hospital   III

WISCONSIN
Appleton
* St. Elizabeth Hospital   III
Eau Claire
   Luther Hospital   III
   Sacred Heart Hospital   III
Green Bay
   St. Vincent Hospital   II
Janesville
   Mercy Hospital of Janesville   III
La Crosse
   La Crosse Lutheran
      Hospital   II
   St. Francis Hospital   III
Madison
   Madison General Hospital   II
   Methodist Hospital   III
   University of Wisconsin
      Hospitals   I
   Veterans Administration
      Hospital   III
Manitowoc
   Holy Family Hospital   III
Marinette
   Marinette General Hospital   III
Marshfield
   Marshfield Clinic   S

Milwaukee
   Milwaukee County General
      Hospital   I
   St. Francis Hospital   III
   St. Joseph's Hospital   II
Watertown
   Watertown Memorial
      Hospital   III
Wood
   Veterans Administration
      Center   II

WYOMING
Casper
* Memorial Hospital of Natrona
      County   III
Cheyenne
* De Paul Hospital   III
* Memorial Hospital of Laramie
      County   III
Laramie
* Ivinson Memorial Hospital   III

PUERTO RICO
Ponce
   Clinica Oncologica Andres
      Grilasca   II
   Hospital De Damas   III
San Juan
   I. Gonzales Martinez Hospital   II
   University District Hospital   I
   Veterans Administration
      Center   III

IV. Breast Cancer Demonstration Projects

At each of the institutions listed below, women aged 35 and older are being examined annually for 5 years (with further follow-up for another 5 years) to determine the best strategy for detecting breast cancer in its early, most curable stages. The demonstration projects, which include manual examination by a physician, thermography (a heat-sensitive picture of the breast), and mammography (a special breast X-ray), are supported by funds from the American Cancer Society and the National Cancer Institute. Although the projects have finished recruiting, women interested in obtaining such a breast examination should contact the nearest center for information on where to get one.

ARIZONA
University of Arizona
Arizona Medical Center
Tucson 85724
(602) 882-7401 or 7402

CALIFORNIA
Los Angeles County, University of
    Southern California/John
    Wesley Hospital
Los Angeles 90033
(213) 748-5379

Samuel Merritt Hospital/Breast
    Screening Center
384 34th Street
Oakland 94609
(415) 658-8525

DELAWARE
Wilmington General Hospital
Chestnut & Broom Streets
Wilmington 19899
(302) 428-4815

DISTRICT OF COLUMBIA
Georgetown University Medical
    School
3800 Reservoir Road, N.W.
Washington, D.C. 20007
(202) 625-2183

FLORIDA
St. Vincent's Medical Center
Barrs Street & St. Johns Avenue
Jacksonville 32204
(904) 389-7751, ext. 8491-2

GEORGIA
Georgia Baptist Hospital
340 Boulevard N.E.
Atlanta 30312
(404) 525-7861

Emory University
Atlanta 30322
(404) 355-4940

HAWAII
Pacific Health Research Institute, Inc.
Alexander Young Building, Suite 545
Hotel & Bishop Streets
Honolulu 96813
(808) 524-4337

IDAHO
Mountain States Tumor Institute
215 Avenue B
Boise 83702
(208) 345-3590

IOWA
Iowa Lutheran Hospital
University at Penn
Des Moines 50316
(515) 283-5678

KANSAS
University of Kansas Medical Center
Rainbow Boulevard at 39th Street
Kansas City 66103
(913) 342-1338

KENTUCKY
University of Louisville School of
   Medicine
601 S. Floyd Street
Louisville 40402
(502) 583-2894

MICHIGAN
University of Michigan Medical
   Center
396 W. Washington Street
Ann Arbor 48103
(313) 763-0056

MISSOURI
Cancer Research Center
Business Loop 70th & Garth Avenue
Columbia 65201
(314) 442-7833

NEW JERSEY
College of Medicine and Dentistry of
   New Jersey
15 S. 9th Street
Newark 07107
(201) 484-9221

NEW YORK
Guttman Institute
200 Madison Avenue (at 35th
   Street)
New York 10016
(212) 689-9797

NORTH CAROLINA
Duke University Medical Center
3040 Erwin Road
Durham 27705
(919) 286-7943 or 383-1060

OHIO
University of Cincinnati Medical
   Center
Eden & Bethesda Avenues
Cincinnati 45229
(513) 872-5331

OKLAHOMA
Oklahoma Medical Research
   Foundation
800 N.E. 8th Street
Oklahoma City 73190
(405) 235-8331, ext. 241

OREGON
Breast Cancer Screening Project
2222 N.W. Lovejoy
Portland 97210
(503) 229-7292

PENNSYLVANIA
Temple University
3401 No. Broad Street
Philadelphia 19140
(215) 221-3832

Albert Einstein Medical Center
York & Tabor Roads
Philadelphia 19141
(215) 567-0559

University of Pittsburgh School of
   Medicine/The Falk Clinic
3601 Fifth Avenue
Pittsburgh 15213
(412) 624-3336

RHODE ISLAND
Rhode Island Hospital
Rhode Island Department of Health
Eddy Street
Providence 02908
(401) 831-6970

TENNESSEE
Vanderbilt University School of
    Medicine
Nashville 37322
(615) 322-2501

TEXAS
St. Joseph's Hospital

1919 LaBranch
Houston 77002
(713) 225-3131, ext. 301

WASHINGTON
Virginia Mason Medical Center
911 Seneca Street
Seattle 98101
(206) 624-1144

WISCONSIN
Medical College of Wisconsin
8700 W. Wisconsin Avenue
Milwaukee 53236
(414) 257-5200

V. Rehabilitation Programs

I. Breast Cancer:

Reach to Recovery. Contact your local unit or state division of the American Cancer Society.

II. Larynx Cancer:

International Association of Laryngectomies
American Cancer Society
777 Third Avenue
New York, New York 10017

Also, contact your local unit or state division of the American Cancer Society for referral to the nearest Lost Chord, Anamilo, or New Voice Club.

III. Colon-Rectal or Bladder Cancer:

Ostomy Rehabilitation Program of the American Cancer Society. Contact your local unit or state division of the American Cancer Society.

Also,

United Ostomy Association, Inc.
1111 Wilshire Boulevard
Los Angeles, California 90017

Index

The Authors

JANE E. BRODY has been a science and medicine writer at *The New York Times* since 1965. In addition to covering major developments in medicine and biology for *The Times,* she has written numerous magazine articles on health issues and coauthored a book with her husband, Richard Engquist, called "Secrets of Good Health."

A native of Brooklyn, New York, Miss Brody majored in biochemistry at the New York State College of Agriculture and Life Sciences at Cornell University and received a master of science degree in journalism from the University of Wisconsin. She came to *The Times* after two years as a general reporter for the *Minneapolis Tribune.* She has received numerous awards for excellence in medical writing.

She and Mr. Engquist live in Brooklyn with their twin sons, Lorin and Erik.

ARTHUR I. HOLLEB, M.D., is Senior Vice President for Medical Affairs and Research at the American Cancer Society. He is editor-in-chief of *Ca,* a cancer journal for clinicians that is published by the American Cancer Society.

A native of New York City, Dr. Holleb is a graduate of Brown University and New York University College of Medicine. As a board-certified surgeon, he specialized in the treatment of breast cancer at Memorial Hospital for Cancer in New York City. He has held numerous teaching appointments. After a year as Associate Director for Education at the M.D. Anderson Hospital and Tumor Institute in Houston, he joined the full-time staff of the American Cancer Society in 1968.

Dr. Holleb is a member of many professional societies and serves on the cancer commissions of the American College of Surgeons and the American College of Radiology. He is also Vice President for the section on cancer of the Pan American Medical Association.

Dr. Holleb and his wife, Carolyn, a former nurse, are also the parents of twins, David and Susan. They live in Larchmont, New York.